Psychosocial Approaches to Child and Adolescent Health and Wellbeing

Jennifer M. Waite-Jones
Alison M. Rodriguez

Psychosocial Approaches to Child and Adolescent Health and Wellbeing

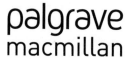

Jennifer M. Waite-Jones
School of Healthcare
University of Leeds
Leeds, UK

Alison M. Rodriguez
School of Healthcare
University of Leeds
Leeds, UK

ISBN 978-3-030-99353-5   ISBN 978-3-030-99354-2   (eBook)
https://doi.org/10.1007/978-3-030-99354-2

Cover illustration: @eStudioCalamar

This Palgrave Macmillan imprint is published by the registered company Springer Nature Switzerland AG.
The registered company address is: Gewerbestrasse 11, 6330 Cham, Switzerland

With love to Stephen, Justin, Julie, Heather, Sam, Ellen, Kate, Erin, Oscar, and Lila. And, also, with love to Yoan, Iris, Albi, and Seren.

Preface

The focus of this book is on the influence of the social environment on the wellbeing of children and adolescents. Whilst acknowledging, and explaining where appropriate, the indisputable biological basis of behaviour, the aim of writing this book was to familiarise or re-familiarise readers with stages of psychosocial development and how theories and studies within psychology and sociology can be used to address questions of current concern. It was felt necessary to adopt a truly psychosocial approach to appreciate the interactive nature of such experiences. As it proved impossible to do full justice to the many existing theories, it was decided to focus on those most useful in introducing readers to the dynamic process of individual development within a highly, socially structured environment.

Central, overlapping elements of biological, psychodynamic, cognitive/social cognitive, and behavioural theories within psychology were selected to explain individual behaviour. Sociological theories chosen include interactionism as it explains the bridge between meeting individual needs and social restraint. A feminist perspective was also adopted as greater gender awareness benefits for both males and females, and despite its shortcomings, functionalist theory was used to illustrate the complex, powerful structures influencing the lives of children and adolescents.

For readers new to this topic, the early chapters focusing on the impact of social context on early child development will be particularly helpful. These explain the development of attachment, sociability, play, and learning and how different theories can explain the conditions needed to foster children's wellbeing during their early life. This is important as early experiences impact on psychosocial development during adolescence and later life.

The critical assessment of current concerns about childhood, adolescence, and parenting within later chapters offers the opportunity for graduate and post-graduate students to appreciate the value of different explanations of influential social forces. Ambiguity in family life, concepts of deviance, and medicalisation are considered as major social influences which can be detrimental to wellbeing. These influences are then considered in terms of long-term conditions, including developmental delay, illness, and disability.

Finally, key elements of what has been previously covered are considered in terms of vulnerability and resilience. Such knowledge of seminal and contemporary theory as well as up to date, empirical evidence within psychology and sociology can, therefore, be used to help identify vulnerability during childhood and adolescence and abilities which can be harnessed to facilitate resilience.

As the focus of this book is on the influence of the psychosocial context into which children within current multicultural Western society are raised, studies from other cultures are utilised where appropriate. Readers are encouraged to reflect on central concepts within each chapter by considering questions asked about the 'virtual family' described in the appendix. Further, more general reflective questions are also offered at the end of each chapter.

Overall, this book should help general readers as well as students on nursing and health and social care courses and nurses, social workers, teachers, and psychologists already working with children and adolescents to develop a critical appreciation of social factors influencing the lives of those in their care.

Acknowledgements—We would like to thank all our students past and present, whose enthusiasm and commitment to our subject suggested a need to write this book.

Leeds, UK   Jennifer M. Waite-Jones
                                                                           Alison M. Rodriguez

Contents

About the Authors

Jennifer M. Waite-Jones   PhD, MSC, PGCE, BA (Hons), is Visiting Lecturer in Psychology in the School of Healthcare, University of Leeds, specialising in child and adolescent health and development. Prior to a lengthy career in higher education, she taught psychology and sociology within schools, colleges, and the voluntary sector. Her past work with national charities helped inform her qualitative research into the psychosocial impact of child and adolescent long-term conditions on carers and family life. She has specialised in ways to reduce the effects of stress on family members through self-management, patient–professional partnerships, promoting peer-support and using mobile technology. In addition to teaching health and developmental psychology and qualitative research methods at graduate and post-graduate levels, she has also supervised and examined the work of PhD students. Jennifer's previous publications include contributing to *Health Psychology in Context* (2009), as well as numerous articles relating to chronic illness in childhood and adolescence. She is a member of the International Family Nursing Association and her previous membership included The British Psychological Society (BPS), Children and Adolescent Psychology, Association of Teachers of Psychology, and Arthritis Care. She is a reviewer for the *Journal of Family Nursing*, *Journal of Disability and Rehabilitation*, *International Journal of Nursing Studies*, *Rheumatology Advances in Practice*, JMIR Publications, DOVE Publications, and a variety of other journals concerned with child, adolescent, and family health. See relevant website: https://www.researchgate.net/profile/Jennifer_Waite-Jones, linkedin.com/in/jenny-waite-jones-88b6a766, Publons https://publons.com.

Alison M. Rodriguez   PhD, MSc, PCPD, BSc (Hons), is Lecturer in Child and Family Health in the School of Healthcare, University of Leeds. She is a psychologist (with a background in health psychology) and Fellow of the Higher Education Academy with extensive teaching, research, and research supervision experience in health and critical health psychology. Alison has provided research supervision to children's nursing and psychology undergraduates and psychology and healthcare postgraduates at master's and doctoral levels and has internally and externally examined several PhD theses. Having used and supervised a range of methods, Alison's methodological passion is phenomenology. Alison's current work focusses on the health and wellbeing of children and young people with long-term, life-limiting, and life-threatening conditions, their needs, and those of their carers. Her externally funded research focuses on improving wellbeing, behaviour change, communication, support, and quality of care for service users and providers. This involves developing complex psycho-therapeutic and self-management interventions. Alison is a grant reviewer for the National Institute for Health Research and charitable organisations. She has presented and published numerous papers on the health and wellbeing of children, adolescents, young people, and older adults with health care and support needs. Alison has also written several research methods articles. She is an associate editor for the *Journal of Child Health Care* and has peer reviewed articles for the following periodicals: *Journal of Pediatric Nursing, Journal of Advanced Nursing, Health Psychology Open, British Journal of General Practice, International Journal of Palliative Nursing, BMJ Open, Journal of Forensic Psychiatry, Archives of Psychiatry & Mental Health, Qualitative Research in Psychology, Journal of Translational Paediatrics, The Indo-Pacific Journal of Phenomenology, Palliative Care and Social Practice, Teaching and Teacher Education, Journal of Teacher Education.* See Twitter—ARodriguez339.https://scholar.google.co.uk/citations?hl=en&hl=en&pli=1&user=NTlRRHAAAAAJ

List of Figures

List of Tables

Introduction

It is not easy to define what is meant by wellbeing as there is little agreement within published texts and practice. The following suggestions offer a useful starting point: 'a person's sense of satisfaction with their life and the level of positive and/or negative emotions they are feeling at a particular time' (Stiglitz et al., 2009), and 'an individual's ability to thrive within an environment which offers enough support and resources for them to meet the challenges and demands of living' (Smith and Hamer 2019). Both suggestions reflect the need to adopt the psychosocial approach adopted within this book rather than concentrate purely on physical wellbeing.

Attempting to ensure the wellbeing of children and adolescents becomes particularly complex as, although there are recognised stages in human development, perceptions of these can vary due to class, religion, ethnicity, geographical area, and economic needs (Marten, 2018). The convention of children's rights (United Nations General Assembly (UN), 1989) proposes that childhood (birth to twelve years) and adolescence (thirteen to nineteen years) with an overlapping period of youth (fifteen to twenty-five years) should be officially recognised as stages, with account taken of the impact of the social environment on wellbeing within each life stage. Wellbeing is, therefore, seen as an ecological concept determined by influences from family life, community, and wider society (McAuley & Rose, 2010).

Although there are specific physical and mental stages within childhood and adolescence where significant, recognisable development occurs, the social context in which a child or adolescent is raised can facilitate or inhibit this development. This is particularly important for children and adolescents' sense of wellbeing. As social animals, being a member of a supportive group is essential for human existence. Children and adolescents need to feel a sense of 'normality' in that they fit in reasonably well with, and conform to, the expectations of the social group in which they are raised.

Across cultures successful emotional development of children and adolescents is, therefore, influenced by means of the family, kinship patterns, and larger social network to which they belong. At times physical and emotional ill health can result from difficult relationships between children and adolescents and these institutions. Such difficulties can be caused and compounded by complex differences in the distribution of power and resources. For example, within the UK the most socio-economically, disadvantaged children and adolescents suffer the worse physical and mental health. Despite overall long-term improvements in infant mortality, the death rate for those born in England's most deprived areas is over twice as high as those from the least deprived areas. Infants from the most deprived areas are also more likely to have a low birthweight and during childhood can be three times more likely to suffer tooth decay and obesity (Public Health England, 2018, 2014–2016 figures).

The origin of the ethnic group to which children and adolescents belong also influences their health and potential wellbeing. For example, higher infant mortality rates have been found within families originating from the Caribbean and South Asia compared to white British families. Children from these families are also more likely to suffer discrimination, to experience disadvantage, and to live in poverty. Moreover, children from Black African and Black Caribbean ethnic groups are more likely to be overweight or obese (Public Health England, 2018. 2016–2017 figures).

Pearce et al. (2019) point out how changes at the macro-level of society through government initiatives in education, employment, social care, and public health are urgently needed to reduce child poverty and improve future opportunities for children and adolescents. It is important that educationalists and health and social care professionals appreciate the powerful social determinants of wellbeing and work towards providing more equitable, child- and adolescent-focussed services. The aim of this text is therefore to use theories and studies within psychology and sociology to help inform the professional practice of those concerned with the wellbeing of children and adolescents within current Western society. Chapter 2 outlines how concepts of 'childhood' and 'adolescence' can differ between different cultures and historical periods. A brief introduction to some theories within psychology and sociology is offered in Chap. 3, as these will be used within the following chapters to explain the psychosocial influences on specific aspects of child and adolescent wellbeing. As a child's first experience of the social world is with early caregivers, the importance of emotional attachments with significant others is considered within Chap. 4. The focus in Chap. 5 is then on the links between good early attachments and a child's sense of self and ability to relate successfully to others. Theories of cognitive and social development during childhood and adolescence are discussed in Chap. 6, with specific emphasis on the importance of play.

The emotionally charged nature of relationships within families (usually described as having some form of kinship and/or living in the same household) is discussed in Chap. 7, whilst in Chap. 8 an outline is offered of theories which may explain the process by which children and adolescents become labelled 'deviant' and responded to negatively within Western society. Current concerns with the increased power of the medical profession to monitor and control the ever decreasing boundaries of what is considered typical emotional as well as physical development in childhood and adolescence are explored in Chap. 9. The impact of being diagnosed with a long-term or complex condition within childhood or adolescence is discussed in Chap. 10. As some children and adolescents manage to achieve well-being in adulthood despite vulnerability to the potential long-term consequences of early adverse experiences an examination of what may promote resilience is offered in Chap. 11.

It has not been possible to devote specific chapters to the influence of gender, ethnicity, class, socio-economic status, and the impact of new technology on the lives of children and adolescents. However, such influences have been integrated throughout this book and will be found to be recurring themes within each chapter. In addition, it is consistently acknowledged that this book has been written during a time of unprecedented, world-wide health concerns due to the spread of the COVID-19 virus (coronavirus) which causes life-threatening, acute respiratory problems. The virus was first identified in December 2019 in the Chinese city of Wuhan. The speed at which this virus spread meant that in 2020 the World Health Organization (WHO) described it as a Public Health Emergency, and it has since become one of the most life-threatening pandemics in history.

The virus can be transmitted through airborne particles and touching contaminated surfaces or fluids. Prior to effective vaccines being developed (which have been administered since December 2020) the only preventative measures possible included wearing face masks and social distancing in public, continual washing and sanitising hands, disinfecting surfaces, and isolating those who had been exposed to the virus or displayed potential symptoms of having caught it.

Different countries have adopted strict measures to help contain the spread of the virus, with often detrimental effects on their economy. Within the UK various, often confusing, and contradictory emergency laws were passed which enforced some lengthy periods of public 'lockdowns' These included closure of public venues, working at home where possible, compulsory mask wearing in public, restricted access to private indoor and public outdoor spaces, school and nursery closures, and severe restricted visiting to hospitals, doctors, and care homes. This has meant that many loved ones could not be with those who died, and only a very restricted number of family members could meetup during festivals and funerals.

Vaccinations have currently helped reduce the number of deaths from this virus. At the time of writing this text they are being offered to secondary school–aged children regardless of parental consent. Despite evidence that children are unlikely to develop severe symptoms from the virus, potential, future, plans include the possibility of vaccinating younger children. It is difficult at this time to accurately assess the devastating long-term effects this pandemic will have on the psychological, social, and physical wellbeing of children and adolescents. However, what is known about some of the short-term consequences is consistently examined throughout this text.

Each chapter concludes with questions relating to a family case study (offered as an appendix), which are accompanied by further reflective questions to help stimulate critical discussion of the psychosocial impact on children's and adolescents' wellbeing.

References

Marten, J. (2018). *The History of Childhood: A very Short Introduction*. Oxford University Press.

McAuley, C., & Rose, W. (Eds.). (2010). *Child Well-being: Understanding Children's Lives at home, School and in the Community*. Jessica Kingsley Publisher.

Pearce, A., Dundas, R., Whitehead, M., & Taylor-Robinson, D. (2019). Pathways to Inequalities in Child Health. *Archives of Disease in Childhood, 104*, 998–1003. https://doi.org/10.1136/arc hdischild-2018-314808

Public Health England, Research and Analysis, Health Profile for England. (2018). Chapter 5: Inequalities in Health. Published September 11. Retrieved March 16, 2020, from https://www.gov.uk/government/publications/health-profile-for-england-2018/chapter-5-inequalities-in-health

Smith, J., & Hamer, J. (2019). *A System Mapping Approach to Understanding Child and Adolescent Wellbeing*. Research Report. July 2019. Department for Education 2019. Reference: DFE-RR945. A System Mapping Approach to Understanding Child and Adolescent Wellbeing: Research Report—Social Care Online (scie-socialcareonline.org.uk).

Stiglitz, J., Sen, A., & Fitoussi, J.-P. (2009). *Report of the Commission on the Measurement of Economic Performance and Social Progress*. Report of the Commission on the Measurement of Economic Performance et Social Progress (europa.eu).

United Nations General Assembly (UN). (1989). https://www.un.org/en/ga/62/plenary/children/bkg.shtml

Changing Concepts of Childhood and Adolescence

2

Currently the development of children and adolescents is assessed in relation to physical, cognitive, and emotional/social domains. These include physical health and motor development; intellectual abilities including attention and memory; and self-regulation, temperament, and interpersonal skills. However, growth in one domain influences the other areas and each can be influenced by environmental factors. For example, conflict, trauma, and neglect can seriously impact on children's early development which may have long-term detrimental physical and emotional consequences (Cecil et al., 2017).

The reaction of children and adolescents will depend on different factors, including their age, individual characteristics, and temperament, as well as the quality of care and support they receive from their family and others in their social environment (Rees & Bradshaw, 2018). Therefore, it is important to understand the social context in which children are raised to appreciate how it impacts on their ability to develop within the three domains outlined above and may promote optimal wellbeing.

The social environment experienced by children and adolescents changes over time and between cultures. This means that various beliefs about rights, responsibilities, and appropriate behaviour dominated different periods within history. Attitudes towards ethnicity, class, and gender behaviour have also differed, depending upon the views of those in power within specific societies (Keith, 2011). The way that attitudes towards children and adolescents have changed within Western society is explored within the following section of this chapter.

2.1   The Social Construction of 'Childhood' and 'Adolescence'

That different 'childhoods' are evident from historical and cross-cultural studies suggests that 'childhood' and 'adolescence' are socially constructed concepts created by adults (James & Prout, 1997; Heywood, 2017). Children and adolescents

J. M. Waite-Jones, A. M. Rodriguez, *Psychosocial Approaches to Child and Adolescent Health and Wellbeing*, https://doi.org/10.1007/978-3-030-99354-2_2

have no power to do this themselves. To appreciate the experiences of children and adolescents within current Western society it is necessary to examine how these periods of human development have been perceived over time.

2.1.1 Pre-industrial Concepts of Childhood

Although evidence about the lives of children and adolescents from pre-history is extremely limited, it appears that children were valued as toys were placed with their bodies during burials. Their value became more evident as increasingly complex communities dependent on agriculture developed. In many cases children and adolescents were ascribed clearly defined gender roles within a patriarchal society (Marten, 2018). However, despite being valued, throughout the history of Western society there appears to have been a tension between the need to control and yet nurture offspring. This was particularly evident within Christian religion. The Catholic church struggled to reconcile the view of children as innocent (given that they were cherished by Christ) with the concept of original sin, for which cleansing was necessary through baptism. Interestingly, Heywood (2017) relates further ambiguities within early religious views on childhood in relation to gender differences, which do not seem too distant from some contemporary prejudicial attitudes. He describes how it was thought that boys could be 'excitable and unstable' whilst girls were criticised as 'extravagant, wilful, jealous, docile, lazy, sharp and sly!'

The tension created by seeing children as innocent yet, having the potential to become out of control is evident throughout later historical periods and influenced approaches within psychology and sociology. Aries (1962) suggests that concepts of childhood and adolescence are a relatively 'recent invention'. He points out that prior to the fifteenth century, after about seven years of age European children were often treated the same as adults regarding their type of clothing, work, marriage, imprisonment, and punishment. Although Aries (1962) did not deny that some emotional ties existed between parents and their children, he insisted that a rigid demarcation between childhood and adulthood did not exist. Although Aries has been criticised for ignoring earlier sources and applying modern French concepts of childhood to children of all Western cultures (Tsar et al., 2016) his ideas stimulated further research. This has revealed past examples of strong parental affection towards their children. For example, Marten (2018) cites evidence of children at play in Bruegel's paintings and past Chinese embroidery which suggests that at least those from wealthy families were indulged. However, it appears that children have generally been viewed in terms of the economic contribution they offer. This, along with high mortality rates and the instability and uncertainty of family life, has influenced the amount of affection and concern expressed by parents.

The shift in attitudes towards children during the sixteenth and seventeenth centuries identified by Aries (1962) meant greater concern with the need to protect yet control children. For example, within philosophy, Hobbes (1588–1679) judged children as essentially evil and savage due to original sin, whilst Locke (1632–1704) suggested that they were born like 'blank slates' (*tabula rasa*) with their personalities created by environmental experiences. According to Locke's view, children required educating by parents and others to become useful members of society (Tsar et al., 2016). Locke's views were not entirely new, as the saying 'Give me a child until he is seven and I will give you the man' has been attributed to both the early philosopher Aristotle (384–322 BC) and the founder of the Jesuit Priesthood Saint Ignatius of Loyola (1491–1556). However, perceiving children as passive, 'empty vessels' into which knowledge requires 'pouring' can be seen to reinforce adults' sense of power to judge their behaviour and shape their moral development.

By the eighteenth century (considered an 'Age of Reason') the view of the 'child as innocent' became influential due to the work of Rousseau (1712–1778). He argued that children represented the perfect state of nature and essential goodness and, therefore, were 'noble savages', born with an innate sense of morality and a 'knowing innocence' that became lost in adulthood (Tsar et al., 2016). The roots of modern attitudes towards childhood are evident in the work of Rousseau as he viewed children as having an intrinsic worth independent of their potential economic contributions and rejected adult interference with their natural stages of development (Marten, 2018).

This 'nature versus nurture' debate still dominates current attitudes towards what is considered appropriate childcare. Children's inherent 'natural' qualities and 'innocence' are still valued, but also their potential for anti-social behaviour is feared and constantly monitored. These opposing views also underpin different theories within psychology and sociology and contemporary attempts to grapple with the thorny issue of children and adolescents' rights and responsibilities. They have been used at different times to define children and adolescents' legal and moral status and justify the way they should be reared and treated.

2.1.2 Childhood and Adolescence During the Industrial Revolution

During the late eighteenth and early nineteenth centuries, there was an upsurge in the use of very young children as forms of labour, particularly in industry and also in agriculture, mining, and even preparation for military service. Within the UK child labour was based on a class system, with divisions even within the lower classes. Very young children from skilled fathers were initially less likely to be employed than those from labourers. However, as increased mechanisation undercut the status of skilled workers, eventually their young children were also sent out to work. Humphries (2013) points out that the Industrial Revolution and resulting growth of urbanisation within Britain were only possible due to dehumanising younger and younger children from the labouring poor by making them responsible for the family income, through working long hours in hazardous occupations.

Interestingly, her evidence base (personal accounts supported by official records and statistics) reflects the gender bias of the period. All accounts and records relate to male occupation. Few records were kept of female occupation although women and daughters worked consistently beside men in agriculture, textiles, and other kinds of work. Negative attitudes towards female occupational status are therefore highly evident by their very absence.

Humphries' (2013) findings also suggest parallels between working-class family life then and in present times. Many families struggled due to economic restrictions created by new poor laws. In addition, large numbers of working children came from single-parent families due to fathers' abandonment or deaths caused by war, work, and sickness.

By the nineteenth century the influence of the Industrial Revolution meant increased attention was given to ensuring child workers from the lower classes demonstrated an appropriate work ethic. Although, Locke had believed in individual rights and that children should be raised with thought and care, other doctrines of the time insisted that physical punishment ensured children's appropriate development. This is evident in the saying, 'spare the rod and spoil the child'. Such dictates also reflect contemporary fears of adults that, unless carefully monitored and interventions used, there is a danger that children will become out of control.

Darwin's (1809–1802) theories of natural selection and survival of the fittest were also used to justify inequalities in the treatment of children from different social classes. Darwin was influenced by the work of Malthus' (1766–1834) which suggested that 'human nature' meant poverty for some was inevitable and impossible to alleviate (Rogers, 1972). However, the plight of young working children was gradually recognised as unacceptable. As the anti-slavery movement achieved success with the Slavery Abolition Act in 1833 it had become apparent that working children suffered similar fates and protective legislation was required. Therefore, in 1833 a Royal Commission defined those under thirteen years as children and the 1834 Factory Act limited the use of child labour in mills and factories. In 1847 a further act was passed limiting the working week for women and boys between thirteen and eighteen years to fifty-five hours a week. Although, slow to be implemented these acts demonstrated recognition that there was a need to protect child workers.

Interestingly, there were also other reasons behind the decisions to control the work carried out by children and women. Given the increased mechanisation of the workplace they could carry out similar work to men but were cheaper to employ. Being favoured by owners of mills and factories meant that children and women could achieve greater economic status than males. This threatened the 'normal', 'natural' social, and, inevitably, patriarchal order, as fathers were meant to be the main breadwinners. Moreover, the increased precociousness and potential self-reliance of children, resulting from workplace experiences and their role of wage earner, raised adult concerns (Hendrick, 1997).

The introduction of compulsory education was meant to benefit all children but, it had unintended consequences for children of the labouring poor. It reduced their opportunity to work and changed their economic status within families from economic contributors to economic burdens. Moreover, the use of physical punishment in schools to enforce discipline ensured a future obedient society in line with the ideals of the middle and upper classes.

2.1.3   Concepts of Childhood and Adolescence Since Industrialisation

Changing attitudes towards child labour meant that children were perceived as needing to be nurtured to be able to better contribute to economic prosperity in adulthood. The status of children, thus, changed and they began to be considered as a form of future economic and social investment. This meant that they became particularly worthy of special attention and in need of greater legal protection, as for example, The Education Acts (1870s and 1880s), Age of Consent (1885), Infant Life Protection (1872 and 1897), and Prevention of Cruelty to, and Neglect of, Children (1889).

Greater state intervention into children's lives also brought increased emphasis on the importance of discipline within family life and parents' responsibility for their children's behaviour. Again, this had an unanticipated, potential negative impact on the labouring poor within the UK. The large number of children within families became increasingly economically dependent and less of an insurance policy for parents against poverty and loneliness of old age. Moreover, tensions were experienced which reflect those of current parents, in that complying with new social, legislative, and moral views of child rearing can conflict with economic demands and the emotionally charged nature of family life.

The mass provision of education meant it was possible to address societal concerns with children's development and behaviour through studying their physical and mental health whilst in school. Hendrick (1997) explains how a 'child study' era emerged between the 1880s and1914 such that children and child welfare achieved a new political and social identity. He suggests that the national importance now placed on monitoring children's development differed considerably from the mid-nineteenth century concern with rescuing, reforming, and reclaiming childhood. Nevertheless, as many children were found to live in poverty and be in poor health more preventative medicine and increased public health measures were introduced. Perceiving the care of children as a necessary investment for the future national economy also meant increased national concern with education and responsible parenting. Greater state intervention into the lives of families, therefore, helped to create a national concept of childhood which resulted in further ideas of age segregation and children's separate identity to adults (Hendrick, 1997).

Although childhood has become increasingly recognised as a life stage within Western society, it is only very recently that 'adolescence' has begun to be seen in this way. Smith (2016) explains that in Latin, 'adolescence' means 'growing or coming to maturity' and that in fifteenth-century France it meant 'youth'. There are universal features of physical changes during puberty, but the social importance of the nature and timing of these changes varies between cultures and different historical periods. In the past most cultures acknowledged the transition of girls to womanhood at the onset of menstruation. It is not as easy to seek such a major physical marker in males. Marten (2018) suggests that as young males on the brink of manhood tend to push social boundaries, group rituals and rites of passage were (and still are in some cultures) introduced as a way of controlling potential rebellion. It is interesting to note that such explanations reinforce stereotypical attitudes that females are defined by their individual biology whilst males are defined by social behaviour. Such reflections on how stereotypical gender differences are reinforced during adolescence within a patriarchal society are evident in the quotation from Shakespeare's A Winter's Tale (cited by Smith, 2016:12):

> I would there were no age between, ten and three-and-twenty, or that youth would sleep out the rest; for there is nothing in the between but getting wenches with child, wronging the ancientry, stealing, fighting.

Within Western society adolescence gradually emerged as a separate life stage due to universal schooling, a decline in traditional forms of authority and increased dependence on peer group status. Evidence of earlier concerns that the behaviour of older children threatened social order within the UK can be seen with the passing of the Youthful Offenders Act in 1854 and later, additional versions. The need to control those within this age group became increasingly seen as necessary and created further tensions within families. G. Stanley Hall (1846–1924) has been credited with 'discovering' the way that adolescence is currently perceived within Western society (see Arnett, 2006). He identified this as a time of 'storm and stress' for young people due to the psychological as well as physical changes taking place during puberty. However, the amount of stress experienced during this time is also influenced by culture. For example, adolescents from pre-industrial societies with strong ties to family and community experience less stress than those within post-industrial Western society who are reported to be more creative but less conforming and likely to indulge in risky behaviour (Arnett, 1995).

2.2 Current Concepts of Childhood and Adolescence

Current Western perceptions of 'childhood' and 'adolescence' can be seen to have been influenced by past events including increased industrialisation, education, and a need for greater child protection. As industrialisation increased so did the need for a more educated workforce. This created an expansion of middle-class families. Changing attitudes to family life along with increased use of birth control meant a decline in the birth rate, such that by the twentieth century there was greater parental investment in raising and cherishing their children. Previous harsh, and controlling, parenting practices ensuring a submissive workforce were replaced by indulging, undemanding parents facilitating current consumerism (Gerhardt, 2014). The concept of an ideal family life developed, involving ritualised festivals. For example, Christmas celebrations were enhanced through greater access to material possessions such as cheap, mass-produced toys. Families and child-related institutions, therefore, began to display the child-centred attitudes currently evident.

Children and adolescents were increasingly seen in terms of future social and economic investments and additional consumers. This meant that lengthy periods of nurturing were required so further legislation was introduced, for example, feeding 'necessitous' children in school (1906), school medical inspections (1907), and increased infant welfare (1918).

This new perception of childhood began to be formally recognised through the work of the League of Nations (1924), and within the justice system through greater consideration being given to children's best interests. Unexpected world events, such as the Second World War, also contributed to changes in attitudes towards childhood. Mass evacuation of children to places of safety within the UK made visible the shocking conditions in which large numbers of children were reared. It also drew attention to the intensity of child–parent bonds and damage caused by removing children from their natural family. Children, therefore, began to be seen even more in terms of being a family member and public responsibility.

Hendrick (1997) points out how such attitudes were influenced by medicine, psychology, and education. The influence of psychology increased, creating a child guidance movement based on the psychoanalytically driven work of Isaacs (1885–1948) and standardised testing created by Burt (1883–1971). The concept of the 'problem child' emerged and, interestingly, the three themes identified by Marten (2018) as underlying this movement: controlling the mind of the child, dictating family life, and ensuring the management of children's behaviour are still popular current concerns.

The introduction of the Welfare State after the Second World War helped to improve the health of children and adolescents. Also, the popular youth culture which started to become visible between the two world wars increased massively due to innovations in the media, including cinema, radio, magazines, and the greater purchasing power available for some young people. However, by the 1950s increased poverty and urbanisation meant higher rates of juvenile crime and raised concerns about working-class youths being out of control and lacking obedience (Marten, 2018).

Issues relating to an increasingly rebellious youth culture came to dominate the 1960s as employment and educational opportunities increased for this age group. Despite media hype and the changes in lifestyle for those from middle-class and upper-class families, the same 'liberated' attitudes towards youth were slow to impact on the lives of many working-class adolescents. Nevertheless, children's rights were included within the increased political and social movements in this, and later periods, such that 1979 was designated the year of the child. However, ironically, around this time, and later in the 1980s, adolescents' spending power was drastically reduced through the lack of employment opportunities (Hendrick, 1997). The school leaving age had been extended to sixteen years in 1973 and for those leaving with no chance of work, government funded schemes were introduced. These included the Youth Opportunity Programme (1978) which was heavily criticised as offering poor training so was later developed into the Youth Training Scheme (1983). These schemes were meant to build bridges between education and work and eventually evolved into the modern apprenticeship schemes of 1990s. However, Simmons (2019) explains how the sub-contracting of such schemes established the basis for current privatisation and marketisation of post-compulsory education.

Also, although meant to increase youth employment opportunities, the introduction of such schemes, offering small amounts of money for those taking them up, also restricted the income and expectations of future high paid employment for adolescents. This helped in regulating their behaviour through their reduced spending power. Interestingly, such schemes were specifically promoted as preparing the future generation to successfully compete with Britain's economic industrial competitors (first author's personal experience) reflecting, again, the way children and adolescents had become to be viewed as national economic investments.

Further changes to perceptions of children and adolescents were evident during the 1980s. For example, the rights of adolescents to be responsible for their own bodies were determined by the Gillick judgement (1985) such that doctors could offer girls contraceptive advice without parental consent. There was also greater awareness of the physical and sexual abuse endured by many in these age groups. For example, in1986 Esther Rantzen, a popular television presenter, initiated the establishment of 'Childline' to provide telephone contact for children in distress. Also, one of the main principles within the Children Act (1989) was to make local authorities more responsible for safeguarding and promoting child welfare, particularly in relation to 'looked after children'.

Although Hendrick (1997) suggests this was not particularly effective legislation, it did grant statutory powers to the UK charity National Society for the Prevention of Cruelty to Children (NSPCC). However, the constant ambivalence in attitudes towards controlling and nurturing children became starkly evident with the hardened public response and stiffer legal changes resulting from the Bulger case (1993) which involved the murder of a small child by two older boys.

During the twenty-first century the Children Act (2004) was passed with the aim to further improve the lives of children and adolescents. This covered universal services as well as those necessary for children with special needs. Local authorities were particularly expected to promote the educational achievement of looked after children. Also, greater increased availability of leisure products and new technology, including social media and mobile phones, within Western society during this period has increased child and adolescent consumerism and parental concerns.

Despite increased protective legislation and availability of such commodities the current 'ideal' childhood is very different to lived experiences of many children and adolescents. The continuing informal segregation based on race, class, and gender influences their educational opportunities and standards of living. Currently, the age of first sexual intercourse is becoming increasingly lower amongst adolescents, whilst rates of single motherhood and sexual diseases are rising. Adolescents are also faced with new choices given the greater public acceptance of transgender people and relationships between same sex couples (Marten, 2018) as well as pressure from ever increasing academic expectations.

2.2.1 Current Concerns with Child and Adolescent Protection and Wellbeing

Although within Western society difference exist due to geographical location and class, child mortality has been reduced due to improved sanitation, nutrition, and child welfare measures. However, the greater value placed on children and adolescents has increased concerns about their mental wellbeing which, in turn, has meant further government intervention into their lives. Since the fundamental shift in thinking about children's rights established by the United Nations Convention on the Rights of the Child (The United Nations, 1989) further legislation within the UK has increased, not only to protect, but to promote the wellbeing of children and adolescents. For example, not only did the Safeguarding Vulnerable Groups Act (2006) improve the vetting of those working with children and/or vulnerable adults, the Children and Young Person's Act (2008) identified the Secretary of State as responsible for promoting the wellbeing of children (under eighteen years) and young people (under the age of twenty-five years). Also, the Education Act (2011) was not only concerned with the provision of schools but also academies, institutions within the further education sector, post-16 education including vocational apprenticeships, and student finance for higher education.

The now firmly established view of children and adolescents within a family setting is evident in The *Children and Families Act* (2014) which reformed services for vulnerable children, extended parental working rights to leave and pay, streamlined the adoption process, and increased separated child–parent contact through improved court processes. However, that the *Children and Families Act* (2014) increased the role of the Children's Commissioner with specific regard to immigration demonstrates concerns with issues not previously experienced within the UK. The greater numbers of immigrant families from different cultures within the UK include a minority whose childrearing practices differ significantly from those acceptable within Western society. For example, the aim of the Forced Marriage Act (2007) and Forced Marriage Unit (FMU) is to protect adolescents from being pressurised to marry against their wishes. Also, the Female Genital Mutilation Act (2003) was passed as a response to family practices of taking girls abroad to undergo female genital mutilation (FGM). That genital mutilation has been condemned by the World Health Organization (WHO) and criminalised by all members of European Union but is still practiced in some other countries demonstrates a conflict between respecting cultural traditions and maintaining human rights.

The lives of children and adolescents have, therefore, improved dramatically. However, to some extent, this can be seen at the cost of previous freedom. For example, the lives of children are increasingly monitored due to greater concerns about the increasing numbers of single-parent families, mothers working outside the home, and reported crimes against children. This has put pressure on parents to ensure they provide more organised child-focused activities and accept the advice of 'experts' on how to rear the 'ideal' child. Adolescents' lives have been further restricted due to the raising of the leaving age of compulsory education or training.

This has restricted their ability to earn an income and gain a sense of freedom and self-esteem from contributing to a family income which they are now still dependent upon.

2.2.2   Experience of Childhood and Adolescence—Improved or Deteriorating?

There is disagreement about whether, in Western societies in general and the UK in particular, the experience of childhood and adolescence is 'better' or 'worse' than in the past. For example, Moffat (2010) points out how children's diet is still a concern, although now more likely to be because of obesity rather than starvation. Also, Gram et al. (2018) maintain that the striving to create the 'ideal' family, producing 'perfect' children can create emotional overload. Moreover, Humphries (2013) suggests that balancing economic demands with a stable family life can create 'dysfunctional' families with unhappy, neglected, and abused children.

There appears to be a deterioration in the subjective wellbeing of some children and adolescents (Rees & Bradshaw, 2018) with the onset of mental health disorders usually becoming evident during these periods. That child mental health difficulties have become more common and affect educational progress, later social relationships and future mental health were reported by Sellars et al. (2019). Linked to such concerns is a generalised fear that the ideal childhood is disappearing due to increased consumerism and parental spending on children. Not only are parents subjected to 'pester power' due to advertising but, according to Hendrick (1997), children are viewed as an emotional indulgence with their pleasure reflecting the success of parent's emotional investment.

Postman (1982) suggested that the origin of childhood and the reasons for its decline lie in changes in communication technology. He saw that prior to the invention of the printing press, when societies depended upon oral traditions for passing on of cultural norms, childhood ended once speech had been mastered. He insisted that literacy, made possible by the printed word, increased children's potential for greater knowledge of the adult world as well as that outside their communities. Montag and Diefenbach (2018) point to similarly unintended side-effects of technology use by questioning its impact on human nature given that constant interaction with virtual realities may reduce the opportunity for emotional needs to be met. Smith (2016) also points out the ambivalence of increased internet experience, as offering greater support from adolescent peers but also the possibility of reinforcing problematic behaviour such as eating disorders.

Palmer (2007) argues that recent technological and cultural changes cause psychological and physical damage to children and adolescents. She points out how the resulting decline of outdoor play is linked to increased obesity and children are at risk of exploitation from advertisers. Palmer (2007) also believes that 'over schooling' reduces the past independence of children and adolescents whose attention span is becoming shorter due to increased 'screen saturation'. However, Furedi (2008) criticises the increased fears for children's safety and resulting child protection measures. In his book, 'Paranoid Parenting' he argues that children are currently overprotected, or too controlled due to an automatic assumption of their vulnerability.

However, the views of both Palmer (2007) and Furedi (2008) may be guilty of over-emphasising the extent to which children are controlled and exposed to rapid technological changes. For example, Bennett (2006) describes the heavily disciplined 'ideal' styles of child rearing common during the 1950s which Palmer (2007) may have in mind. She points out that currently more children experience family outings and tailored leisure activities and that the past greater exposure to lengthy unsupervised outdoor play in the 'fresh air' could lead to bullying and other unpleasant behaviour and, thus, was not always beneficial.

Bennet (2006) also compares the educational experiences offered today with the harsh and undignified way pupils were often treated in the past. She responds to current concerns with paedophiles with accounts of how such dangerous individuals also were known to exist in the past. Nevertheless, Palmer's (2007) concerns cannot be completely dismissed. For example, the report into Rotherham council, covering 1997 to 2013 (Jay, 2014), demonstrated a woeful lack of response to known groups of males abusing vulnerable young girls. This practice has also been found to exist in other areas of the UK. Such accounts suggest a need to take child protection issues very seriously.

2.2.3   Improving the Lives of Children and Adolescents

Those caring for children and adolescents strive to learn from the complex and often conflicting views of modern childhood and adolescence to ensure the promotion of the 'best interests of the child' established by the UN (1989). The need to be aware of the maturational, psychological, and social needs of children and adolescents means that it is appropriate to utilise a bio-psycho-social framework in practice. For example, findings within neuroscience demonstrate different rates of development between neural networks in the frontal cortex during adolescence (Blakemore & Mills, 2014). This, together with social control theory (Hirschi, 1969), can help in understanding their increased self-focussed and risk-taking behaviour and underpin interventions which promote a sense of belonging and reduce anti-social behaviour.

Increased use of digital technology by children and adolescents, so criticised by Palmer (2007), can also be harnessed to promote their wellbeing. For example, Poyntz and Pedri (2018) point out the positive impact it has on education and online learning. However, they, too, caution against the potential it creates for greater monitoring and interventions by corporations, governments, and predatory individuals. Nevertheless, the use of such technology can also be seen to have provided education and a lifeline for self-isolated children and adolescents, as well as kept educational institutions, businesses, and governments running, during restrictions caused by the COVID-19 virus pandemic in 2020.

New technology has also been found useful in promoting and maintaining the health of children and adolescents, contributing to the current ideal of child-centred care identified by Ford et al. (2018). Further innovations within child and adolescent health include involving them more in decisions made about their care. For example, O'Hara et al. (2019) point out that although this can be challenging given the responsibilities and traditional practices with healthcare, involving patients means creating better quality and safer care. Also, Lawton et al. (2019) suggest the involvement of child and adolescents as ambassadors when creating health policies and within health research as another step in improving their care.

Greater improvement of children and adolescents' mental health can also be achieved through recognising the damaging impact of early adverse experiences on their later development and promoting greater resilience. For example, Sciaraffa et al. (2018) suggest core protective measures including offering safe and healthy environments allowing children to play and explore. This helps to maximise interpersonal capacities associated with resiliency, such as self-efficacy and self-regulation. They also state that extra support is necessary for these children in times of stress and protective measures should be offered at national and community levels.

Having reflected on changes on the lives of children and adolescents, including improved recognition of their needs over time within the UK, it is important to avoid complacency as many children and adolescents are still disadvantaged through their class, ethnic background, and gender. For example, Martin (2018) states that, despite legislation such as the Sex Discrimination Act (1975), gender codes are still transmitted within schools conveying stereotyped views of femininity and masculinity. She also points out that most boys and girls choose 'gender-appropriate' subjects, and when boys do take those normally expected of girls, their efforts are given more credit than the girls in the class, who are expected to find learning such subjects easier as this should 'come naturally'. Martin (2018) argues that such perceptions provide a basis for how boys, girls, men, and women are expected to behave within the family and workplace, which is not always to their advantage.

In addition, there still exist increased high levels of infant mortality, low birth weight, and dental decay in childhood in those born in the most deprived areas including those from different ethnic groups (Public Health England, 2018). Although the links between social deprivation and poor health outcomes are complex, the differences in distribution of power and resources determine the material and psychosocial conditions in which children grow up. Pearce et al. (2019) stress the need for radical changes at a macro level of society, including improved social security systems, employment, and childcare provision.

Moreover, the COVID-19 virus pandemic (2020) has demonstrated the shrinking nature of the world. Increased immigration means that practitioners within the UK are caring for more children and adolescents with varied past cultural experiences which may, even, have involved extreme violence. Despite greater world regulation on child labour, in areas of extreme poverty economically distressed families still rely on their child or adolescent's income. Moreover, Marten (2018) states that in 2017 it was estimated by a child advocacy group that a quarter of the over 40 million people (mostly female) involved in sex trafficking and slavery were children.

Having offered, here, a very brief overview of the many changes regarding childhood and adolescence within Western society, and the UK specifically, it will be seen that many issues covered are expanded upon and further explored in later chapters. Specific emphasis is placed on conflicting concerns introduced within this chapter such as fears of increased child exposure to an adult world yet increased criticisms of overprotection. Concerns about overprotection currently mean that children and adolescents now face humiliation in being referred to within the media as 'post-millennium snowflakes'. However, it is well worth remembering the view of Marten (2018) who concludes that despite economic class and other societal pressures, children still manage to be 'children', and add to this that adolescents will still remain 'adolescents'.

Summary

- The cognitive, social, and emotional stages evident in children and adolescents' development are heavily influenced by the social context in which they are raised.
- It is necessary to distinguish between children and adolescents, who have always existed, and 'childhood' and 'adolescence' which are socially constructed concepts based on how childhood and adolescence have been perceived during different historical periods and between different cultures.
- The modern idea of childhood in the UK stems from legal changes during and since industrialisation such as: excluding children from employment, establishing, and extending periods of compulsory education, recognising children and adolescents' rights, and creating a juvenile justice system.
- Despite additional safeguarding policies and child-centred attitudes offering greater protection for children and adolescents, evidence suggests that their wellbeing is not necessarily improving. Social inequalities, new technology, increasing mental health problems, and reported cases of child abuse are current concerns.

Case Study Questions

Read the family case study on page 265 and consider the following:

- How might the different experiences of this family have impacted upon the lives of Gemma, Ben, Liam, and Chrissy?
- How would have Gemma, Ben, Liam, and Chrissy have been seen and treated within the pre-industrial and industrial past?
- Suggest the different kinds of support needed for each member of the family and how the COVID-19 'lockdown' has made the provision of such support more difficult.

Reflective Questions

- Do current child/adolescent-centred attitudes create indulged, 'infantilised', 'snowflakes'?
- Should parents and agencies responsible for the wellbeing of children and adolescents be more protective or allow them more individual freedom?
- How may early experiences affect the future life-course of children and adolescents today in comparison to those of their parents?

References

Aries, P. (1962). *Centuries of Childhood: A Social History of the Family*. Vintage Books.

Arnett, J. (1995). Broad and Narrow Socialization: The Family in Context of Cultural Theory. *Journal of Marriage and the Family, 57*, 617–628. https://doi.org/10.2307/353917

Arnett, J. J. (2006). G. Stanley Hall's Adolescence: Brilliance and Nonsense. *History of Psychology, 9*(3), 186–197. https://doi.org/10.1037/1093-4510.9.3.186

Bennett. (2006, September 14). So, our 'Toxic' Culture is Bad for Children? In the Good Old Days, We Just Had to Endure Days of Boredom and Beatings. *The Guardian*.

Blakemore, S-J., & Mills, K. L. (2014). Is Adolescence a Sensitive Period for Sociocultural Processing? *Annual Review of Psychology, 65*, 1870–207. https://doi.org/10.1146/annurev-psych-010213-115202115202

Cecil, C. A. M., Viding, E., Fearon, P., Glaser, D., & McRory, E. J. (2017). Disentangling the Mental Health Impact of Childhood Abuse and Neglect. *Child Abuse & Neglect, 63*, 06–119. https://doi.org/10.1016/j.chiabu.2016.11.024

Children and Families Act. (2014). http://www.legislation.gov.uk/ukpga/2014/6/notes/division/2

Children and Young Person's act. (2008). https://www.legislation.gov.uk/ukpga/2008/23/notes/division/2

Female Genital Mutilation Act. (2003). https://www.gov.uk/government/publications/female-genital-mutilation-resource-pack/female-genital-mutilation-resource-pack

Forced Marriage Act. (2007). https://webarchive.nationalarchives.gov.uk/20081105214212/http://www.justice.gov.uk/docs/consultation-31-07.pdf

Ford, K., Campbell, S., Carter, B., & Earwaker, L. (2018). The Concept of Child-Centered care in Healthcare: A Scoping Review Protocol. *BI Database System Review Implement Rep., 16*(4), 845–851. https://doi.org/10.11124/JBISRIR-2017-003464

Furedi, F. (2008). *Paranoid Parenting: Why Ignoring the Experts May be Best for your Child*. Continuum.

Gerhardt. (2014). *Why Love Matters: How Affection Shapes a Baby's Brain*. Routledge.

Gram, M., Therkelsen, A., & Larsen, R. K. (2018). Family Bliss or Blitz? Parents' and Children's Mixed Emotions Towards Family Holidays. *Young Consumers, 19*(2), 185–198. https://doi.org/10.1108/YC-06-2017-00703

Hendrick, H. (1997). *Child Welfare: England, 1872-1989*. Routledge.

Heywood, C. (2017). *A History of Childhood*. Polity Press.

Hirschi, T. (1969). *Causes of Delinquency*. University of California Press.

Humphries, J. (2013). Childhood and Child Labour in the British Industrial Revolution. *Economic History Review, 66*(2), 395–418. https://www.jstor.org/stable/42921562

James, A., & Prout, A. (1997). *Constructing and Reconstructing Childhood*. Falmer Press.

Jay, A. (2014). Independent Inquiry into Child Sexual Exploitation in Rotherham. 1997–2013 Alexis Jay OBE (2014). https://www.rotherham.gov.uk/downloads/file/279/independent-inquiry-into-child-sexual-exploitation-in-rotherham

Keith, K. D. (2011). *Ed.* Cross-Cultural Psychology Contemporary Themes and Perspectives, Wiley.

Lawton, J., Blackburn, M., Breckenridge, J. P., Hallowell, N., Farrington, C., & Rankin, D. (2019). Ambassadors of Hope, Research Pioneers and Agents of Change-Individuals' Expectations and Experiences of Taking Part in a Randomised Trial of an Innovative Health Technology: Longitudinal Qualitative Study. *BMC Research, 20*, 289. https://doi.org/10.1186/s13063-019-3373-9

League of Nations. (1924). https://treaties.un.org/Pages/Content.aspx?path=DB/LoNOnline/pageIntro_en.xml

Marten, J. (2018). *The History of Childhood: A very Short Introduction*. Oxford University Press.

Martin, J. (2018). Gender and Education. Perspectives through time. In M. Cole (Ed.), *Education, Equality and Human Rights* (4th ed.). New York. Routledge.

Moffat, T. (2010). The "Childhood Obesity Epidemic": Health Crisis or Social Construction? *Medical Anthropology Quarterly, 24*(1), 1–21. https://doi.org/10.1111/j.1548-1387.2010.01082.x

Montag, C., & Diefenbach, S. (2018). Towards Homo Digitalis: Important Research Issues for Psychology and the Neurosciences at the Dawn of the Internet of Things and the Digital Society. *Sustainability, 10*, 415. https://doi.org/10.3390/su10020415

O'Hara, J. K., Aase, K., & Waring, J. (2019). Scaffolding our Systems? Patients and Families 'Reaching In' as a Source of Healthcare Resilience. *BMJ., 28*, 3–6. https://doi.org/10.1136/bmjqs-2018-008216

Palmer, S. (2007). *Toxic Childhood*. Orion.

Pearce, A., Dundas, R., Whitehead, M., & Taylor-Robinson, D. (2019). Pathways to Inequalities in Child Health. *Arch. Dis. Child, 104*, 998–1003. https://doi.org/10.1136/archdischild-2018-314808

Postman, N. (1982). *The Disappearance of Childhood*. Cornet.

Poyntz, S. R., & Pedri, J. (2018, January). Youth and Media Culture. Education and Society, Technology and Education, Languages and Literacies. Online Publication Date. https://doi.org/10.1093/acrefore/9780190264093.013.

Public Health England, Research and Analysis, Health Profile for England. (2018, September 11). *Chapter 5: Inequalities in Health*. Retrieved March 16, 2020, from https://www.gov.uk/government/publications/health-profile-for-england-2018/chapter-5-inequalities-in-health

Rees, G., & Bradshaw, J. (2018). Exploring Low Subjective Well-Being Among Children aged 11 in the UK: An Analysis Using Data Reported by Parents and by Children. *Child Indicators Research, 11*(1), 27–56. https://doi.org/10.1007/s12187-016-9421-z

Rogers, J.A. (1972). Darwinism and Social Darwinism. *Journal of the History of Ideas, 33*, 2. University of Pennsylvania Press Stable. http://www.jstor.org/stable/2708873

Safeguarding Vulnerable Groups Act. (2006). (c 47) https://www.southglos.gov.uk/documents/cyp120032.pdf

Sciaraffa, M. A., Zeanah, P. D., & Zeanah, C. H. (2018). Understanding and Promoting Resilience in the Context of Adverse Childhood Experiences. *Early Childhood Educ. J., 46*, 343–353. https://doi.org/10.1007/s10643-017-0869-3

Sellars, R., Warne, N., Pickles, A., Maughan, B., Thaaper, A., & Collinshaw, S. (2019). Cross-Cohort Change in Adolescent outcomes for Children with Mental Health Problems. *The Journal of Child Psychology and Psychiatry, 60*, 813–821. https://doi.org/10.1111/jcpp.13029

Simmons, R. (2019). Time to Revisit the Youth Training Scheme? *Post 16 Educator, 97*, 16–17. ifyoucan.org.uk

Smith, P. K. (2016). *Adolescence. A Very Short Introduction*. Oxford University Press.

Tsar, M., Rodreguez, S., & Kupferman, D. W. (2016). Philosophy and Pedagogy of Childhood, Adolescence and Youth. *Global Studies of Childhood., 6*(2), 169–176. https://doi.org/10.1177/2043610616647623

United Nations General Assembly (UN). (1989). https://www.un.org/en/ga/62/plenary/children/bkg.shtml

Psychosocial Theories of Childhood and Adolescence

3

3.1 Childhood and Adolescence and the Psychosocial Approach

Although perceptions of childhood and adolescence have varied historically and cross-culturally there are some universal elements common within these stages of development which can be explained by adopting a psychosocial approach. This approach also helps to explain the often, diverse range of experiences within childhood and adolescence across different cultures, ethnicities, genders, sexualities, and physical abilities, and is useful for ensuring that children and adolescents receive appropriate care.

To understand child and adolescent wellbeing, it is important to consider their physical, emotional, and cognitive development as well as how this interacts with the environment into which they are born. The psychosocial approach adopted within this book, therefore, draws from work within psychology including biologically based theories, psycho-dynamic theories, behavioural/social learning theories, and theories of cognitive development. These are integrated with sociological theories including interactionism and feminist theories as they concentrate on the interactions between humans and their societies. Functionalist theory is also considered as a way of identifying the social structures in which these interactions occur. It is beyond the scope of this book to include other important structural theories, such as Marxism, or the diverse explanations offered within post-modernism.

The aim within this chapter is, therefore, to offer a brief explanation of the theories identified above and how they can be usefully combined within a bio-psychosocial framework to help understand how to best promote the wellbeing of children and adolescents.

3.2   Theories Within Psychology

3.2.1   Biology-based Theories

Awareness of the influence of children and adolescents' biological inheritance moulded by interactions with their environment is essential when attempting to promote their wellbeing. However, this also means grappling with the age-old concerns about the role of the 'mind' and consciousness, as thoughts can create physiological changes and physiological changes can affect thinking.

Box 3.1 Examples of Mind/Body Interactions

Mind affecting body: Those unfortunate enough to have experienced old-fashioned, insensitive methods within dentistry may find that they turn pale, and their heart rate increases at the mere thought of an impending dental appointment.

Body affecting mind: Severe, painful scratching from a previously loved cat may create a strong dislike of cats in their owner, who may then give away the pet they once adored.

Although the location and substance of the mind remain a mystery, even to some current psychologists, those who take a biological approach firmly see the 'mind' and the 'brain' as one and the same. Much has been learned about the functions of the brain through studies of mental and physical trauma (Lewis-Williams & Pearce, 2005) and new techniques within neuroscience, such as Magnetic Resonance Imagery (MRI) and Positron-Emission Tomography (PET) scanning. These have proved useful in demonstrating the rapid growth of the brain during early development, as well as later changes during adolescence which continue into adulthood (Lebel & Beaulieu, 2011).

Brain and behaviour are assumed to be a product of human evolution and include specific neuro-chemical activities created by brain function and specialisation. The brain and nervous system appear to form a complex communication system involving electrical impulses ('messages') transmitted via a network of nerve fibres. These electrical 'messages' are inhibited or amplified by means of chemicals (hormones and neurotransmitters) which bind with specific receiving neurones situated at regular gaps (synapses) between the nerve fibres.

Although inherited chromosomes (thread like structures) containing genes carry a 'blueprint' (DNA) of an individual's potential development, stimulation from the environment is required to establish a complex network of neural connections as the child develops. As the network increases a pruning process occurs in which those connections that do not correspond to repeated forms of experience will die away. Those connections which reflect consistently repeated experiences are eventually coated with a myelin sheath to improve and ensure the strength of the electrical impulse being transmitted (Robinson, 2008).

Psychologists, such as Gesell (1880–1961), developed a theory of maturation as they believed that a universal predetermined biological timetable exists for human development, including the brain. Franke et al. (2012) point out how such a time-table includes specific periods of rapid, highly coordinated neural development leading to different stages of brain maturation between infancy and late adolescence. Cross-cultural studies have also confirmed universal timing in the acquisition of skills such as pointing, crawling, walking, and talking as well as physiological changes such as those during puberty (Robinson, 2008).

The brain appears to operate through genetically coded programmes within specific regions which eventually interconnect such that the whole brain is involved. However, the bi-directional nature of neural activity responding to, and changing the individual's environment within a person's different life stages, creates a highly complex system. Studies suggest that maturation occurs when myelination is complete, but this occurs at different times within the numerous regions of the brain. For example, the frontal lobe formation, one of the four lobes within the cerebral cortex, is not fully formed until adulthood (Blakemore & Mills, 2014). Also, there appears to be sensitive periods for optimal development of different sections and sub-sections within the brain.

The limbic system, along with the brain stem, is responsible for controlling emotions as well as, to some extent, cognition (LeDoux, 1998). This system also includes the hippocampus, thalamus, hypothalamus, pituitary gland, and amygdala. The hippocampus is often considered as the 'gateway' to memories. The pituitary gland controls many of the processes within the limbic system through production of hormones but, in turn, is controlled by hypothalamus which also affects appetite, mood, and sex hormones. The hypothalamus also acts as a kind of thermostat in responding to environmental stimuli by controlling levels of cortisol which in turn sets off a chemical chain reaction impacting upon the immune system. The important role of the amygdala has become increasingly recognised as it acts upon stimuli from the sensory systems and creates a quick response to uncertainty, fear, and danger (Robinson, 2008).

There are also two distinct hemispheres within the brain placed above and around the brain stem, which is a primitive area vital for life and tapers down to the spinal cord. There appears to be a 'division of labour' between the two hemispheres. The left hemisphere is responsible for language production and seems to seek order and reason. The right hemisphere is more involved with sensory perception and adopts a more 'global', integrative, and holistic style of processing adding emotional depth to experiences. Despite initial dominance of the right hemisphere during early infancy the left hemisphere is the most 'dominant' in most people, particularly once language develops.

The two hemispheres are joined by the corpus collosum, a bridge made up of bundles of nerve fibres, which is the most influential of the three communication routes between the two hemispheres. Keshavan et al. (2002) demonstrated that even here, development continues through childhood and adolescence into early adulthood. Damage to the corpus collosum has revealed the role of visual processing in the right hemisphere and control of language ability within the left hemisphere. However, over time the two halves of the brain adapt, and other areas of the brain compensate such that the patient appears to function relatively normally.

Box 3.2 Example of Research Demonstrating the Separate Roles of Right and Left, Brain Hemispheres

Sperry (1913–1994) studied a patient whose epilepsy had been reduced by cutting the corpus collosum. He found that this person could name an image of an object within his right visual field (processed by the left hemisphere) but could not acknowledge an image in the left visual field (processed by the right hemisphere).

However, when asked to draw what he could see in this left visual field, the patient easily achieved this, demonstrating his actual awareness of its existence but difficulty in articulating such knowledge.

Studies of brain injury have also helped to identify areas of the brain responsible for specific aspects of personality.

Box 3.3 Early Evidence of the Influence of Brain Damage on Personality

Phineas Gage (1823–1860), a railway employee, received a blow from a 'tamping iron' during an accident when using dynamite. The tamping iron entered through his cheek bone and exited through the top of his skull.

After recovering and returning to work it appeared that Gage's personality had changed. Although previously a polite and conscientious worker, he now lacked concentration, could not hold a job down, and was insulting to women.

It is also thought that inherited personality characteristics such as extraversion, impulsivity, and novelty-seeking are linked to a person's physiological and genetic make-up (Tudorache et al., 2018). Individual differences in temperament were studied by Chess and Thomas (1977) as this forms the basis of personality. They identified a neurological basis for three types of temperament (later divided into subtypes) suggesting recognisable personality characteristics, such as those people who react quickly to negative stimuli, those more tolerant, and those who react after a certain threshold of tolerance has been reached.

Box 3.4 Study of Neurologically Based Temperament (Chess & Thomas, 1977)

Through dipping new-born babies' toes in ice cold water Chess and Thomas (1977) found three different types of responses to the unpleasant stimuli. They saw these as the basis of later personality differences.

Easily aroused temperament—babies reacted by crying immediately to the unpleasant stimuli.

Placid temperament—babies took much longer to notice the change in temperature.

Slow to warm up temperament—babies took longer than the first group to react but were equally distressed.

Gender differences within brain development have been identified which influence thinking and behaviour. Robinson (2008) suggests that as, on average, girls are so much quicker to acquire language and reading skills may mean that the current methods used in schools can disadvantage boys.

Recent findings within psychoneuroimmunology suggest how complex interactions between neural and immunologic processes impact on health. For example, stress may cause inflammation, whilst inflammation impacts on mental health (Slavich, 2019). The inherent plasticity of the brain, with inherited timing and sensitivity to respond to environmental stimuli, enables constant building of existing structures, creating a 'sculpture' best adapted to survive within the situation in which a child is raised. However, Anderson (2003) points out that eventually, as the person matures, environmental influences begin to outweigh inherited characteristics although positive and negative experiences prior to adolescence can be harder to change than those after this period. For example, the impact of early social deprivation can inhibit the capability of the brain to develop to its full inherited capacity.

Those taking a biological approach have even tried to seek the location of the 'sense-of self' in humans which makes them unique amongst other living creatures. For example, Northoff et al. (2006) identified cortical midline structures within the brain which they think constitute a person's feeling of 'self' and are responsible for concepts of 'me' and 'mine'. Nevertheless, despite this and the amazing amount that has been learned about the development and function of the brain, the biological explanation for human thinking and behaviour still has limitations. Studies such as those by Northoff et al. (2006) and others may well have identified areas within the brain where feelings of 'self' may exist, but they are still unable to tell from these what it 'feels like' to be 'someone' who not only perceives something, but also behaves differently to others and may even change their perception and response at different times and in different situations. Returning to a previous example, it cannot explain what it 'feels like' for any individual to love or dislike cats. More seriously, it cannot explain what it 'feels like' to be a survivor of child abuse or neglect.

Although studies of the brain can indicate links between behaviour and adverse experiences, there is a need to consider other theories of human thought and behaviour to try and understand wellbeing in childhood and adolescence. As people's behaviour often seems to result from unconscious feelings and desires it is useful to consider work from psychodynamic theories.

3.2.2 Psychodynamic Theories

Whilst biological explanations cannot fully explain just what constitutes the 'mind', psychodynamic theories, based on the work of Freud (1920, 1923), describe it as psychic energy and offer explanations of how it functions. Freud attempted to transcend biology and neurology and seek explanations of what constituted 'personhood' through suggesting that it is formed through a dynamic process primarily experienced in early childhood. Freud acknowledged that being a social animal, responding to the needs of others appears to have promoted the survival of humans as a species. However, he recognised that this creates a constant internal struggle with individual aggressive instincts. Survival requires suppressing personal desires and conforming to social conventions. According to Guntrip (2018), this demonstrates how, by emphasising instincts and drives, Freud 'hovered' between the view of 'personhood' and biology.

Freud's theories were influenced by his medical training and experiences of treating patients whose symptoms had no apparent physical cause. He used observations of patients' incongruent behaviour, 'slips of the tongue' (saying things they had not meant to), and accounts of their dreams. He also analysed humour, Greek myths, and Western fairy tales to develop a psychodynamic theory which he and others have modified over time.

Freud concluded that the 'mind' operates at three levels: a conscious level (of which a person is aware), an unconscious level (which the person can never access), and a pre-conscious level (information laying below consciousness but can be retrieved when needed). Freud saw the 'mind' as a dynamic process seeking to reconcile the conflicting demands of a person's individual desires and social needs to achieve satisfaction and survival. This process included the formation of an 'ego' (part conscious and part unconscious) to keep the unconscious instinctual survival drive ('id') satisfied in ways that appear socially acceptable. Freud suggested that strict, early moral teaching of parents and caretakers becomes internalised, creating a third part of the 'mind', the 'superego' (part conscious and part unconscious). To maintain wellbeing the 'ego' is then responsible for balancing both the demands of the 'id' and the 'superego' in ways that the person is not fully conscious of.

Box 3.5 A Personal Example of How Freudian Theory Can Be Used to Explain Behaviour

An example of how certain incidents can be explained in terms of Freud's theory can be offered from the following direct experience of the first author.

After arriving to teach psychology in a building which used to be an old school and making a drink of tea to take into the classroom, she noticed a notice on the door which stated boldly *No food or drink to be taken into the classroom*. Despite this she proceeded to enter the room with cup of tea in hand. However, before having time to greet the rows of students gathered there, she slipped backwards onto the floor and the tea flew up in the air, landing on top of her!

She has since related this incident to many psychology students to illustrate how such an undignified entrance could be explained in Freudian terms. It could be said that unconsciously, despite the prohibiting sign, her 'id' desired tea. However, her 'superego' had internalised the need to obey such social rules. On entering the classroom, her 'ego' resolved the conflict by making her trip up. Resolution was achieved in that the 'id' never had to sacrifice its desire for tea whilst the 'superego' was satisfied that the prohibited tea was not drunk in the classroom!

Freud believed that these three parts of the mind develop as the child passes through psychosexual stages where instinctual energy in the form of pre-sexual feelings dominates specific areas of their body. Adverse experiences at any one of these stages can influence later personality development. This process was also thought to eventually include a desire for the opposite parent/caretaker and jealousy of the same sex parent/caretaker, termed the 'Oedipus' complex.

According to this theory secure parenting enables successful transition through these stages such that the 'ego' can balance the demands of both 'id' and 'superego' in ways which allow the child to later function well within their society. However, psychological energy used to deal with early hurtful parenting/caretaking experiences inhibit the 'ego's' ability to achieve such a balance.

If the 'ego' cannot succeed in repressing unacceptable thoughts a person will experience anxiety and their 'ego' will be forced to activate defence mechanisms. These can be used in positive ways. For example, sublimation involves the energy created by internal conflicts being released through a socially acceptable activity such as sport, music, or art. However, difficult early experiences can result in blocking, inhibiting, or distorting conscious awareness of disturbing thoughts through using of other defence mechanisms.

Box 3.6 Examples of Defence Mechanisms

Purposeful forgetting—an adolescent may forget the date of an unwelcome test.

Rationalisation—an explanation of being too busy is given by the adolescent for missing the test which does not ring true.

Displacement—the adolescent blames the teacher for not having reminded them about the date of the test.

Projection—the adolescent feared failure if took the test so accuses the teacher of not wanting them to pass by not reminding them of the date of the test.

Freud used 'free association' to gain access to his patients' unconscious thoughts. His aim was to relieve tension by uncovering and making patients consciously aware of their unconscious desires. This could involve a form of transference where patients' past thwarted relationships were mirrored and then worked out within the relationship between Freud and his patients. He also thought that a counter transference occurred within his own response to his patients' reactions. In the past therapists using Freud's methods were told to be wary of counter transference, but more recently they are expected to analyse their own feelings to offer insight into their client's position (Gallup & O'Brien, 2003) (Fig. 3.1).

Freud often found his patients to have experienced early sexual abuse and theorised that their 'illnesses' were a result of their ego's struggle to repress memories

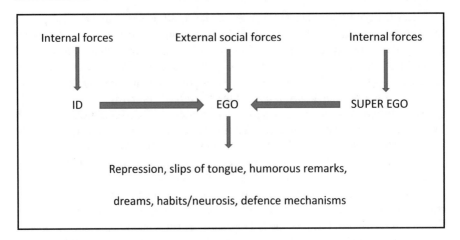

Fig. 3.1 Psychodynamic explanation of forces influencing a person's behaviour

of such trauma. However, Freud modified his theory in response to adverse reactions from colleagues who could not believe that such abuse existed and instead suggested that his patients were recalling fantasies about desiring such activities. As these strange illnesses were reported mainly by female patients, Freud thought it must also be connected to their reproductive system and termed the condition 'hysteria'. As 'hysteria' literally means 'wandering womb' and later work found no such related abnormalities the term was changed to 'neurotic'.

Freud's later interpretation has been criticised for hiding and compounding the effects of real cases of sexual abuse. It is now recognised that sexual abuse as well as other less traumatic events including insensitive parenting can create hard to manage tensions leading to maladaptive behaviour.

Freudian theory has been modified to form object relations theory which concentrates on the importance of identification with and separation from parents/caregivers. Deal (2008) explains that children create subjective, internal representations of themselves and others. These representations become 'objects' which influence how later experiences are perceived. Positive caregiving allows infants to internalise and develop a sense of stable relationships with others and ability to influence their environment whereas those who internalise negative experiences are at risk of pathology. Analysts try to understand their clients' real relationships as well as their internalised representation of such relationships.

Similar modifications to Freud's work are evident in intersubjective theory. Psychologists such as Stern (1985) stress how the child and caregiver are two subjects coming together in mutual experiences and shared emotional states. Such emotional connections create empathetic relationships through which the child can gain a sense of self and understanding of others. Both theories suggest that the child develops a self-identity through the responses of those near to them.

The influence of Western culture is particularly evident in the development of Self psychology which also has roots in psychodynamic theory. It reflected the period in which it was promoted (1990s) by American psychologists such as Kohut

(1913–1981) through emphasising a need for self-fulfilment. Kohut suggested that during childhood the actions of others are internalised with empathy, a key environmental condition for healthy, secure development.

Attachment theory is the most currently influential development from Freudian theory which also emphasises the importance of early childhood experiences. It was developed by Bowlby, who also trained within Freudian psychology, and has been popular since the 1940s. At the core of this theory is an assertion that the child needs to develop a secure attachment with at least one significant other during first two years of life or risk emotional suffering and difficulty in future relationships. Despite early criticism of over-emphasising the role of the mother in this process, it has remained highly influential and, as Bowlby saw attachment and loss as 'two sides of the same coin,' also underpins current models of grieving used within counselling and healthcare (Bowlby, 1969; Kubler-Ross, 1969). Attachment theory will be discussed in much more detail within Chap. 4.

Theories based on the work of Freud may share similar criticism, including cultural and ethnic bias; they often rely on interpretations of retrospective accounts taken from clinical populations. It is, also, hard to assess the therapeutic effectiveness of psychoanalytic-based therapies given the length of time they often take and difficulties in controlling influences, such as the personality of the analysts. However, support has been found for some elements of Freudian-based theories, for example, Fongay and Target (2000) found evidence from neurological studies to support unconscious preferences and prejudice.

Psychodynamic theory proved particularly useful in the formation of play therapy and family therapy. For example, Bettlheim (1903–1990) achieved some success when using a modified version of play therapy with child survivors of concentration camps. Despite Freudian ideas often being deemed common sense or folk psychology, it must be remembered that those within the West now live in a post-Freudian society which has absorbed many of Freud's ideas into popular thinking and expressions. For example, few people would not recognise the term 'Freudian slip' which is often expressed after saying something unintended. We are, thus, placed in a position of evaluating Freud's theory using many of his own ideas! It cannot be ignored that when Freud bravely attempted to identify the workings of the unknown world within the elusive 'mind' he had no access to modern techniques but could only make inferences from patients' accounts.

It will now be useful to examine current theories within cognitive psychology which do have the advantage of findings based on techniques within neuroscience as well as the work of previous environmental and developmental psychologists.

3.2.3 Cognitive Theories

Cognitive theories also attempt to explain the 'mind' but envisage it as an information processor. Cognitive theorists see the 'mind' as creating an internal model of the world based on stimuli from the environment. This model is created through memory and imagination to enable problem solving and other higher mental capacities. Eisser (2014) sees this as a constructive process operating in two stages. First information is taken in quickly to see 'the big picture' (involving primitive survival mechanisms) and then, secondly by a more detailed appraisal (involving higher order mental functions). Both stages include information processed by areas of the brain linked to specific sense organs, such as vision and hearing. Thinking, concept formation, and other higher order mental functions create and are created by such processes in a highly complex way.

Box 3.7 Example of How Driving a Car Involves Conscious and Unconscious Decision Making Based on Suggestions Made by Lachman et al. (2015)
Past experiences of driving a car are coded and stored within the driver's nervous system. Current driving involves a constant process of matching what is perceived to what is already known and registering anything out of the normal that needs to be given more attention.

This results in conscious control of decisions such as speed, parking, and changing gear. However, much processing operates at an unconscious level. For example, the driver may not even be aware of 'seeing' the key landmarks being matched to stored memories along with other, related information when making appropriate turns.

Eisser (2014) points out how 'beauty really is in the eye of beholder' as the brain creates coherent meaning by interpreting, transforming, and elaborating on stimuli using imagination. Despite fundamental differences, this theory shares similarities with Freudian theory in that information from the senses is transformed and changed before appearing as consciousness or action. Cognitive theory, therefore, also sees the basis of much behaviour operating at an unconscious level.

Memory is, therefore, a key function in cognitive processing which enables humans to function. For a person to lose their memory means they lose their very sense of their own existence. It has been found that speed of normal memory processing declines with age. However, Park and Festini (2017) describe how more areas of older people's brains are used during memory tasks, reflecting their use of mental strategies to counter difficulties in memory processing. Current practical interventions to maintain memory function (particularly in relation to dementia) involve memory training, learning new skills, and even suggestions of applying mild electric neuro-stimulation.

Conners and Halligan (2020) attempt to explain higher order cognitive processing involved in beliefs by studying disruptions to normal processing (cognitive deficits) such as delusions. Beliefs provide a stable depiction of a person's experiences enabling them to create a framework from which to interpret sensory experience as well as make decisions and carry out actions. Beliefs also regulate emotional experience, define identity, and coordinate group behaviour. Models of normal cognition have been developed from patterns of behaviour observed during brain injury studies. For example, Capgras, a false belief that a familiar person has been replaced by an imposter, could reflect damage to the autonomic response system in face processing; Inter-metamorphosis, the belief that a person has changed physically and psychically into someone else, could be due to stimulation of inappropriate face recognition units within the brain; and Cotard, the belief that one is dead, could arise from loss of autonomic responsiveness. As not all patients with the same physical damage appear to have such delusions, it is thought that a secondary process takes place within other areas of the brain which integrate information into a coherent form and this may or may not be damaged (Conners & Halligan, 2020).

Brain imaging has helped create visual mapping of brain functions which complement existing theories of cognitive development within childhood and adolescence. Although cognitive development in childhood and adolescence will be discussed further within Chaps. 4, 5 and 6 it will be useful to offer a brief overview here as cognitive theory has changed how children and adolescents are now perceived as active participants in learning.

Current theories and studies relating to cognitive development are based on original work carried out by Piaget (1896–1980) and Vygotsky (1896–1934). Their work suggests that humans build up mental constructs, termed 'schemas' (models), of their world which are coded in neural networks within the brain and develop to record experiences of interactions with the environment. Schemas once formed are constructs used to understand experiences but are also consistently changed as new neural connections are formed due to new experiences. Amended schemas are then used to interpret future experiences, and again they may change when further neural connections are formed to record these new experiences, and so the process continues. This indicates the flexible way the brain is constantly adapting to allow the person to survive within their environment.

Piaget believed that each of a child's actions (he termed operations), such as sight, sound, taste, smell, touch, is recorded and categorised by specific neural connections within the brain. These categories (schemas) change slightly as new information is added (assimilation) and new schemas are created when experiences are very different and include sub-categories of related information (accommodation). Piaget explained this constant developmental process in childhood as including periods where sufficient schemas are formed to aid understanding of the current environment (state of equilibrium) interspersed with new experiences (state of disequilibrium) requiring adaptation of existing schemas or creation of new ones.

Piaget's work suggests that cognitive development occurs in a kind of spiralling process within which stages are evident. He saw the first, sensory motor stage exists for about the first two years in which the child's thinking is dominated by physical mastery of their world and they are egocentric, as have no concept of other's thoughts or needs. The second, pre-operational stage experienced by children about two to seven years old involves the ability to carry out one step logical thinking and some reduction in egocentric thinking in social situations. The third, concrete-operational stage is experienced about seven to eleven years of age and involves the ability to recognise general principles if aided by concrete examples and enables further reduced egocentricity. The final, formal-operational stage is thought to exist from about eleven years old and involves the ability to think more abstractly and greater ability to see from another's point of view (Piaget & Inhelder, 1977). New findings, such as those by Blakemore and Mills (2014), demonstrate how some egocentricity continues and full intellectual abilities may not be reached until a person is in their early twenties.

Vygotsky's theory of cognitive development is compatible with the work of Piaget, to a great extent; however, he emphasised the role of socio-cultural influences on cognitive development. He was heavily influenced by Marxist philosophy which purports that 'historical changes in society and material life produce changes in human nature' (see Blake & Pope, 2008, p. 60) and stressed how social interaction facilitates the development of mental functions. Vygotsky recognised that a gap exists between what children and adolescents can do independently and what they may need help with when learning new tasks and concepts. He termed this the 'Zone of Proximal Development (ZPD)' and emphasised the need for those interacting with children and adolescents to provide appropriate support (scaffolding) to aid their development.

Differences between Piaget and Vygotsky were, therefore, based on the way they emphasised the individual or social roots of learning. Piaget was more influenced by biology, particularly maturation. He believed that children inherit a natural tendency to explore their environment which provides the experiences necessary to ensure the process of cognitive development. Vygotsky, like Piaget, advocated active, hands-on methods to facilitate learning, but he saw that negotiation and interaction with others are necessary to develop cognitive abilities. He saw that non-verbal communication and language enabled the learner to successfully integrate their experiences within their unique set of thought processes.

Vygotsky suggested three types of speech exist: social, private, and internal. He saw that social language was used to give information to children by those older and more experienced. This form of communication was translated by the child into their private language to help them process what has been said and apply what learned to similar situations. Internal or inner speech was then thought to occur as the child carried out a silent, abbreviated form of dialogue which forms the essence of conscious mental activity. Vygotsky was, therefore, suggesting that thinking equals social speech which has been transformed into private speech and become internalised (Blake & Pope, 2008).

Support has been found for the theories suggested by both Piaget and Vygotsky. For example, Fongay and Target (2000) report how children transform early interactions with caregivers into schemas of themselves and others and create internal working models of their world through their unique constructions. A safe environment allows them to develop a sense of identity and autonomy, whereas an unsafe environment can create psychopathology. Also, such egocentricity in early childhood can mean that a child can think difficulties experienced, such as divorce, are created by their own wishes. The work of Piaget and Vygotsky revolutionised techniques within education and have influenced approaches within all forms of child and adolescent care.

Nevertheless, Piaget has been criticised for adopting a cultural bias, including some inconsistencies, under estimating children's knowledge and not taking enough account of children's social context. Cognitive theories generally have also been criticised as mental processing can only be inferred from what a person says or does and using experiments involving memory tests or problem-solving tasks. Also, Eisser (2014) suggests that such abstract theories still fail to explain the 'mind'.

Despite such criticism, cognitive theories have been successfully used as a basis for therapeutic interventions which attempt to change a person's maladaptive negative perceptions. For example, rational emotive therapy (RET) developed by Ellis (1980) involves challenging a person's negative thoughts and replacing them with positive ones. However, currently the most popular way of using cognitive theory within therapy is to combine it with other theories within psychology. For example, cognitive behavioural therapy attempts to change a person's maladaptive perceptions by rewarding and reinforcing them for displaying more appropriate thinking and behaviour. As this involves a form of associated learning, an explanation is now required of the behaviourist approach within psychology.

3.2.4 Behavioural Theories

Behaviourism, founded by Watson (1913), denies any existence of the 'mind' or consciousness, explaining that the 'behaviourist cannot find consciousness in the test tube … [but] … does however find an ever widening stream of behaviour' (Watson, 1926, p. 456). Watson thought that eventually all forms of behaviour, including 'thinking' (which he saw as merely sub-vocal movements of the larynx), could eventually be understood in terms of chemistry. He was influenced by the work of Pavlov (1849–1936) who studied the conditioning of animal behaviour through the process of association (classical conditioning). Watson believed that reflexes reacting to stimuli from the environment created more complex behaviour in humans as it could lead to a variety of possible associated consequences (Watson, 1926).

Whilst studying animal digestive systems Pavlov had found that dogs would start to salivate at the sight of the assistants bringing their food or the sound of the buckets in which the food was normally carried. He realised that the saliva was stimulated through these sights and sounds being associated with the arrival of food. He termed these unconditioned stimuli (sight of assistant) and unconditioned response (saliva) as occurred unintentionally. He then purposefully created learned behaviour through association by constantly pairing the food with different stimuli, such as a bell, until eventually just hearing the bell alone caused the dogs to salivate. Salivation this time was a conditioned response.

Box 3.8 Classical Conditioning of Dogs Based on Pavlov's Work (1927)

Stimuli	Response
Ringing bell alone	No salivation
Food	Salivation—unconditioned
Food + ringing bell paired together over time	Salivation
Ringing bell alone	Salivation—now conditioned

Whilst on most occasions it took numerous pairings before the animal salivated to the bell or other such stimuli, Pavlov found that if the event was intensely pleasurable or painful associations could be formed after one pairing. He also found that dogs would salivate to similar stimuli to the original pairing (generalisation), but also discriminate differences between different stimuli such as squares and circles printed on cards. Over time after the pairings had been discontinued the conditioned response also ceased (extinction). However, Pavlov was surprised to find that under certain (particularly stressful) occasions the conditioned response would reappear (spontaneous recovery).

Watson (1926) described how classical conditioning can be used to understand and control human behaviour, particularly in relation to phobias. He cited examples from his previous experiments in using classical conditioning to create fear in infants (which today would be considered highly unethical). For example, he described his (infamous) studies with his assistant, Rayner in 1920, in which 'little Albert' was conditioned to fear the white fluffy animals and objects he previously liked, due to the loud noise of an iron bar being banged each time he attempted to touch the original animal or those with similar qualities.

The basic elements of classical conditioning were gradually developed into more complex theories of operant conditioning. Rather than just create biological reactions, operant conditioning attempts to shape the actions of animals and humans through associated learning involving gaining pleasure or avoiding pain.

Through shaping the behaviour of cats, Thorndyke (1898) had developed a 'law of effect' which says that any act associated with pleasure or avoiding pain will be repeated. Skinner (1948–1987) utilised this theory to develop a process of behaviour shaping using reinforcements. One of his methods was to develop a 'Skinner box' in which he conditioned rats to press a lever to obtain food. He classed the food as a primary reinforcer as it represented a basic (primary) need. Skinner then paired the presentation of the food pellet only when a green light was on. Eventually the rats would press the lever in response to the green light even when no food was offered. The green light had become a secondary reinforcer as it was associated with the original primary reinforcer (food).

When applying Skinner's work to humans it is easy to see examples of his conditioning techniques within current childcare practices. For example, the tick, sticker, or smiley face offered to pupils in schools is associated with pleasure gained from gaining the teachers' approval and is intended to ensure that the pupil will continue such work.

Skinner preferred the use of positive reinforcement but realised that negative reinforcement, where an act will be repeated to avoid pain, was a particularly effective way of controlling behaviour. For example, drivers obey speed restrictions to avoid the penalties if caught driving too fast. Skinner preferred the use of positive and negative reinforcement to create required responses rather than punishment to stop undesirable behaviour as this can have unintended consequences. If the punishment is not clearly linked with the act the person may not make the required association. Also, the process can create unhelpful negative feelings towards the punisher.

To ensure that the desired behaviour was continued Skinner tried various schedules of reinforcement. He found that the most effective was to use partial reinforcement, where acts are rewarded randomly once the association has been made. The desired behaviour is continued as the person or animal knows the reward will come but not when. A very common example of the highly successful use of such behaviour shaping is gambling. The user of the fruit machine will keep adding money and pressing the lever of the machine to gain the reward, as consistently as any rat in a Skinner box!

Skinner's work has also influenced education in many ways. The learning machines he developed established methods recognisable in current online teaching aids. His machines were designed such that learning was broken down into small tasks and, by starting with relatively easy tasks and immediately rewarding the success of these, the learner was positively reinforced to move on to further, more challenging tasks. However, concerns of over use of such teaching methods have been raised by Knox et al. (2019) who caution against what they see as 'learnification' and 'datafication,' based on behaviourism, inflicted upon humans through digital technologies. They fear that such machine learning systems impede autonomy and participation and shape the learner's behaviour in ways that can inhibit creativity and generation of new ideas.

Pasquale and Cashwell (2018) are also concerned about the use of digital technology based on behaviourist principles being used to predict cases of law and sentencing. The fear that predictions based on models following Skinner's concepts of inputs and corresponding outputs ignores changes in human behaviour and social attitudes.

However, therapies based on behaviourist techniques have been found to be particularly effective, particularly in relation to phobias. Watson (1926) had argued that therapy must involve action and not just talking, and Skinner (1988) stated that troublesome behaviour was just due to troublesome associations which need adjustment. Nevertheless, ethical concerns have been raised about the lack of control and dehumanisation clients may experience when exposed to behaviourist-based therapies. For example, token economy can involve withdrawing basic rights and using them to reward desired behaviour.

Skinner (1988) recognised the ethical implications of his work but insisted that control is ethical if executed for the good of those controlled. He recommended solutions to world environmental problems using behaviourist techniques to reduce some of the self-destructive behaviour of humankind. However, Skinner's assumption that humans can know what is good and what is harmful in every situation has been doubted.

It appears that the core base of 'stimulus response' theory, concentrating only on observable variables and denial of any inner intentions, within behaviourism denies free will and consciousness. However, some behaviourists are beginning to acknowledge elements of cognition within the process of learning through association (Eisser, 2014).

3.2.5   Social Cognitive Theory

Bandura modified and improved on the behaviourist approach by first developing social learning theory and later social cognitive theory which both include cognition. However, he does not equate the 'mind' with computers insisting that: 'Consciousness cannot be reduced to a non-functional by-product of the out-put of a mental process realised mechanically at non-conscious lower levels' (Bandura, 2001, p. 3).

Social cognitive theory links elements of previous theories given that it acknowledges how complex human behaviour includes associated learning (basis of behaviourism) but also involves making choices (a cognitive element) along with observation, imitation, and identification (psychodynamic concepts). Bandura developed his theories from his studies which included measuring increased aggression in children's play after they had witnessed aggressive acts carried out on large, inflatable, weighted 'bobo' dolls, painted as clowns which returned upright when knocked down (see Bandura et al., 1961, 1963; Bandura & Walters, 1963).

Bandura's work has demonstrated the power of observational learning and modelling through vicarious reinforcement. It suggests that specific qualities of role models can influence the extent to which their behaviour will be copied. For example, children are more likely to copy the behaviour of those who are warm and loving, hold positions of authority, are famous, or share similarities to the child such as age and gender. It also explains how spontaneous learning with no explicit reinforcement occurs, the influence of actions rather than words and impact of family and peer behaviour.

Social cognitive theory has been particularly influential in explaining the potential power of the media in promoting aggression. Studies have shown links between violence depicted in the media and increased aggression, anti-social behaviour and desensitisation to violence as well as increased fear of being the victim of violence. However, Bandura's studies also demonstrate the potential for curbing aggression, as children were less likely to copy the behaviour of adults shown to be punished for behaving aggressively.

A particularly concerning element of observational learning identified by Bandura's work is latent learning, as children may not immediately copy behaviour to which they have been exposed but do so later when it proves useful. For example, although girls were less likely than boys to copy the aggression witnessed towards the bobo dolls, they did so later after seeing the boys being rewarded with sweets for such behaviour.

Nevertheless, social cognitive theory does not merely see humans as passive responders to environmental stimuli or observed behaviour. Despite limitations set by the environment people make choices which may set the course that their life-path will take. Bandura identified the ability to make such choices as 'human agency' which is linked to consciousness and includes, for example, self-referencing, self-reflection, intentions, and forethought (Bandura, 2001).

Bandura saw that such cognitive processing created a sense of meaning, direction, satisfaction, and self-efficacy through success in achieving desired goals. He recognised the unique faculty of metacognition within humans which enables them to reflect on their own reflections and evaluate the effectiveness of their actions, promoting adaptation and change at individual and collective levels. Graham and Arshad-Aya (2016) point out that humans naturally internalise the cultural tools available. They stress how Bandura's work demonstrates the processes involved in conforming as well as deviant behaviour, reflecting the internalisation of culturally approved emotional practices.

Social cognitive theory explains not only individual behaviour but also certain social processes. Bandura sees that human agency exists in three modes. The first mode is direct 'personal agency' where people pursue their individual goals. The second mode is 'proxy agency' where a person recognises the greater expertise of others and relies on them to secure their goal (e.g. allowing the dentist to extract a tooth to relieve toothache). The final mode is 'collective agency' which involves the person belonging to a group to use socially coordinated means of achieving the desired goal (e.g. joining a union to achieve better working conditions). Bandura, therefore, reflects on the 'complex interplay between intrapersonal, biological, interpersonal and socio-structural determinants of human functioning' and points to the currently increasing use of digital technology which affects the environment at both individual and societal levels. He insists that a psychosocial approach is necessary to promote human development' (Bandura, 2001, p. 18).

3.3 Theories Within Sociology

To achieve the psychosocial approach advocated by Bandura (2001) it is necessary to combine theories from sociology with those from psychology. As, within this book it is not possible to do full justice to all theories within sociology a selection has been consciously made, here, to include those which will prove most pragmatically useful for those caring for children and adolescents.

3.3.1 Interactionist Theories

Interactionist theories include shared interconnected ideas and influences rather than form a single discipline. They take a micro, 'bottom-up' approach in trying to understand the patterns formed by people's interactions with others which, when combined, shape societies. Symbolic interactionism is particularly useful as it creates a bridge between social psychology and social structuralism. It has roots in social action theory founded by Weber (1864–1920) as, although he adopted a macro approach in attempting to explain societies, Weber recognised the importance of acknowledging social context and individual points of view. He suggested empathising with individual behaviour to understand the impact of social structures and appreciated that there could be no truly objective way of studying society.

The work of G.H. Mead (1863–1931) was particularly concerned with how individuals socially collaborate. Influenced by the concept of the 'looking glass self' developed by Cooley (1864–1929), Mead saw that it was through social experience that individuals developed a sense of self. He saw childhood as dominated by learning social roles through imitation in the same way as rules of a game are learned. Mead thought that once gaining a sense of self, people were constantly attempting to modify their actions to fit with socially acceptable behaviour. However, he also suggested that once their identity is formed people have the power, collectively to change society. Mead's theories reflect Bandura's third mode of 'collective agency', by emphasising group behaviour which Bandura stated was 'more than the sum of its parts'.

This approach was called symbolic interactionism as symbols within the structure of society were seen by Mead to provide messages of meaning which indicate appropriate behaviour. For example, in Western society lighting candles in Church is easily recognised as respecting the memories of loved ones or other important people who are deceased. Therefore, such patterns of behaviour are studied within symbolic interactionism to see how, once combined, they create a mosaic of shared actions carried out by different groups, communities, and institutions.

Blumer (responsible for producing Mead's work from his notes) was instrumental in developing the 'Chicago School' which specialised in studying individual and group actions within urban areas. Also, the 'Iowa School' was developed to find ways of incorporating empirical testing within a symbolic interactionist framework. A further 'Indiana School' was developed in the 1960s which also used quantitative methods to study the patterns emerging from data collected using a symbolic interactionist approach (see Blumer, 1980).

Goffman (1923–1982) took an interactionist approach when studying the impact of being confined in total institutions such as mental hospitals and prisons. He also saw socialisation as a form of 'social drama' with the roles people took on, defined by their appearance, including dress and uniforms. Goffman found that often people used 'impression management', including dress and behaviour, to ensure their actions were socially acceptable (frontstage behaviour), whilst often engaging privately in socially unacceptable ways (backstage behaviour). Becker (1986) also used an interactionist stance when investigating the social context of deviance and how people experience social exchange and collaboration.

Although the interactionist approach may not explain the power of social institutions and structures such as class, gender, and race as well as is done within the macro theories, this approach does help to capture their effects on people. Interactionist theories can help explain issues such as social inequality through identifying the way people's emotions shape and constrain social behaviour. People are born into societies which have clearly defined expectations of what is socially acceptable behaviour which if transgressed leads them to feel shame, guilt, and embarrassment. Therefore, negative emotions as well as positive ones, such as a sense of pride when conforming to social expectations, ensure that established social order and hierarchies are maintained.

Gidden's (1979) structuration theory attempts to fuse macro (structural) and micro approaches. Despite being criticised for over emphasising the ability of individuals to influence change, Giddens maintains that structures make social action possible but social action also creates structures. The bottom-up approach within interactionism suggests a role for individual agency in that accumulation of views which challenge established social rules may reach a peak which then creates change within social institutions. However, change may also occur due to new, unanticipated events. For example, the current effects of the COVID-19 virus on social life across the world are yet to be understood, as is the impact of the related and rapid use of new technology.

Fine and Tavory (2019) suggest that although past methods within the micro approach meant that crucial elements were forgotten, taken for granted, or seen as mundane, currently some of the essential elements are re-emerging. For example, adopting an interactionist approach is particularly useful in understanding the emergence of new forms of socio-technical life experienced by children and adolescents due to different types of media which have the power to change social relationships and consumption. Digital information is now produced, and analysed by states, corporations, and cities with virtual worlds and new social media platforms developed. Housley and Smith (2017) stress how digital technology offers new ways of acting and perceiving the self and creates new forms of social stratification exploiting individuals and making 'real' different forms of social stigma and prejudice.

Such digital technology and communication systems mean that the world is much more interconnected. A distressing recent example is how the mishandling of the unlawful death of a person of colour in one country (USA) once reported through social media created mass protests across the Western world. Interactionist approaches offer one way of attempting to understand the impact of the current fast-changing social landscape within the UK due to world events, health issues, and new digital technology, which are recurrent themes, throughout this text.

3.3.2 Feminist Theories

Feminism is commonly seen as developing in three waves, originating as early as 1792 with Mary Wollstonecraft's work: *The Vindication of the Rights of Women*. Nevertheless, traditional sociology has taken the male perspective for granted seeing gender as due to natural differences with men influenced more by culture and women by nature. Although Karl Marx (1818–1883) recognised gender inequality, he saw it embedded within class, cultural, and ethnic differences rather than an issue of its own right (Giddens, 2000). However, sociological approaches changed considerably within the 1960s as a second wave of feminism became evident, which attempted to promote women's views as equally as valuable as the taken for granted male perspective.

Having lived through this period, it is hard for the first author to fully describe the powerful impact of feminism on the lives of women during the 1960s, 1970s, and 1980s. That, in 1974 Ann Oakley (see Oakley, 2018) should choose to study 'the sociology of housework' may seem banal to modern readers, but at the time it was revolutionary. It brought to common consciousness the taken for granted work of women. The importance of 'invisible' female labour started to be acknowledged in contrast to the belief that: 'housework is only noticed if it is not done!' For those readers who wish to gain more awareness of what it was like to be a woman at that time, it would be useful to read the novel, *The Women's Room*. Written by Marilyn French (1977), it explores the humiliating experiences of an American housewife, returning to study in an attempt to forge a career. The impact it has on women is evident, even in current times. For example, the actress Kate Mosse reported: 'They said this book would change lives—and it certainly changed mine'.

The work of Lopata (1973) links symbolic interactionist and feminist approaches. Although, a fellow contemporary of Becker and other males taking a symbolic interactionist approach within their research, Lopata appears to be less well known because she chose to apply this approach to female experiences, such as the 'occupational housewife' and widowhood. Over time her work became increasingly influenced by contemporary feminism and she began referring to 'male dominance'. Lopata pointed out that although there are no clear 'sex/gender roles' any more than there are 'race roles' or 'class roles', sexism has never been taken as seriously as race and class inequality. Her work on the status of females within patriarchal societies has helped influence the way the changing roles of women are recognised within Western culture.

Given the different experiences of women, over time different forms of feminism have developed. As a result, the current 'third wave of feminism' is rather fragmented. It, also, often now includes elements of other perspectives such as Marxist feminism. Some examples of current feminist perspectives, as defined by Marcionis and Plummer (2012), are offered below.

Liberal feminists warn against the danger of women becoming ethnocentric 'male-clones' and suggest using education and legislation to ensure equality between the sexes. However, Burman and Stacey (2010) add a note of caution to this approach as in some cultures, education is used by those in power to avoid tackling established conventions of early marriage. Also, keeping girls in school longer can ensure that they are taught 'approved' ways of behaving.

Radical feminists see that power imbalances within social structures and institutions based on gender dominate all cultures and class. Men are seen to have a monopoly on sex which they use to denigrate women. However, this approach includes clear divisions between those such as Millet (1970) who see gender resulting from socialisation and can be changed and others such as Rich (1977) who stress the importance of promoting motherhood and other biological differences which males fear and attempt to control.

Some feminists of colour argue that their experiences differ from those of white feminists. They insist that inequalities of class, race, and gender, creates for them a qualitatively different way of life. Marxist-feminists base female inequalities on class and economic relationships. They believe that inequalities exist within family roles which help to perpetuate female oppression. Patriarchy is seen to cover up violence within the private lives of women and limit the kind of paid work and positions of importance they can hold.

Some of the over zealousness of feminists and resistance from powerful forces within society (such as mainstream media), along with the emerging divisiveness within feminism, have made this approach vulnerable to the misconception that feminists are 'man haters, refusing all male help' (Yuill, 2012). However, as a movement it has been particularly successful in raising awareness of the prevalence of child sexual abuse and domestic violence. Interestingly, at the time of writing this book, a new 'Me Too' movement has emerged, initially exposing sexual harassment and abuse within the film industry. It has proved successful in bringing to account powerful males guilty of sexual abuse of both men and women within the entertainment industry.

Feminist approaches have also proved particularly useful in relation to women's health. Yuill (2012) points to the male-dominated areas of midwifery and health which have marginalised women within practice and research. She refers to how this has been responsible for the forced institutionalisation of childbirth which in turn has often been responsible for the depression experienced in early motherhood which was then diagnosed and treated as the illness 'post-natal depression'. Within health research feminist approaches, questioning assumed validity, valuing subjectivity, and identifying gaps through their marginalised standpoint have helped both male and female patients.

Feminist approaches are relevant to the wellbeing of children and adolescents particularly as they will be influenced by their mothers' experiences. Burman and Stacey (2010) state that the colonial-based requirement of male protection still dominates women and children, placing them both in a state of dependency. They also suggest that even the current trend to 'listen to the voice of the child' represents Western, masculine concepts of individualism and ignores the diverse socio-economic situations in which children and adolescents are placed. Burman and Stacey (2010) maintain that the 'child' is perceived as needing an ideal-typical white, middle-class childhood that is also culturally masculine. This ignores economic situations where children and adolescents must earn a living.

It can, therefore, be seen how adopting a feminist approach can be useful in considering issues of equality applicable to males as well as females. Both are confined by established views based on gender divisions influenced by class, ethnicity, and disability. It will now be useful to contrast this perspective with how functionalism attempts to explain and may appear to justify some of the established social structures constantly shaping the lives of children and adolescents.

3.3.3   Functionalist Theory

Feminist theorists would point to the influence of Harriet Martineau (1802–1876) on the development of theories and methods within sociology. She published research on marriage, children, religious life, and race relations, and thought that in addition to observing and reporting their findings, sociologists should also work to benefit society. Martineau insisted that the study of society must be comprehensive, including important key elements such as politics, religion, and other social institutions (Giddens & Griffiths, 2006, p. 20). This approach was adopted by the, better known, male 'founding fathers' of sociology, who, sadly, ignored her belief that it was also important to include the lives of women. Influenced by the work of Herbert Spencer (1820–1903), Martineau and others felt that it was possible to study 'social facts' in same way as physical facts. This belief particularly influenced the development of the functionalist approach which saw that society needed to be studied as a whole unit made up of interrelated parts.

Functionalism, therefore, attempts to examine how different social structures fit together and function for the good of society. This approach can be taken to analyse small and larger scale societies, as well as their component parts. Within Western society sub-systems have been identified including political parties, industry, communication strategies binding members in shared cultural beliefs, and kinship networks. Analysis of elements of each subsystem is thought to help explain the function they and their component parts provide for wider society. For example, the family can be studied as part of the kinship sub-system to help understand how industrialisation and urbanisations have impacted upon traditional family structures, and the implication of this for the rest of society.

Box 3.9 Agriculturally Based Kinship Sub-system (Henslin, 2010, p. 27)
The past agricultural system on which Western society was based meant that marriage provided an important function in maintaining the family unit which, in turn, contributed to the successful economic functioning of society. The function of roles attributed to all family members ensured continued existence of the family and their economic and emotional survival. Wives, daughters, and other related, resident females were responsible for household work, childcare, care of small animals such as chickens, milking cows, dairy produce, baking and sewing. Husbands, sons, and any other resident male relatives were responsible for larger animals, planting, harvesting, building, and maintenance. This provided an economic unit in which all members depended upon each other for survival.

Henslin (2010) points out how, in terms of functionalist theory, current economic and socially accepted independence of spouses has resulted in the family unit becoming more fragile as there are less interdependent functions binding family members together.

The functionalist approach was originally based on work carried out by Durkheim (1858–1917) who was also responsible for formally establishing sociology as an academic discipline in universities. He recognised that as humans are social animals, they need to live in groups to ensure survival. He suggested that this becomes possible through members sharing core values. Being a member of a group means submitting some individual differences and conforming to what is good for the whole group rather than pursuing any conflicting, individual desires. The group, therefore, represents a distillation of common beliefs and behaviour that members need to follow to maintain membership. Durkheim (1938) identified this as the 'collective conscience' (which, when translated, can mean conscious as well as conscience). As this approach assumes that the shared core values and beliefs enable humans to function in groups it is known as a consensus. These core values are maintained through religious beliefs, rituals, laws, and customs passed on through generations and, if necessary, modified for the continued good of the group. However, using such an approach to study the continued existence of small communities is easier than when trying to understand the complex structures and functions within Western society.

Functionalist theory sees society as an organic system, very much like the human body, in that it is made up of separate but interrelated systems, with some providing more important functions than others. Like the body, societies emerge, grow, and may wither away. Durkheim believed that, as societies need to be kept in state of balance, order is maintained through the division of labour and complimentary roles. He identified the function of religion in helping to maintain solidarity, cohesion, and bind people together. Although religion has declined in Western society, Punch et al. (2013) explain that those adopting a functionalist explanation would point out that other forces, such as nationalism, socialism, and hero worship of certain leaders, now offer a similar function.

Even the continued existence of crime, despite assumed agreement of core values, can be explained in functionalist terms. These would refer to how when a rule is broken, it can provide a positive function in reinforcing these rules and bringing the majority of people closer by shared responses of outrage.

Functionalism came to dominate sociological approaches in the first half of the twentieth century, particularly due to the way it was interpreted by Talcott Parsons (1951). Parsons synthesised the classic works of Durkheim and others into a descriptive framework which influenced the development of later forms of functionalist theories. Ormerod (2019) likens this process to an hourglass depicted in Fig. 3.2.

Parsons' contribution to the functionalist approach was influenced by his own past experiences within biology as well as work from psychology, economics, anthropology, and sociology. From this he created an analytic framework and categorising process useful for studying the interacting set of system elements and subsystems making up a society. The influence of Freudian theory is evident in Parsons' concepts of cognitive, catharsis, and evaluation processes involved in the individual actions creating change and maintaining social stability. He also pointed out how shared understanding and acceptance of varied status were evident in the meaning behind many symbols, such as wedding rings, tattoos, flags, and logos. Parsons identified compatibility, conformity, and cultural patterns as pre-requisites necessary for any society to survive.

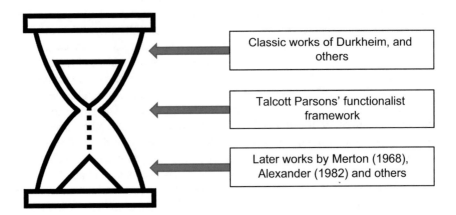

Fig. 3.2 Parsons' synthesis of classic works influencing later functionalist theories

---

Box 3.10 Pre-requisites Required for Societal Survival Identified by Parsons

1. Elements of the social system must be compatible enough to meet the individual members' survival needs.
2. Enough members must conform to social rules to make deviance obvious and unacceptable.
3. Cultural patterns (acceptable forms of behaviour) must be achievable to avoid generating conflict and too much deviance.

Parsons recognised how the plasticity of human nature facilitated learning from experience and being influenced by others and created a ready willingness to conform to the rules required by different institutions within society, such as medicine and education. The interaction of these institutions ensures survival at a societal level. For example, interactions between education, economics, and politics mean that students are prepared for the types of work required to ensure the existence of the whole society (Henslin, 2010).

However, the functionalist approach has been severely criticised as too static, supporting the status quo. It justifies social inequalities as necessary to provide leadership and ensure order, although cautions that if inequalities become too extreme the resulting social instability could threaten the existence of society. For example, the functionalist view would see too few members of the population being very wealthy, whilst the majority who were poor would threaten social stability leading to mass disagreement about current norms and governing strategies. However, it is obvious that societal processes are much more complex given that Western society continues to survive despite such huge amounts of wealth held by so few people.

Functionalism has also been criticised as not satisfactorily explaining major structural changes. It attempts to explain changes in terms of an evolutionary 'structural differentiation', which develops as societies gradually become more complex with greater specialisation in their component parts. For example, the education plays a limited role within simple societies, but as they develop in complexity, the function of education gains in importance and becomes more formalised (Henslin, 2010). However, this sort of explanation falls short in explaining the fast pace of some radical changes, such as those created by new technology.

Later sociologists attempted to address some of shortcomings within the functionalist analysis. For example, Merton (1968) developed a 'middle range' theory which adopts a more focussed approach and is less grand scale. Others, such as Alexander (1982), created neofunctionalism to include work from other disciplines and adopt a multidimensional approach. Neofunctionalism has been used to explain global issues through stressing the growing economic interdependence between nations, international legal regimes, and supranational rules encouraging political and market integration and welfarist objectives.

However, a consensus-based view of societies still cannot adequately explain the inherent conflict between individualism and collectivism which exists within Western society. There is a consistent, underlying tension between concern for others and individual gratification. Within the UK this has become more starkly obvious within the government's response to the pandemic created by the COVID-19 virus. The tension between meeting the cost of saving human life and protecting the population whilst ensuring the comfortable position of the very wealthy few has meant the government oscillating between protective measures for fear of a public outcry and making economic-based decisions in line with capitalist principles. It has been interesting to see how the government has appealed to the altruistic nature of individuals and over-used the terms 'caring for others' whilst, at the same time further wealth was accumulated by those who saw the advantages to be gained by investing in supplying the new resources required, such as protective clothing and testing procedures.

3.4 Developing a Bio-Psychosocial Approach

3.4.1 Systems Theory

As no one theory can fully explain the impact of childhood and adolescent experiences it is useful to include elements of each within the 'biopsychosocial' approach suggested by Bandura (2001, p. 4). This approach is reflected in the work of Bronfenbrenner (1979) which describes a series of interrelated systems, creating a 'Russian doll' type structure, with parent–child dyads influenced by family relationships, structure, and social setting (Fig. 3.3).

At the centre of this model, the actual experiences of the child, including interactions with parents, school, friends, and others, make up a 'microsystem'. As the relationships between parents, teachers, religious leaders, and social services within the child's life may be compatible or include conflict these relationships can be identified as a 'mesosystem'. The wider set of influences, including social institutions affecting children indirectly such as parents' work settings and local authority policies, mass

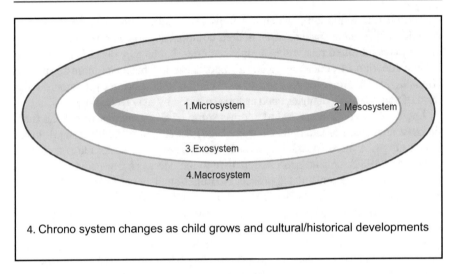

Fig. 3.3   Model of Bronfenbrenner's (1979) bio-ecological theory

media, community resources, are classed as an 'exosystem'. The even broader influence of cultural values, laws, and governmental resources is identified as a macrosystem. Bronfenbrenner also recognised that the impact of changes within families (such as birth of a sibling) and society (such as war) will be determined by the child's age and life stage; hence, he identified this as a 'chronosystem'.

The influences identified by the bi-directional interactions within this model in conjunction with the theories from psychology sociology outlined above will be evident within the rest of this text.

Summary

- Some universal elements of needs at stages of development during childhood and adolescence can be understood by applying theories from psychology and sociology. Biologically based theories explain how the structure and function of a complex brain govern human thought and action. Psychodynamic theories attempt to make invisible, unconscious mental processes intelligible. Cognitive theories use the computer as an analogy to convey the way the brain processes information, whilst behavioural theories reduce all human thought and action to learning based on association. Social cognitive theory adds the role of observational learning to elements of previous theories and acknowledges the impact of social processes.
- Sociological approaches including interactionist theories, feminist theory, and functionalism offer insight into how interactions between individuals and existing social structures impact upon children's and adolescents' wellbeing. The bottom-up approach of symbolic interactionism not only identifies patterns created by individual behaviour which mould people's self-concept and behaviour but also allows room for human agency. Feminist theory is particularly helpful in highlighting the power of gender socialisation for male as well

as female wellbeing. Despite its weaknesses as a grand theory enabling analysis of different societies, functionalism helps identify important social structures and their impact on individuals.

- Systems theory offers a bio-psychosocial model which can help capture the dynamic processes of human development and socialisation which the psychosocial theories outlined within this text attempt to explain.

Case Study Questions

Read the family case study on page 265 and consider the following:

- According to feminist theories, what challenges may Gemma face in attempting to pursue a future medical career?
- How would social cognitivists explain potential links between Stuart living in the family home and Ben's later behaviour?
- What elements of different psychological theories underpin the play therapy suggested as a way of helping improve Liam's behaviour?

Reflective Questions

- How well does functionalist theory explain recent developments within Western society?
- What are the strengths and limitations of behaviourist theory?
- Why is there a need to adopt a bio-ecological approach to understanding the impact of early experiences across an individual's lifespan?

References

Alexander, J. C. (1982). *Positivism, Presuppositions, and Current Controversies (Vol. 1 of Theoretical Logic in Sociology)*. University of California Press.

Anderson, S. L. (2003). Trajectories of Brain Development: Point of Vulnerability or Window of Opportunity? *Neuroscience & Biobehavioral Reviews, 27*(1–2), 3–18. https://doi.org/10.1016/S0149-7634(03)00005-8

Bandura, A. (2001). Social Cognitive Theory: An Agentic Perspective. *Annual Review of Psychology, 52*, 1–26. https://doi.org/10.1146/annurev.psych.52.1.1

Bandura, A., Ross, D., & Ross, S. A. (1961). Transmission of Aggression through Imitation of Aggressive Models. *Journal of Abnormal and Social Psychology, 63*, 575–582. https://doi.org/10.1037/h0045925

Bandura, A., Ross, D., & Ross, S. A. (1963). Imitation of Film-mediated Aggressive Models. *Journal of Abnormal and Social Psychology, 661*, 3–11. https://doi.org/10.1037/h0048687

Bandura, A., & Walters, R. H. (1963). *Social Learning Theory and Personality Development*. Holt, Rinchart & Winston.

Becker, G. S. (1986). *Human Capital: A Theoretical and Empirical Analysis with Special Reference to Education* (3rd ed.). The University of Chicago Press.

Blake, B., & Pope, T. (2008). Developmental Psychology: incorporating Piaget's and Vygotsky's Theories in Classrooms. *Journal of Cross-Disciplinary Perspectives in Education, 1*(1), 59–67.

Blakemore, S.-J., & Mills, K. L. (2014). Is Adolescence a Sensitive Period for Sociocultural Processing? *Annual review of Psychology, 65*, 1870–1207. https://doi.org/10.1146/1nnurev-psych-010213-115202

Blumer, H. (1980). Mead and Blumer: The Convergent Methodological Perspectives of Social Behaviorism and Symbolic Interactionism. *American Sociological Review, 45*(3), 409–419. https://doi.org/10.2307/2095174

Bowlby, J. (1969). *Attachment & Loss: Vol. 1 Attachment*. Hogarth Press.

Bronfenbrenner, U. (1979). *The Ecology of Human Development: Experiments by the Nature of Design*. Harvard University Press.

Burman, E., & Stacey, J. (2010). The Child and Childhood in Feminist Theory. *Feminist Theory, 11*(3), 227–240. https://doi.org/10.1177/1464700110376288

Chess, S., & Thomas, A. (1977). Temperament and the Parent-Child Interaction. *Pediatric Annals, 6*(9), 26–45. https://doi.org/10.3928/0090-4481-19770901-07

Conners, M. H., & Halligan, P. W. (2020). Delusions and Theories of Belief. *Consciousness and Cognition, 81*, 102935. https://doi.org/10.1016/j.concog.2020.102935

Deal, K. H. (2008). Psychodynamic Theory. Advances in Social. *Work, 8*(1), 184–195.

Durkheim, E. (1938). *The Rules of Sociological Methods*. Free Press.

Eisser, U. (2014). *Cognitive Psychology*. Psychology Press.

Ellis, A. (1980). Rational-Emotive Therapy and Cognitive Behavior Therapy: Similarities and Differences. *Cognitive Therapy and Research, 4*, 325–340. https://doi.org/10.1007/BF01178210

Fine, G. A., & Tavory, I. (2019). Interactionism in the Twenty-First Century: A Letter on Being-in-a-Meaningful-World. *Symbolic Interaction, 42*(3), 457–467. https://doi.org/10.1002/symb.430

Fongay, P., & Target, M. (2000). The Place of Psychodynamic Theory in Developmental Psychopathology. *Development and Psychopathology, 12*, 407–425. https://discovery.ucl.ac.uk/id/eprint/134129/1/download9.pdf

Franke, K., Luders, E., May, A., Wilke, M., & Gaser, C. (2012). Brain Maturation: Predicting Individual *BrainAGE* in Children and Adolescents using Structural MRI. *Neuro Image, 63*(3), 1305–1312. https://doi.org/10.1016/j.neuroimage.2012.08.001

French, M. (1977). *The Women's Room*. Hachette Digital Press. www.hachette.co.uk

Freud, S. (1920). *A General Introduction to Psychoanalysis*. Boni & Liveright.

Freud, S. (1923). *The Ego and the Id* (Standard ed., Vol. 19). : Hogarth.

Gallup, R., & O'Brien, R. N. (2003). Re- establishing Psychodynamic Theory as Foundation Knowledge for Psychiatric/Mental Health Nursing. *Issues in Mental Health Nursing, 24*, 213–227. https://doi.org/10.1080/01612840305302

Giddens, A. (1979). *Central Problems in Social Theory: Action, Structure and Contradiction in Social Analysis*. University of California Press.

Giddens, A. (2000). *Sociology*. Polity Press.

Giddens, A., & Griffiths, S. (2006). *Sociology*. Polity.

Graham, P., & Arshad-Aya, A. (2016). Learned Unsustainability: Bandura's Bobo Doll Revisited. *Research, Centre for Environment Education, Ahmedabad, Gujarat (Los Angeles, London, New Delhi, Singapore, Washington DC and Melbourne), 10*(2), 262–273. https://doi.org/10.1177/0973408216650954

Guntrip, H. Y. (2018). *Personality Structure and Human Interaction: The Developing Synthesis of Psychodynamic Theory*. Routledge.

Henslin, J. M. (2010). *Sociology, a Down to Earth Approach*. Pearson.

Housley, W., & Smith, R. J. (2017). Interactionism and Digital Society. *Qualitative Research, 17*(2), 187–201. https://doi.org/10.1177/1468794116685142

Keshavan, M. S., Diwadkar, V. A., DeBellis, M., Dick, E., Kotwal, R., Rosenberg, D. R., Sweeney, J. A., Minshew, N., & Pettegrew, J. W. (2002). Development of the Corpus Callosum in Childhood, Adolescence and Early Adulthood. *Life Sciences, 70*(16), 1909–1922. https://doi.org/10.1016/S0024-3205(02)01492-3

Knox, J., Williamson, B., & Bayne. S. (2019). Machine Behaviourism: Future Visions of 'Learnification' and 'Datafication' Across Humans and Digital Technologies. *Learning, Media and Technology, 45*(1), 31–45. https://doi.org/10.1080/17439884.2019.1623251

Kubler-Ross, E. (1969). *On Death & Dying*. Tavistock/Routledge.

Lachman, R., Lachman, J. L., & Butterfield, E. C. (2015). *Cognitive Psychology and Information Processing*. Psychology Press.

Lebel, C., & Beaulieu, C. (2011). Longitudinal Development of Human Brain Wiring Continues from Childhood into Adulthood. *The Journal of Neuroscience, 31*(30), 10937–10947. https://doi.org/10.1523/JNEUROSCI.5302-10.2011

LeDoux, J. (1998). Fear and the Brain: Where Have We Been, and Where Are We Going? *Society of Biological Psychiatry, 44*, 1229–1238.

Lewis-Williams, D., & Pearce, D. (2005). *Inside the Neolithic Mind: Consciousness, Cosmos and the Realm of the Gods*. Thames & Hudson.

Lopata, H. Z. (1973). Self-Identity in Marriage and Widowhood. *The Sociological Quarterly, 14*(3), 407–418. Published online: 15 Dec 2016. https://doi.org/10.1111/j.1533-8525.1973.tb00869.x

Marcionis, J. J., & Plummer, K. (2012). *Sociology. A Global Introduction* (5th ed.). Pearson Educational Ltd..

Merton, R. K. (1968). *Social Theory and Social Structure* (Enl. ed.). Free Press.

Millet, K. (1970). *Sexual Politics*. University of Illinois Press.

Northoff, N., Heinzel, A., Greck, M., Dobrowoiny, H., & Panksepp, J. (2006). Self-Referential Processing in our Brain—A Meta-Analysis of Imaging Studies on the Self. *NeuroImage, 31*(1), 440–445. https://doi.org/10.1016/j.neuroimage.2005.12.002

Oakley, A. (2018). *The Sociology of Housework*. Polity Press.

Ormerod, R. (2019). The History and Ideas of Sociological Functionalism: Talcott Parsons, Modern Sociological Theory, and the Relevance for OR. *Journal of the Operational Research Society, 7*(12), 1–24. https://doi.org/10.1080/01605682.2019.1640590

Park, D. C., & Festini, F. C. (2017). Theories of Memory and Aging: A Look at the Past and a Glimpse of the Future. *Journal of Gerontology: Psychological Sciences, 72*(1), 82–90. https://doi.org/10.1093/geronb/gbw066

Parsons, T. (1951). *The Social System*. Routledge and Kegan Paul.

Pasquale, F., & Cashwell, G. (2018). Prediction, Persuasion, and the Jurisprudence of Behaviourism. *University of Torono Law Journal, 68*(Suppl. 1), 63–81. https://doi.org/10.3138/utlj.2017-0056

Pavlov, I. P. (1927). *Conditioned Reflexes*. Oxford University Press.

Piaget, J., & Inhelder, B. (1977). *The Psychology of the Child*. Routledge & Keegan Paul.

Punch, S., Marsh, I., Keating, M., & Harden, J. (2013). *Sociology. Making Sense of Society*. (5th Edition). Harlow. Pearson Educational Ltd.

Rich, A. (1977). *Of Woman Born: Motherhood as Experience and Institution*. W. W. Norton.

Robinson, M. (2008). *Development from Birth to Eight. A Journey through the Early Years*. Open University Press.

Skinner, B. F. (1988). The Operant Side of Behaviour Therapy. *Journal of Behaviour Therapy and Experimental Psychiatry, 19*(3), 171–179.

Slavich, G. M. (2019). Psychoneuroimmunology of Stress and Mental Health. In K. Harkness & E. P. Hayden (Eds.), *The Oxford Handbook of Stress and Mental Health*. Oxford University Press. https://doi.org/10.1093/oxfordhb/9780190681777.013.24

Stern, D. (1985). *The Interpersonal World of the Infant*. Basic Books.

Thorndyke, E. L. (1898). *Animal Intelligence*. New York. Mac Millan.

Tudorache, C., Slabbekoorn, H., Robbers, Y., Hin, E., Meijer, J. H., Spaink, H. P., & Schaef, M. J. M. (2018). Biological Clock Function is linked to Proactive and Reactive Personality Types. *BMC Biology, 16*, 148. https://doi.org/10.1186/s12915-018-0618-0

Watson, J. B. (1913). Psychology as the Behaviourist Views it. *Psychological Review, 20*, 158–177.

Watson, J. B. (1926). Behaviourism: A Psychology Based on Reflex-action. *Philosophy, 1*(4), 454–466. Royal Institute of Philosophy. https://doi.org/10.1017/S003181910002581X

Yuill, O. (2012). Feminism as a Theoretical Perspective for Research in Midwifery. *British Journal of Midwifery, 20*(1), 36–40. https://doi.org/10.12968/bjom.2012.20.1.36

Attachment, Parenting, and Culture

4

4.1 Origins of Attachment Theory and Its Impact on Early Child Development

As explained in Chap. 2, the concept of attachment, developed by Bowlby (1907–1990), stresses the importance of early childhood experiences and has proved essential in understanding child and adolescent wellbeing. Attachment has been defined as an intense, emotional relationship between two people enduring over time. Stress is experienced when those within the relationship are separated for a long period (Kagan, 1995).

A child's attachment, usually to its primary caregivers, is particularly evident by about eighteen months of age, when children stay physically close to their caregivers when in a new environment. They also become distressed when these caregivers are absent. However, Schaffer (1996) found that the attachment process starts from birth and can be seen to develop in the following four stages (Table 4.1).

A strong attachment provides a secure base from which children can explore their environment and other relationships as well as a 'safe-haven' to which they can return when feeling threatened. Attachment theory maintains that a child needs to develop a secure attachment with at least one significant other during the first two years of life or risk emotional suffering and difficulty in future relationships. To appreciate the impact of attachment theory on the current care of children and adolescents, it is important to examine how it was developed by Bowlby and influenced by other work within psychology at the time, including psychodynamic, biological, and cognitive-based theories.

4.1.1 Influences on Attachment Theory

Bowlby proposed that human infants are born with an attachment behavioural system embedded in their central nervous system and, therefore, 'hard wired' to seek

J. M. Waite-Jones, A. M. Rodriguez, *Psychosocial Approaches to Child and Adolescent Health and Wellbeing*, https://doi.org/10.1007/978-3-030-99354-2_4

Table 4.1 Stages of Attachment Development identified by Schaffer (1996)

Attachment stage	Approximate age	Behaviour
Stage 1 Pre-attachment	From birth to about six months	Attracted to human faces but comfortable with any caregiver
Stage 2	Three to six months	Smiles at familiar faces but can tolerate any caregiver meeting their needs
Stage 3	Seven or eight months	More comfortable with familiar carers and may display reticence when held by strangers
Stage 4	Nine months onwards	A strong attachment to a primary caregiver becomes obvious but also displays attachment behaviour towards other carers

out relationships with those who offer a sense of security. Babies possess innate abilities to suck, nestle into a person's body, gaze, smile, and cry which all illicit a response from their caregivers. When receiving sensitive responses to such cues, babies become securely attached to those caring for them (Schaffer, 2004). This process can be seen to be in line with Darwinian theory of evolution as it ensures protection for young humans whilst they are vulnerable. If attachment continues in a healthy way throughout life, it can also mean that vulnerable, elderly parents are protected by their now adult offspring.

As a psychoanalyst Bowlby was particularly concerned about the mental health of the many young children who had suffered separation from their families and/or death of their parents during Second World War. He researched such effects by studying children in his own clinic and those spending long periods in a sanitorium. Bowlby was also influenced by ethological studies carried out by Lorenz (1935). It was Lorenz who first used the term attachment to describe the 'imprinting' process he, and others, observed in young geese and other birds which involved following their mother after hatching. Imprinting appeared to involve an innate readiness for the young birds to follow the first bright, moving object seen after hatching which was usually their mother. Initially it was thought that there was only a short 'critical period' after hatching for imprinting to develop. However, further studies found that imprinting could develop later, but may take longer and more effort to establish. It was concluded that the period after initial hatching was a 'sensitive' time for imprinting to occur rather than 'critical'. Bowlby saw a similar sensitive period within the first two years of human infants' lives facilitating the establishment of secure attachments with primary caregivers to provide protection.

In addition, Bowlby was impressed by the findings of the work carried out on monkeys isolated from birth by Harlow (in 1959, and later with other colleagues). These studies observed the behaviour of young monkeys reared with two 'surrogate mothers', one made of wire mesh with a feeding bottle and the other covered by cloth with no food provided. Harlow and his fellow experimenters found that the young monkeys spent much longer clinging to the cloth covered 'mother' than with the one that provided food. Such findings challenged the accepted 'cupboard love' explanation of why very young birds and animals continued to stay close to their mother purely for food. It became evident from the studies that contact with the soft texture of the cloth covered 'mother' was more important than the food provided by the wire 'mother'. It was also found that, when older, the monkeys used in these studies had difficulties in interacting with other monkeys. They were also incapable of mating and, after artificial fertilisation, had difficulty in successfully rearing their offspring.

Bowlby recognised that findings from such studies offered a new way of thinking about human infant-mother attachment. He rejected the psychodynamic 'cupboard-love' explanation for infants' motivation to seek proximity with those who met their basic needs. Bowlby rather began to see such attachment as a psychological bond influenced by the environment into which the child is born and impacting on their later behaviour. He used the concept of 'maternal deprivation' to explain the disturbed behaviour, including 'affectionless psychopathy' (evident by lack of guilt and inability to maintain stable relationships), exhibited by some children in his own studies who had suffered early separation from their mothers (Bretherton, 1992).

However, later work by those such as Rutter (1972) suggested the need to differentiate between deprivation and privation. Deprivation means loss or separation of a caregiver and if short term can cause distress but, long term can create 'separation anxiety'. In contrast privation was experienced by monkeys in Harlow's experiments as they never experienced any interactions with a real 'mother figure'. It is possible that such a lack of any kind of attachment may be experienced by children being raised in a poorly staffed institution or suffering parental abuse. Rutter believed that affectionless psychopathy was more a result of privation rather than deprivation. Also, further work by Schaffer and Emerson (1964) challenged the child–mother bond as the single most important influence. They found that children were able to form multiple attachments and that the strongest bond evident was not always with the mother, even when she was the main caretaker.

Despite an initial over emphasis on the mother–child attachment, Bowlby has been particularly influential in pointing out how early relationships provide the child with an internal working model of their world and adaptive ways of behaving which provide a 'blueprint' for future relationships. Caregivers who respond sensitively to their child's needs ensure that such a model will provide a secure base. However, when caregivers are inconsistent or regularly fail to respond sensitively the child will develop a model of an insecure world and behave in ways which may prove maladaptive as they mature. The intergenerational influence of such a process was also noted by Bowlby (1969) as caregivers' own long-established internal working models can influence the ways in which they react to their own children.

The influence of Piaget's (1896–1980) work on cognitive development is also evident within attachment theory as Bowlby saw that secure attachment figures provide the security of the familiar from which the child can seek out novel experiences (Steele et al., 2017). This means that they can mentally try out alternative forms of behaviour using their past knowledge to understand and respond to present and future experiences (Bretherton, 1992). Studies by Klaus et al. (in 1972 and later) allowed mothers greater contact with their newborn babies during their stay in maternity hospitals which demonstrated the power of longer, close proximity on the security of future relationships between mothers and their infants. Not only were these children more likely to display secure attachments but also enhanced cognitive skills when older.

4.1.2 Attachment Theory and Separation Anxiety

Bowlby recognised the infant's need for tender bodily contact, particularly with its main caretaker, usually its mother. He noted a consistent three-stage pattern of behaviour exhibited by young children when separated from their mother for any length of time which involved protest, despair, and detachment. During the first 'protest' stage, young children would outwardly show their bewilderment and fear by vigorously screaming, crying, kicking, and struggling to escape. They often clung to the mother to try and stop her leaving. A second stage of 'despair' was then evident as children appeared to calm down and appear apathetic. They suppressed feelings of anger and fear and rejected offers of comfort from others, often displaying attempts to self-comfort by rocking and thumb sucking. Over time in the third stage, 'detachment' was apparent and such children began to respond to others, but all rather superficially. They often rejected their mother if eventually reunited with her and had to develop a new relationship with her.

Ainsworth, who worked with Bowlby and other colleagues, developed the 'Strange Situation' method of identifying different types of attachments between mothers and their infants (see Ainsworth, 1979). This method involves observing how, when playing in the same room as their mother, a young child reacts to interactions provided in Table 4.2.

Ainsworth identified three types of attachments between the infants and their mothers. She found that 70% of the infants displayed secure attachments as, although upset at their mothers' departure, once comforted they soon resumed play. However, 15% of attachment styles exhibited were classed as 'insecure/avoidant' as these children appeared to take little notice when their mother left or returned, and 15% were classed as 'insecure/ambivalent' as these children sought contact with their mother but then rejected it and were hyper vigilant of her further movements.

Ainsworth's studies provided the basis of future work in identifying attachment styles and the extent to which they may influence a child's relationships in later life. In addition, Main and Hesse (1990) later noted that some children exhibited a mixture of avoidant and ambivalent behaviour including 'freezing' or stereotyped

Table 4.2 Interactions observed within the strange situation test by Ainsworth (1979)

1 Mother and child are together in a playroom. A stranger enters and attempts to engage with the child.
2 Mother leaves the room. Stranger attempts to comfort the child.
3 Mother returns, comforts the child, and the stranger leaves.
4 Mother leaves again. Stranger enters and attempts to comfort the child.
5 Mother returns, picks up the child, and the stranger leaves.

actions and even fear when reunited with their mother which they classed as 'disorganised attachment'.

The 'strange situation' test has demonstrated the importance of parental sensitivity in meeting the needs of their child. Stern (1977) used the term 'interactional synchrony' to describe the finely tuned dynamic created when parents recognised and responded sensitively to the emotional cues within their child's behaviour. Such responses ensure that the child's needs are met and provide them with a sense of wellbeing. A lack of synchrony inhibits the child's ability to internalise a stable, self-concept and regulate their emotions (Steele et al., 1999). The child may doubt itself and feel shame, constantly attempting to secure connectiveness and prevent humiliation and rejection from others (Ko et al., 2019).

Infants displaying anxious-avoidant attachments have been found to have parents who frequently ignore their need for proximity and tend to encourage greater autonomy than is developmentally appropriate for the child. Later, these children often present with a false sense of independence and cease to seek parents out for comfort or safety. Parents of infants displaying anxious-ambivalent attachments tend to be inconsistent in meeting their child's needs and discourage exploration. The lack of predictability of their parent's responses means that such children become hypervigilant, displaying both hostile and 'clingy' behaviour. Parents of children who develop a disorganised attachment have been found to act in frightening, frightened, sexualised, or other ways atypical of expected parental behaviour. Often such parents have unresolved issues including a history of loss and abuse which can influence the way they see their relationship with their own child. For example, Zeegers et al. (2017) found that the mental representation of attachment described by expectant mothers influenced their child's attachment security as well as their later understanding of emotion and social cognition. Interestingly, the mental representations of attachment described by expectant fathers influenced their child's attachment behaviour and later mental wellbeing.

Methods of assessing adult attachments, such as the Adult Attachment Interview (AAI) (see George et al., 1996; Main & Goldwyn, 1987), also suggest that early attachment security may influence adult relationships and parenting. For example, the descriptions of the four different patterns of adult attachment, Dismissing, Autonomous, Preoccupied and Unresolved, are provided in Table 4.3.

However, the impact of parents' own levels of attachment security on their child's attachment behaviour is not always predictable as Barbaro et al. (2017) suggest that

Table 4.3 Adult attachment styles identified by George et al. (1996) and Main and Goldwyn (1987)

Dismissing	Adults work hard to protect an unrealistic positive (idealised) image of their parents and childhood and dismiss the significance of their childhood relationships
Autonomous	Adults have felt loved and supported by their parents
Preoccupied	Can result from having early attachment needs denied and/or having experienced early role reversal in having to care for their parent
Unresolved	Involves continued grief from past childhood trauma and loss for which a sense of responsibility is felt even though it is not the case

there are also genetic and environmental influences. As a psychoanalyst, Erikson (1959) also recognised the impact of the social and cultural environment on emotional development. He believed that to achieve wellbeing individuals need a supportive environment to successfully complete psychosocial stages during specific phases of their life. He suggested that each stage requires successful negotiation of psychological conflict. Resolution cannot be achieved if a child suffers emotional and social deprivation in one stage and this leaves them less able to deal with conflicts faced in the next phase of their development. For example, such children will not be able to develop a sense of trust in themselves and others necessary to achieve the autonomy, sense of initiative and industry necessary in the following stages of their development. As a result of this, when older such children may be prone to feelings of shame, guilt, and inferiority.

4.1.3   Attachment Theory and Parenting Styles

Attachment patterns have been found to be associated with different parenting styles which impact on the child's sense of wellbeing. For example, Baumrind (1971) suggested three styles of parenting based on the extent to which parents sought to control and/or accept their child's behaviour. She suggested an authoritarian parenting style exists in which parents are unaware of the developmental needs of their child and establish a rigid set of rules with little provision of emotional support. Such parenting can create low self-esteem in children who have difficulties in developing positive social skills and may act aggressively.

In contrast the permissive parenting style, identified by Baumrind, involves parents who have relaxed social attitudes, accept all aspects of their child, and make little attempt to control their behaviour. Although this style has been found to produce more self-confident children, they often have low self-control, have greater emotional problems, and are more likely to drop out of education and be drawn to crime.

Baumrind found the third, authoritative, style of parenting to be the most conducive for children's wellbeing. This involves warm parent–child relationships as parental demands are reasonably high, but children are consulted rather than dictated to and encouraged to become involved in decisions about their future progress. This has been found to help develop increased self-regulation, confidence, and compliance. Baumrind's original description of the authoritative, authoritarian, and permissive parenting styles was based on dimensions of demandingness and responsiveness but further studies have identified a fourth style based on parental rejection and neglect (Smetana, 2017).

Support has been found for these forms of parenting styles. For example, Kooraneh and Amirsardari (2015) identified ways in which different forms of parenting influenced early internal models children create and use to understand their world. However, Smetana (2017) points to the flexibility within parenting styles and the extent to which they demonstrate moral, social, prudential, and personal core concerns. These are explained in Table 4.4.

Table 4.4 Domains of core parenting concerns identified by Smetana (2017)

Moral	Nurturing their child's sense of justice and awareness of the needs of others
Social	Their child is aware of and adheres to social conventions within their society
Prudential	Creating comfortable and safe environment for their child
Personal	Recognising the child's individual needs during their development

Smetana (2017) offers the example of how mothers convey such concerns through their tone of voice when interacting with their toddlers. When responding to moral transgressions mothers tend to use an angry, intense tone of voice. If responding to prudential or potentially harmful behaviour they will use a fearful tone, but, if the child's action is prudential mothers merely respond in a playful tone.

Compatibility of styles between parents is important. For example, Berkien et al. (2012) suggest that distress experienced by infants receiving conflicting emotional responses from two caregivers can lead to disorganised attachments. However, the impact of negative parenting styles can also be buffered by relationships with significant others. For example, Akhtar et al. (2016) found that emotional closeness to grandparents was positively associated with children's psychosocial wellbeing and particularly effective in compensating for the effects of parental conflict and unconducive parenting styles.

4.2 Influence of Attachment During Adolescence

As seen within Chap. 1, the concept of adolescence, as a transition period between childhood and adulthood, is relatively new and refers to those aged between ten and nineteen years of age. Within Western culture, transition to adulthood appears to take longer than in the past due to the longer periods in which adolescents are expected to stay in education and training. This means that this age group spend longer periods relying on parents for economic support. As a result, many do not consider themselves, and are not considered by parents, to be fully adult until at least twenty-five years of age (Padilla-Walker & Nelson, 2012).

4.2.1 Attachment and Adolescent Emotion Regulation

Psychological theories try to explain why adolescence is seen as an increasingly stressful period involving difficulties in appreciating the perspectives of others. For example, biological theories explain how neurological and hormonal changes, with rapid maturational rates, are responsible for adolescent behaviour, such as stressful mood swings and increased risky behaviour. Although secure attachments have been found to help to regulate emotions, neurochemical development during adolescence means that reward systems within the brain develop faster than self-regulatory systems. This may explain the increased self-absorbedness and risk taking during this period, as the emotional rewards outweigh potential negative results of risks (Blakemore & Mills, 2014).

As adolescents are expected to display greater independent emotion regulation and self-control such deficits may become particularly apparent if not mediated, at least to some extent, by secure attachments (Stepp, 2001). Connections between the pre-frontal cortex, amygdala, and hippocampus may be one mechanism responsible for the 'internal working model' which Bowlby believes to develop in infancy through attachment which becomes consolidated during adolescence. Interestingly, Fearon et al. (2014) point out that this will also have been influenced by a genetic inheritance which begins to become more influential on personality during late childhood and adolescence This means that any newly modified working model includes parents' response to their adolescent's now more obviously inherited personality traits, which will continue into adulthood. However, according to Fraley (2002), the extent to which working models developed in infancy can be radically changed depends on specific interpretations within psychology. Those who adopt a revisionist view accept that changes can be made to the original working model. However, those taking a prototype stance believe that there will always remain a core, established in infancy which influences later behaviour, particularly when under stress.

4.2.2 Psychosocial Changes During Adolescence

Although neurochemical and genetic inheritance influences adolescents' development, such impact upon individuals will also be determined by expectations of others within their social environment. Despite greater restrictions on ways to achieve economic independence, adolescents are expected to take on new social roles which involve more responsibility and accountability for their actions. Erikson believed that during this period adolescents need to be allowed to experiment with different social roles to establish an individual identity. He saw that a lack of secure, supportive relationships within this period can result in a failure to achieve a stable identity and leave adolescents in 'role confusion'.

Authoritative parenting involving affection, consistent rules, but low levels of control and monitoring the adolescent's whereabouts has been found most conducive to adolescents' wellbeing. However, other adolescent attachments become influential during this period. For example, peer relationships can also provide a safe base from which different social roles can be explored to foster identity formation. Meeus et al. (2002) see peers and parents as offering complimentary support, with parents more influential regarding education and career choice whilst peers provide leisure opportunities and friendships. However, inherited temperament can still be influential on both relationships with parents and peers (Patterson et al. (2017). For example, an inherited social reticence can mean that an adolescent withdraws from peers which limits opportunities for socialisation and increases the potential for peer rejection.

In addition, the effect of both temperament and parenting styles will be influenced by the adolescent's environment. Shared environmental effects can include the characteristics of parents, neighbourhood, and culture. For example, overprotective and authoritarian parenting is more likely to be experienced by those in poverty and living in areas with high crime rates (Dash, 2013), whereas high levels of social cohesion within neighbourhoods can act as a buffer from such adverse effects (Kingsbury et al., 2019).

4.2.3 Attachment and Vulnerability During Adolescence

The stressful nature of adolescence as a life stage appears to be increased due to difficulties in forming early attachments. For example, high levels of cortisol, influential in stress responses, have been found in personality disordered adolescents suffering attachment difficulties through early neglect and abuse (Lyons-Ruth et al., 2011). Such findings also mirror animal studies which report high levels of cortisol to be found in offspring suffering poor maternal care. Sensitive parenting can offer a form of 'emotional scaffolding' to reduce some of the stress experienced by adolescents and help to ensure that independence is gradually established by this period (Coleman & Hagell (2007).

Adolescents' wellbeing may be compromised when parents do not adapt well to their adolescent's desire for independence. For example, Padilla-Walker and Nelson (2012) identified a form of 'helicopter' parenting, involving parents' continued, well-meaning but misplaced psychological and behavioural control. This may have been helpful during early childhood but is detrimental to adolescents' developing autonomy. Such parents become over involved, constantly checking on their adolescent's educational progress and social life. This form of parenting can create anxiety, depression, and low self-worth, in adolescents who lack satisfaction with their relationship with their parent and disclose less to them.

Parental wellbeing may also influence their adolescents' development. For example, Pratt (2019) points out that lack of mother–child synchrony predicts poor emotion regulation and mental health in children and adolescents. Pratt (2019) found that depressed mothers' lack of ability to tune into their infants' cues impacted upon children's early neurological development and pre-adolescent emotional control. Also, the work of Garcia et al. (2017) demonstrates the interrelated nature of attachment and different adverse life events. They identified and studied different forms of early trauma impacting upon adolescent wellbeing including separation and loss; domestic violence; emotional, sexual, and physical abuse; neglect; community violence and illness/medical trauma. Their findings suggest that that separation due to youth hospitalisation is closely linked to increased behavioural problems amongst adolescents who also suffered domestic violence, neglect, and community violence.

Adoption may also form a further risk to wellbeing during adolescence. Negative pre-adoption experiences were found by Pace et al. (2017) to be linked to adolescent psychiatric problems, attachment insecurity, and emotional regulation difficulties. Behavioural problems were more prevalent in those who had been adopted later in childhood. However, although adolescents initially raised in institutions were found to have greater emotional regulation difficulties overall, those with highly competent adoptive parents were found to be able to form secure attachments. Pace (2017) points out that the plasticity of adolescent brains can offer the potential for reframing emotional regulation strategies through such adopted family experiences.

A current concern about problems during adolescence is the susceptibility of this age group to addiction. This can be explained to some extent, as due to adolescents' difficulty in self-regulation due to attachment difficulties. For example, Ching and Tak (2017) found links between smartphone addiction, parenting styles, attachment, and self-regulation. They point out how during adolescence, mobile phones become to reflect self-identity, individuality, and autonomy, but can also result in bullying, social anxiety, low self-esteem, and problematic behaviour. Ching and Tak (2017) suggest that less impulse control resulting from insecure attachments through restrictive parenting proves a predictor of possible problematic smartphone use. They found that positive parenting styles, promoting secure attachments have the potential to promote resistance to overuse of mobile phones. Such findings are important as mobile phone addiction is only one example of vulnerability to other forms of addictive behaviour during adolescence. For example, Hamilton-Giachritsis and Fairchild (2020) identified adolescents' vulnerability to alcohol addiction and online gambling when in the presence of peers as well as potential sexual exploitation through digital technology when alone.

4.3   Parenting and Culture

Although biology plays a highly important role in the formation of attachments, the ability to form secure parent–child relationships is also influenced by the environment in which they develop. Removing mothers and children from poor socio-economic living conditions can improve attachment security which is important as child and adolescent antisocial behaviour is more prevalent in socio-economically deprived areas (Kobak et al., 2009). To fully appreciate the impact of attachment theory it is useful to understand the historical and political reasons why it has come to dominate the care of children and adolescents within Western society.

4.3.1   Historical Context of Attachment Theory and Parenting

Many psychologists have developed new theories which have proved to be of little significance. However, the acceptance of Bowlby's work may well have been due to the prevailing 'zeitgeist', a coming together of moves within intellectual, moral, and cultural thinking creating conditions for radical change within a given era. As seen within Chap. 2, responses to inhumane conditions created by rapid industrialisation included philanthropic movements and government concerns with the poor physical health. This was particularly noted when recruiting soldiers for war and led to greater state intervention on the nations' physical health. Investment in children's health began to be considered as particularly beneficial for the future of the nation. The status of psychology as a discipline increased as it offered the opportunity to improve and control minds as well as bodies. Freudian theory had established a theoretical foundation for understanding the impact of early experiences on later mental health. All this, as well as chance encounters, paved the way for Bowlby to develop attachment theory and for it to begin to dominate the future wellbeing of children and adolescents.

Chance appears to have played a part in Bowlby's career as a psychoanalyst and his development of attachment theory. His post-graduate, voluntary work at a school for maladjusted boys offered him first-hand experience of the effects of lacking a stable mother figure on children, particularly in relation to two boys whose behaviour was very difficult to control (Bretherton, 1992). Increased interest and research in childhood psychology across Europe and the USA also provided fertile ground for Bowlby's work. When he was asked by the World Health Organisation (WHO) to report on the effects on children of the loss and separation many had experienced because of the Second World War, Bowlby consulted and drew together eminent researchers including Erikson, Lorenz, and Harlow. He also benefited from experienced and dedicated collaborators including Ainsworth, Robertson, and others. However, it may be surprising to know, given the current dominance of attachment theory on child/adolescent development, that many of Bowlby's colleagues within the psychoanalytic community were highly critical of his theory (Bretherton, 1992).

Nevertheless, Burman (2008) questions the studies on which attachment theory is based. For example, she asks how studying children damaged through war experiences can offer a 'natural experiment' and, therefore, be applicable to all children? She criticises the strange situation test as unethical and not reflecting the influence of working mothers on the children who accepted comfort in the absence of their mother. Burman rather sees the basis of attachment theory dominated by US ideals of autonomy and biased in relation to gender and class. She also points out the difficulties of generalising from animal behaviour, particularly that exhibited by 'tortured' monkeys to humans.

Within her feminist critique of developmental psychology, Burman warns how research findings are often used to promote social movements and social policy without taking account of the social context in which they are developed. She also points out how Bowlby's ideas were popularised through use of the media, such as radio and newspapers, and insists that they should be seen in terms of the constant controversy regarding women's employment.

The points made by Burman need to be acknowledged as the political ripeness for Bowlby's theory cannot be overstated. During the Second World War, women without children, or with those over fourteen years of age, had been conscripted into work such as nursing, factory work, munitions, farming, and elements of the armed forces. The prime minister at the time had also asked for volunteers to work, particularly in bomb shell-filling factories, and arranged free day care facilities for those with young children through expanding local authority-run nurseries and registered child minders. Those mothers who already worked outside the home were offered help with the cost of childcare (reported by the Manchester Guardian, 10.3.1941).

At the end of the war Bowlby's work, with its original stress on the important mother–child bond (monotropy), provided an ideal solution to avoid potential mass male unemployment. Interpreting Bowlby's theory in ways to suggest links between mothers working outside the home and children's later delinquency offered the UK post-war government an ideal justification for forcing mothers to return to their 'natural' roles of mothers and homemakers. This meant that there were now jobs available for the male soldiers returning from the war. Burman notes that using Bowlby's work to justify the post-war closure of nurseries also exaggerated the glorification of motherhood and 'celebration of home and hearth'.

There was a distinct feeling of déjà vu within the early 1980s as attempts were made by the Conservative government to reduce unemployment by popularising attachment theory once again. Advertisements were created which claimed that working mothers should be at home looking after their children. It was an ironic move as the prime minister at the time, Margaret Thatcher, was herself a working mother. However, the movement was short lived due to the need for both parents to work, given the government's conflictingly previous drive towards greater home ownership which had created a need for two family wages.

Although Burman's criticisms cannot be ignored, in fairness to Bowlby, much of his work has been misrepresented by later summaries (Bretherton, 1992). In his original work he had not only cited mother but also mother substitute, and he also later retracted the overemphasis of such figures, accepting that other attachment figures can also be important (Clarke & Clarke, 1998). However, this retraction was never popularised as, obviously, it did not fit with the political and social climate of the time.

Although aware that the whole family needed to be researched Bowlby was forced to concentrate on the mother–child relationships for practical reasons and through pressures within his own clinic. Bowlby was aware of the intergenerational transmission of attachment relations and the possibility of helping children by helping both parents. He also understood that poor social, economic, and health factors influenced attachments and likened therapists to gardeners taking account of the soil by noting parents' interactions within their community (Bretherton, 1992). Sadly, as Clarke and Clarke pointed out in 1998, Bowlby's call to society to provide support for parents is still not adequately heeded within the UK today.

Bowlby's work on loss, and subsequent depression after prolonged parental separation, has formed the basis for theories of grief now used to understand both child and adult bereavement (Bretherton, 1992) and attachment theory is integral to current concepts of compassionate child and adolescent care.

4.3.2 Impact of Attachment Theory on Parenting and Family Life

Attachment theory can be seen to have had a lasting impact on family life as, although within Western culture children may now be economically worthless, they have become emotionally priceless (Burman, 2008). It is also important to note that Bowlby's ideas were popularised at a time when, due to improved communication and geographical mobility, accelerated by the Second World War, the 'nuclear' family became increasingly common. This meant less opportunity for support from extended family members and greater emphasis on mothers as homemakers and fathers as 'family-breadwinners'.

The feminist explanations offered by Burman (2008) and Enoch (2012) help in understanding how the use of attachment theory by the government and other powerful bodies, who took no account of socioeconomic status, shaped popular 'taken for granted' ideas (hegemony) about the role of motherhood. Ideals of home and motherhood were first used to entice mothers into war work and the use of state provided childcare which offered to 'protect and safeguard their children' as it would 'preserve their family life' (cited by Enoch, 2012, p. 430). Once the war was over, to ensure work was available for the returning male soldiers, the same ideals were used to force mothers to return to their 'natural' role of homemaker as 'useful, well-adjusted citizens are the most valuable possession a country has, and good mother care during early childhood is the surest way to produce them' (Dr Spock, cited by Enoch, 2012, p. 435). Women as full-time homemakers were considered essential to their working husband's wellbeing and avoiding raising juvenile delinquents.

Although many working mothers protested, nurseries were closed with little or no notice. No consideration was given to the attachments the children may have formed with the nursery staff, despite Bowlby using the terms mother/substitute within his original work. Those mothers who previously needed to work to provide for their families were placed under economic and emotional stress as made to feel guilty if unable to become full-time homemakers. Mothers who did return to this role felt guilty at the potential damage their working may have caused. Their overprotective reaction and sole, continuous care could have meant that separation distress identified within psychology became a 'self-fulfilling prophecy' given that their children were less used to being looked after by others. This whole process reinforced patriarchy and constrained female roles. An idealised view of motherhood was created, yet women became responsible for preparing children for a world from which they, themselves, were marginalised (Burman, 2008).

Mothers had little option but to accept their roles of full-time child carers and homemakers due to social stigma as well as financial and legal constraints. Being financially dependent on their husbands prevented them from obtaining a lengthy and costly divorce. However, although still risking social censure, some mothers could attempt to raise their children alone after the changes made to the divorce law (1969) and Equal Pay Act (1970).

Fathers also suffered from the emphasis on mother-child relationship, as despite further attachment studies, such as those by Schaffer and Emerson (1964) demonstrating the value of other family bonds, it, unintentionally, relegated them to mere providers of economic, social, and emotional support. By the 1980s other works such as that by Lamb (1977) began to recognise the complimentary nature of both parents but fathers were still seen as more necessary for play than caring. However, later the demand for both parents to work outside the home, due to increased home ownership and male unemployment, has meant that fathers are now more involved in childcare. Shared responsibility for parental care is currently more apparent within Western families and particularly in current media portrayal of family life.

Whilst there is a need for more research on father–child attachment it appears that fathers provide a safe space and encourage exploration (Cowan & Cowan, 2019) and may influence future peer relationships as well as adolescent behavioural problems. However, Kuo et al. (2019) suggest that even a secure attachment with their father may not be enough to reduce stress reactions in infants insecurely attached to their mothers. Also, within her feminist interpretation of the implications of attachment theory, Burman points to an ambiguity within greater male involvement in children's care. Whilst it may be liberating for women and enable closer bonds between fathers and their children, it could also be interpreted as males taking over the one area of life where women, only relatively recently, gained more power and control. She points out how the status of women into male-dominated work outside the home has not made similar progress.

However, there is also a need to consider the whole network in which children are embedded. Dagan & Sagi-Schwartz, (2018) and Kuo et al. (2019) recommend that future research focusses on different family dynamics that create secure attachments. Current family structures are diverse and can include blended families; single-sex parenting; same-sex parenting; and same-sex, transgender parenting, and the influence of attachment within such families will be discussed in more detail in Chap. 7.

Attachment theory has revolutionised policies and practice within medicine and institutional care through highlighting unintended, unconducive practices. Current maternity practices such as greater involvement of fathers, mothers spending less time in hospital, and staff promoting skin to skin contact as soon as possible after birth are based on attachment theory.

The family-based care currently practiced in child healthcare owes much to the work of Bowlby and, particularly his brave and committed collaborator, James Robertson (see Robertson & Robertson, 1967–1973). Robertson had been alerted to the distressing effects of hospitalisation on young children when his own infant daughter had to spend time in hospital due to gastroenteritis. Working as Bowlby's research assistant, Robertson filmed young children in hospital and was deeply concerned to see the obvious stages of distress, despair, and detachment they experienced as separated from their caregivers. Hospital policies at the time maintained that visits by parents would upset their hospitalised child so were best avoided or, if unavoidable, be of minimal frequency and duration. These films were not received well by the medical establishment which was highly critical of Robertson's work. However, although it took a long time and much persuasion, Robertson persisted in challenging current childcare policies. His films of children's distress when in hospital or other form of institutional care eventually revolutionised the way children and their parents were later treated. The impact of attachment on the physical and mental health of children and adolescents will be discussed later in this chapter as well as in Chap. 9.

Attachment theory also currently dominates adoption and fostering policies. The short-term fostering practices carried out by James Robertson and his wife, which included careful pre-fostering preparation, helped demonstrate how this form of alternative care improved on the use of institutions. However, as the idea that attachment to biological caregivers was important was generally accepted it also, unintentionally, became misrepresented. Those wishing to abolish institutional care focussed on the biological basis rather than taking account of other influences and the policy of 'better a bad home than a good institution' adopted. Indeed, Tizard and others (see Tizard, 1977) demonstrated the need to take account of the quality of care within a child's home. They found that children returned to their poor biological home after spending time in an institution fared less successfully than those who continued to grow up in the institution or were adopted.

Nevertheless, within institutional care the importance of attachment was interpreted in different ways. For example, Hayes (1984) describes her personal work in childcare and how some homes discouraged staff from forming attachments with children whilst others permitted developing attachments so long as procedures were put in place to prevent favouritism and prepare children if existing staff left and new staff arrived. Concerns about attachment difficulties experienced by children in care have led to recommendations by the National Institute of Health and Care Excellence (NICE) in 2015, that such children should be fostered or adopted if possible, to offer them continuity and relationships based on a secure base.

Attachment theory currently underpins many practices within child day care centres. As a result, the National Institute of Child Health and Human Development (NICHD, 1997) found high-quality day care to be particularly beneficial for children of stressed mothers. The implementation of attachment principles in schools has also been found to improve the general wellbeing of students to the extent that for some, they can offer a necessary secure base not always possible at home (Harlow, 2019). Moreover, studies of 'attachment aware schools' by Rose et al. (2019) found significant improvements in pupils' academic achievement and behavioural difficulties.

Further initiatives involving attachment theory include government-run programmes such as Sure Start (now known as Children's Centres). Initially established in the late 1990s to serve disadvantaged families with young children and later offered across England, these programmes provided health, education, and childcare services. Cattan et al. (2019) found that Sure Start proved highly beneficial for children's health and in reducing hospitalisation, particularly in disadvantaged areas. However, despite many successes of the programme many centres were later closed for economic reasons.

Other initiatives based on attachment theory which are currently proving popular are parenting classes. However, the success of these classes is rather mixed. For example, Sutton (2019) suggests that they improve parenting strategies, whilst Lindsay and Totsika (2017) found no improvement in parenting stress or satisfaction of being a parent. Burman (2008) suggests that childhood intervention programmes based around the relationship between child and mother without changing the context in which they live must be viewed with caution. She also points out that small-scale experiments may work but not be generalisable on a larger, wider national scale.

4.3.3   Social Influences on Parenting

Whilst Ainsworth firmly believed that all infants share the basic need for at least one trustworthy, attachment figure, she accepted that, how such a need is expressed and met can differ between cultures (Duschinsky et al., 2020). Indeed, findings from the strange situation studies have found differences in the types of attachment security of infants within European and other countries. For example, in Germany avoidant insecure attachments were reported most often, whilst in Israeli kibbutz and Japan, ambivalent insecure attachments were more common than expected. This was explained as due to a tendency within Germany to value independence, whilst in Japan and Israel children were less likely to interact with strangers.

Although Bretherton (1992) cautions against overinterpreting such cross-cultural studies, it appears that different types of attachment are particularly dependent on the environment in which the child is raised. For example, face-to-face interaction between Tikopian infants and their paternal uncles were deliberately encouraged in preparation for the quasi-parent role uncles provide later in a child's life. In contrast, as Efe infants live in very close, semi-nomadic communities within Africa, they experience 'multiple mothering'. Although by the time they were six months old, Efe babies showed some preference for their biological mother; they were also happily nurtured by many other mothers within their community (Bretherton, 1992).

More recent studies of parenting have identified considerable similarities within the effects of parenting styles across cultures, particularly as children develop towards adolescence. For example, Akhtar et al. (2016) report more social competence in adolescents experiencing authoritative parenting within Pakistani extended families. Similar findings were also recorded by Sorkhabi and Mandara (2013) despite their concerns with Baumrind's original use of high functioning, white families when developing her concept of parenting styles. Sorkhabi (2005) had found that the shaming and demands for obedience within authoritarian parenting were interpreted in similar ways by children and adolescents from various cultures and were also more likely to result in maladjustment.

Also, the influence of the child's environment becomes particularly evident during middle childhood as attachment ties begin to be more complex than those earlier with close caregivers. Peer relationships are now seen to begin to offer potential long-term stability and security (Becke & Bongard, 2018).

Variability in parenting styles has been found within, as well as between, cultures. For example, Smetana (2017) points out how, although, Chinese parenting is often described as authoritarian, including over controlling 'tiger moms', different styles are used within urban and rural regions. Socio-economic status has been found to be particularly influential on different types of parenting within and across cultures. For example, Mooya et al. (2016) found that poverty was mostly responsible for the differences in sensitivity towards caregiving of infants practiced by mothers and siblings from different cultural groups in Zambia. Burman (2008) cautions against using Western ideals to judge parents' lack of sensitivity towards their offspring in other cultures, as this is often influenced by poverty. She offers the example of how in poor communities within South America some mothers may feel compelled to neglect the youngest of their many children to aid the survival of the remaining siblings.

An important influence of parenting style is the extent to which it is seen as normative. For example, Smetana (2017) found that the authoritarian parenting experienced by most adolescents within China had little detrimental effect but, became so when such practices were continued within Chinese immigrant families living in Canada, where authoritative parenting was common. Also, Fuligni and Tsai (2015) found that immigrant adolescents experience similar conflict and cohesion within family life to peers within their host society. However, they also retain a sense of obligation to meet family needs in line with their heritage culture which can inhibit the educational and future economic potential of those from poorer families. Current changes resulting from an increasingly interconnected world and greater numbers of immigrant families make it very important for those responsible for the care of children and adolescents within the UK be aware of such constraining experiences.

4.4   Attachment, Health, and Therapeutic Approaches

4.4.1   Attachment and Health

Bowlby had recognised the influence of family life on both mental and physical illness. He explained how often it is difficult to change the negative, taken for granted patterns of interaction within families because they have become so habitual that family members cease to be aware of them (Bretherton, 1992). Attachment theory offers a framework for understanding how such interpersonal relationships can affect health, for example, delayed achievement of developmental milestones (Wilkinson & Walford, 2001) and psychosomatic disorders (Steele et al., 1999).

Problematic attachments have been found to influence early neural development through impacting on neurological systems responsible for controlling stress, such as the hypothalamic-pituitary-adrenal axis within the brain. This can impair immune system functioning and lead to cardiovascular and autoimmune diseases as well as certain types of cancer. Insecure anxious attached individuals have been reported to be more prone to experiencing strokes, heart attacks, high blood pressure, and ulcers, even when sociodemographic and psychological risk factors were accounted for. However, less consistency was found regarding health risks and avoidant attachments (Jaremka et al., 2013).

Increased production of cortisol has been found to impair immune responses as well as affect memory loss and levels of anxiety as well as cause irreversible neuron damage to humans and animals. Whilst studies have found greater levels of cortisol in young monkeys separated from their mothers, links between elevated cortisol levels and separation distress in children are not as clear given that, ethically, it has only been possible to study short-term separations. Nevertheless, studies have suggested that securely attached children produced lower cortisol levels than those who were insecurely attached (Ahnert et al., 2004).

The inability to develop a secure attachment can make it difficult for children to regulate their emotions and cope with future negative life events. This may mean that those growing up in particularly stressful environments can experience mental health problems. These can be in the form of internalising behaviour, such as depression, anxiety, and self-harm, or externalising behaviour, such as oppositional defiant disorder and delinquency during adolescence (Sutton, 2019).

Some children experience particularly severe, adverse events which can lead to serious, long-term mental health conditions. Cecil et al. (2014) investigated links between different types of early maltreatment, inhibiting secure attachments and mental health disorders. They found some evidence that emotional abuse was particularly influential on mental health, but that many types of abuse occurred together, with worse symptoms depending on the number of types of abuses experienced.

Two specific mental health disorders directly linked to attachment problems are reactive attachment disorder (RAD) and disinhibited social engagement disorder (DSED). Initially these were both seen as aspects of reactive attachment disorders but later recognised as two distinct conditions (DSM-V; American Psychiatric Association, 2013). Diagnostic criteria for both conditions require children to have a cognitive age of at least nine months and have experienced serious social neglect in early life. RAD symptoms are characterised by an absence of attachment behaviours. Such absence usually becomes evident between the ages of nine months and five years. It includes a lack of focused attachment behaviour towards any caregiver as well as an inability to be comforted when distressed or engaged in social and emotional interactions. Children diagnosed with RAD also have problems in regulating their emotions, show aggression, fear, and irritability, even towards attempts to comfort them. They may also experience delay in language and other cognitive abilities as well as additional medical conditions including failure to thrive and skin lesions (Horner, 2019).

In contrast, children diagnosed with DSED (which is slightly more common than RAD) are inappropriately friendly with familiar and unfamiliar adults and lack a wariness of strangers which means they may well wander off with someone they do not know. Such children will have suffered neglect before they are two years old or have experienced disturbed or inconsistent caregiving. Their symptoms may also include language delay and often overlap with those related to attention deficit hyperactivity disorder (ADHD). Their symptoms, even after interventions, persist longer than those within RAD, possibly into adolescence (Horner, 2019).

Some children diagnosed with these attachment disorders have experienced institutional care with poor staff/child ratios. Others may also have suffered the death/loss of a caregiver or have had parents/caregivers who themselves had developed insecure attachments or have mental health problems. In some cases, caregivers may have engaged in drug and alcohol abuse, domestic violence, and sexual abuse. Horner (2019) points out how some children diagnosed with these disorders later develop obesity and nonspecific physical complaints.

4.4.2 Attachment As a Basis for Therapeutic Approaches

Attachment theory has been highly influential in understanding and treating the effects of adverse experiences on children and adolescents. Robertson eventually disagreed with Bowlby's term 'detachment' as the third stage of loss, rather seeing this as 'denial' and a warning sign that children were suppressing deeply held emotions. As mentioned previously, the pioneering films and articles produced by Robertson broadened the focus of care on to the whole family rather than just the individual child. Robertson and his wife recognised the value of one consistent carer rather than numerous care takers within childcare and ways in which separation distress could be reduced by carefully staged preparations for alternative care. In addition, they recognised that, as new attachments may form with foster mothers, staged preparations were also needed when children were reunited with their own mothers (Alsop-Fields & Mohay, 2001).

Attachments can, therefore, be seen, not only in terms of family relationships but also developing with others who may play a significant role in the lives of children and adolescents, such as practitioners, teachers, and peers. These relationships can be used as forms of substitute care as well as help to reduce past insecurities and painful experiences. Current formal therapeutic approaches based on attachment theory take account of family dynamics as well as environmental and biological influences. For example, Holmes and Slade (2019) refer to the biological mechanisms of attachment which can be harnessed within Attachment-Informed Psychotherapy (AIP). They also stress the need for therapists to focus on the early experiences of parents as well as the child/adolescent with a disorganised attachment. As such children/adolescents may have developed self-soothing strategies, such as self-harm, eating disorders, or addictions, therapists try to develop a supportive relationship which offers them the 'safe base' they lack. As disorganised attachments can create quick reactions to feared situations, through working alongside the therapist, the child/adolescent is encouraged to self-reflect and develop a more realistic view of themselves and others, including misunderstandings.

Current, formal therapeutic practitioners, therefore, work with the whole family rather than just the child or adolescent. Such therapeutic work aims to increase the security of the child's attachment relationships with their primary caregivers, and thereby with others, as well as help parents to reflect on their own attitudes and feelings about their child or adolescent's behaviour. The success of preventative measures is suggested by Horner (2019) who found that risks of disorganised attachments can be reduced in prenatally depressed mothers if they are provided with high-quality caregiving and support within the first three months of their child's life.

The Secure Attachment Family Education intervention programme addresses the unconscious influence of parent's past painful experiences on their own parenting and family life. Walter et al. (2019) use the term "ghosts in the nursery" to describe this dynamic. Practitioners help parents reflect on their own past experiences and educate them about attachment theory and child development. Video recording and role play are used to encourage parental sensitivity when interacting with their infants and they are provided with social support (Berkien et al., 2012).

Attachment-based therapies are, also, often used to help children/adolescents cope with bereavement. The whole family is engaged in treatment to reduce parent–child conflict, facilitate grieving, and cope with the absence of the deceased parent (Carr, 2014). Family therapy has also been found to be particularly helpful for families struggling to adapt to the changes required when children enter adolescence. Liddle and Schwartz (2002) describe how family therapy focusses on the extent to which relationships within the family may be dysfunctional rather than any individual's shortcomings. They point out that often there are variations due to culture or context but stress that there needs to be a change in parenting styles during this period. Such strategies reflect how positive psychology has been incorporated into specific forms of family therapy. Therapists attempt to change attitudes within families from focussing on problems to seeking to achieve goals. Rather than expect the 'problem' adolescent to change, therapists adopt a structured process using empathy to explore family rituals, seek examples of the adolescent's helpful behaviour, and encourage positive ways for family members to talk to each other which influence the whole family system (Conoley et al., 2015).

Family-based therapies have been found to reduce the need for institutional care and risks of arrest and recidivism. For example, Carr (2014) cites how family-based therapies have been found to reduce offending by adolescents with conduct disorders and reduce offending by their siblings.

4.4.3   Attachment and the COVID-19 Pandemic

Powerful changes are taking place at the time of writing this text due to the pandemic created by the spread of the COVID-19 virus, which will have serious implications for the future wellbeing of children and adolescents, not only in the UK, but worldwide. It is useful to apply attachment theory as a means of understanding the possible long-term consequences of the drastic measures different countries have had to adopt in attempts to curtail the spreading of this deadly virus.

Rapid introductions of new (often confusing) laws creating 'social lockdowns' in an attempt to prevent the virus spreading have included bans on families meeting together; closure of schools, universities, community facilities, and 'non' essential shops; parents working from home as much as possible; and strict travel restrictions. This has meant that families have had to face extremely long periods without any external forms of support. In addition, 'home schooling' has meant that, as well as being full time childcarers, parents have had to take on a new role of teacher whilst working from home, which has proved particularly hard for single parents.

The 'Stay Home; Protect the National Health Service (NHS); Save Lives' directive promoted by the British government has had serious effects on families as the home is not always the safest place for children to live. (This will be discussed further in Chap. 7.) Stress from continued social isolation has meant unrelieved constant contact within families and less access to supportive networks. This has the potential to increase family conflict and become a catalyst for violence. As a result, an increase in domestic violence has been reported by countries such as, Australia, France, and the UK (Usher et al., 2020). Violence from family members is currently even less visible to those outside the family unit with children more at risk of abuse, particularly those already living with abusive adults (Bradbury-Jones & Isham, 2020). Since such restrictions were established the National Society for the Protection of Children (NNSPC) have reported that, physical abuse of children and adolescents has risen by 53% in England, with adolescents four times more likely to be abused than younger children (Hamilton-Giachritsis & Fairchild, 2020:26).

Another example of the impact of restrictions, due to the virus pandemic, is the increased reliance of children and adolescents on technology for social interactions with others. Although this may offer a way of experiencing some form of social interaction, it also has the potential to exacerbate the existing problems of addiction to digital technology pointed out by Hamilton-Giachritsis and Fairchild (2020). In addition, support by means of technology may not even be possible or helpful for children and adolescents controlled by abusive adults, particularly in families facing socio-economic deprivation (Bradbury-Jones & Isham, 2020). Also, if digital technology is accessible, adolescents from socially deprived areas may lack the privacy to contact support services, due to confined living space (Golberstein et al., 2020).

The above findings are concerning as, during these unprecedented times, children and adolescents are in even greater need of protective, stable family relationships, yet, frustrations from the restrictions placed on family life appear to be continually increasing. Whilst it is too early to appreciate the long-term effects, Moccia et al. (2020) have sought to assess vulnerability, based on attachment styles, to stress created by the COVID-19 virus restrictions in Italy. Interestingly they found females more vulnerable, particularly if they have insecure anxious attachments and are prone to depression, whilst avoidant attachments offer some protective factors.

The influence of attachment as well as genetics and environment within first few years of life can be seen to have a lasting effect, even in adulthood. Appreciating the impact of separation anxiety and ways in which specific parenting styles can promote the necessary stability, security, and continuity required even during adolescence is particularly important, as is the role attachment plays in adolescent emotion regulation. It is necessary to see attachment theory within its historical and cultural context to appreciate the way it has revolutionised hospital provision for parental visiting as well as child patients' education, social contact, and play. Its profound effect on the procedures within nurseries, fostering, and adoption cannot be overstated. This theory also underpins therapeutic approaches to problems within childhood and adolescence, particularly the use of family therapy. Given that Bowlby saw attachment and loss as two sides of the same coin his work has influenced current models of grieving used within counselling and healthcare.

It becomes clear that attachment theory usefully integrates different elements of child development into a unified perspective which can be used to understand social and cognitive development within childhood and adolescence, as well as other influences on their wellbeing covered within further chapters of this book.

Summary

- Attachment theory, developed by Bowlby and based on ethology, psychodynamic, and cognitive theories, stresses the importance of early secure caregiver–child relationships in providing a safe base to aid children's and adolescents' social and cognitive development. Secure attachments allow them to develop an 'internal working model' used to understand future experiences. Attachment theory suggests that if a secure attachment has not been formed with a caregiver within the first years of life, children may have difficulties with future relationships. Removing a child from their attachment figure is seen to create 'separation anxiety' and potential insecure attachments. Sensitivity, stability, and continuity within specific parenting styles can promote secure attachments.
- Secure early attachments serve to support adolescents as they experience rapid biological changes, particularly in emotion regulation. They also aid psychosocial changes and influence choice of peer relationships. Secure attachments can help adolescents deal with change in manageable stages.
- Attachment theory became popularised during a period of growing interest in child psychology at the end of the Second World War. It served a political purpose in avoiding mass male unemployment by forcing women to give up their wartime jobs and deeply affected the roles of mothers and fathers. Feminists believe that it initially reinforced patriarchy with marginalisation of mothers from the 'outer world' and fathers from family life. Over time, the importance of attachments to both parents has been recognised and shared parenting roles become more common. Attachment theory is now integral to policies and practices within hospitals and other forms of alternative care. Given the Western-based nature of attachment theory, caution is needed in applying it to other cultures. Evidence suggests different parenting styles are favoured in different cultures. Nevertheless, similarities in the aims of parenting exist and differences appear to be context driven.
- Attachment theory underpins many therapeutic methods and has shifted focus from individual child/adolescent behaviour to a family-centred approach. It also underpins theories of loss used within counselling and healthcare
- The impact of the COVID-19 virus pandemic (2020) on attachment formation and influence of parenting needs to be considered. Social restrictions imposed to reduce the spread of the virus create stress and frustrations within family life. Abuse of children and adolescents has increased with those already vulnerable most at risk of such abuse remaining undetected. Potential long-term effects need to be monitored and treated.

Case Study Questions

Read the family case study on page 265 and consider the following:

- In what ways may the family circumstances and relationships in the first few years of each child's life have impacted on their ability to form secure attachments?
- How might Gemma's and Ben's early experiences and the biological and psychosocial changes they are currently experiencing be influencing their behaviour?
- What therapeutic approaches could be offered to help Lily and her family?

Reflective Questions

- Why should issues of gender, class, poverty, and race be considered when assessing the importance of attachment theory and parenting?
- In what ways might the restrictions imposed by the UK government due to COVID-19 have impacted on family life and the ability for babies born in this period to form secure attachments?
- How might issues of attachment, parenting, and culture impact across an individual's lifespan?

References

Ahnert, L., Gunnar, M. R., Lamb, M. E., & Barthel, M. (2004). Transition to Childcare: Associations with Infant-Mother Attachment, Infant Negative Emotions, and Cortisol Elevations. *Child Development, 75*(7), 639–650. 009-3920/2004/7503-001.

Ainsworth, M. D. S. (1979). Infant—Mother Attachment. *American Psychologist, 34*(10), 932–937.

Akhtar, P., Malik, J. A., & Begeer, S. (2016). The Grandparents' Influence: Parenting Styles and Social Competence among Children of Joint Families. *Journal of Child and Family Studies, 26,* 603–611. https://doi.org/10.1007/s10826-016-0576-5

Alsop-Fields, L., & Mohay, H. (2001). John Bowlby and James Robertson: Theorists, Scientists and Crusaders for Improvements in the Care of Children in Hospital. *Journal of Advanced Nursing, 35*(1), 50–58.

Barbaro, N., Boutwell, B. B., & Shackleford, T. K. (2017). Rethinking the Transmission Gap: What Behavioral Genetics and Evolutionary Psychology Mean for Attachment Theory. A Comment on Verhage et al. (2016). *Article in Psychological Bulletin, 143*(1), 107–113. https://doi.org/10.1037/bul0000066

Baumrind, D. (1971). Current Patterns of Parental Authority. *Developmental Psychology, 4*(1), pt. 2, 1–103. https://doi.org/10.1037/h0030372.

Becke, S. D., & Bongard, S. (2018). Comparing Attachment Networks During Middle Childhood in Two Contrasting Cultural Contexts. *Frontiers in Psychology, 9*(1201), 1–18. https://doi.org/10.3389/fpsyg.2018.01201

Berkien, M., Louwerse, A., Verhulst, F., & van der Ende, J. (2012). Children's Perceptions of Dissimilarity in Parenting Styles are Associated with Internalizing and Externalizing Behaviour. *European Child and Adolescent Psychiatry, 21,* 79–85. https://doi.org/10.1007/s00787-011-0234-9

Blakemore, S.-J., & Mills, K. L. (2014). Is Adolescence a Sensitive Period for Sociocultural Processing? *Annual review of Psychology, 65*, 187–207. https://doi.org/10.1146/annurev-psych-010213-115202

Bowlby, J. (1969). *Attachment and Loss, Volume 1: Attachment*. Penguin.

Bradbury-Jones, C., & Isham, L. (2020). The Pandemic Paradox: The Consequences of COVID-19 on Domestic Violence. *Journal of Clinical Nursing, 29*, 2047–2049. https://doi.org/10.1111/jocn.15296

Bretherton, I. (1992). The Origins of Attachment Theory: John Bowlby and Mary Ainsworth. *Developmental Psychology, 28*(5), 759–775.

Burman, E. (2008). *Deconstructing Developmental Psychology*. Routledge.

Carr, A. (2014). The Evidence Base for Family Therapy and Systemic Interventions for Child-focused Problems. *Journal of Family Therapy, 36*, 107–157. https://doi.org/10.1111/1467-6427.12032

Cattan, S., Cont, G., Farquharson, C., & Ginja, R. (2019). *The Health Effects of Sure Start. The Institute for Fiscal Studies*. Nuffield Foundation Study. http://www.ifs.org.uk

Cecil, C. A. M., Viding, E., Fearon, P., Glaser, D., & McCrory, E. J. (2014). Disentangling the Mental Health Impact of Childhood Abuse and Neglect. *Child Abuse & Neglect, 63*, 106–119. https://doi.org/10.1016/j.chiabu.2016.11.024

Ching, K. H., & Tak, L. M. (2017). The Structural Model in Parenting Style, Attachment Style, Self-regulation and Self-esteem for Smartphone Addiction. *IAFOR Journal of Psychology & the Behavioral Sciences, 3*, 85–103.

Clarke, A., & Clarke, A. (1998). Early Experience and the Life Path. *The Psychologist, 11*(9), 433–436.

Coleman, J., & Hagell, A. (Eds.). (2007). *Adolescence, Risk and Resilience. A Conclusion*. Wiley & Sons.

Conoley, C. W., Plumb, E. W., Hawley, K. J., Spaventa-Vancil, K. Z., & Hernández, R. J. (2015). Integrating Positive Psychology into Family Therapy: Positive Family Therapy. *The Counseling Psychologist, 43*(5), 703–733. https://doi.org/10.1177/0011000015575392

Cowan, P. A., & Cowan, C. P. (2019). Introduction: Bringing Dads Back into the Family. *Attachment & Human Development, 21*(5), 419–425. https://doi.org/10.1080/14616734.2019.1582594

Dagan, O., & Sagi-Schwartz, A. (2018). Early Attachment Network with Mother and Father: An Unsettled Issue. *Child Development Perspectives, 12*(2), 115–121. https://doi.org/10.1111/cdep.12272

Dash, S. (2013). Parenting Next to the Bogeyman. *The Psychologist, 26*(3), 232–233.

DSM-V. (2013). *Diagnostic and Statistical Manual of Mental Disorders (DSM–5)*. American Psychiatric Association.

Duschinsky, R., Van Ijzendoornb, M., Fosterd, S., Reijmana, S., & Lionettie, F. (2020). Attachment Histories and Futures: Reply to Vicedo's 'Putting Attachment in its Place. *European Journal of Development Psychology, 17*(1), 138–146. https://doi.org/10.1080/17405629.2018.1502916

Enoch, J. (2012). There's No Place Like the Childcare Center: A Feminist Analysis of <Home> in the World War II Era. *Rhetoric Review, 31*(4), 422–442. https://doi.org/10.1080/0735019 8.2012.711199

Erikson, E. H. (1959). *Identity and the Life Cycle: Selected Papers*. International Universities Press.

Fearon, P., Shmueli-Goetz, Y., Viding, E., Fonagy, P., & Plomin, R. (2014). Genetic and Environmental Influences on Adolescent Attachment. *Journal of Child Psychology and Psychiatry, 55*, 10331041. https://doi.org/10.1111/jcpp.12171

Fraley, R. C. (2002). Attachment Stability from Infancy to Adulthood: Meta-analysis and Dynamic Modeling of Developmental Mechanisms. *Personality and Social Psychology Review, 6*, 123–151.

Fuligni, A. J., & Tsai, K. M. (2015). Developmental Flexibility in the Age of Globalization: Autonomy and Identity Development Among Immigrant Adolescents. *Annual Review of Psychology, 66*, 411–431. https://doi.org/10.1146/annurev-psych-010814-015111

Garcia, A. R., Guptab, M., Greesona, J. K. P., Thompsona, A., & DeNard, C. (2017). Adverse Childhood Experiences Among Youth Reported to Child Welfare: Results from the National Survey of Child & Adolescent Wellbeing. *Child Abuse & Neglect, 70*, 292–302. https://doi.org/10.1016/j.chiabu.2017.06.019

George, C., Kaplan, N., & Main, M. (1996). Adult Attachment Interview. Unpublished Manuscript, Department of Psychology, University of California, Berkely (3rd Edition).

Golberstein, E., Wen, H., & Miller, B. F. (2020). Coronavirus Disease 2019 (COVID-19) and Mental Health for Children and Adolescents. Journal of American Medical Association. *Pediatrics, 174*(9), 819–820. https://jamanetwork.com/ on 09/27/2020

Hamilton-Giachritsis, C., & Fairchild, G. (2020:26). *How Safe are our Children? 2020*. NSPCC Learning. https://learning.nspcc.org.uk/media/2287/how-safe-are-our-children-2020.pdf

Harlow, E. (2019). Attachment Theory: Developments, Debates and Recent Applications in Social work, Social Care and Education. *Journal of Social Work Practice, Online Journal, 35*(7), 1–13. https://doi.org/10.1080/02650533.2019.1700493

Harlow, H. (1959). *Love in Infant Monkeys Affection* (pp. 68–74). Scientific American Inc..

Hayes, N. (1984). *A First Course in Psychology*. Nelson.

Holmes, J., & Slade, A. (2019). The Neuroscience of Attachment: Implications for Psychological Therapies. *The British Journal of Psychiatry, 214*, 318–319. https://doi.org/10.1192/bjp.2019.7

Horner, G. (2019). Attachment Disorders. *Journal of Pediatric Health Care, 33*(5), 612–622. https://doi.org/10.1016/j.pedhc.2019.04.017612

Jaremka, L. M., Glser, R., Loving, T. J., Malarky, W. B., Stowell, J. R., & Kiecolt-Glazer, J. (2013). Attachment Anxiety Is Linked to Alterations in Cortisol Production and Cellular Immunity. *Psychological Science, 24*(3), 272–279. https://doi.org/10.1177/0956797612452571

Kagan, J. (1995). On Attachment. *Harvard Review Psychology, 3*, 104–106.

Kingsbury, M., Clayborne, Z., Colman, I., & Kirkbride, J. B. (2019). The Protective Effect of Neighbourhood Social Cohesion on Adolescent Mental Health Following Stressful Life Events. *Psychological Medicine, 50*, 1292–1299. https://doi.org/10.1017/S0033291719001235

Klaus, M. H., Jerauld, R., Kregar, N. C., McAlpine, W., Steffa, M., & Kennel, M. D. (1972). Maternal Attachment: Importance of the First Post Partum Days. *The New England Journal of Medicine, -03-02*(9), 460–463.

Ko, A., Hewitt, P. L., Cox, D., Flett, G. L., & Chen, C. (2019). Adverse Parenting and perfectionism: A Test of the Mediating Effects of attachment Anxiety, Attachment Avoidance, and Perceived Defectiveness. *Personality and Individual Differences, 150*, 109474. https://doi.org/10.1016/j.paid2019.06.017

Kobak, R., Zajac, K., & Smith, C. (2009). Adolescent Attachment and Trajectories of Hostile–Impulsive Behavior: Implications for the Development of Personality Disorders. Development and Psychopathology, 21, 839–851. https://doi.org/10.1017/S095457940900045

Kooraneh, A. E., & Amirsardari, L. (2015, June). Predicting Early Maladaptive Schemas Using Baumrind's Parenting Styles. *Iran Journal of Psychiatry Behavioural Science, 9*(2), e952. https://doi.org/10.17795/ijpbs952

Kuo, P. X., Saini, E., Tengelitsch, E., & Volling, B. L. (2019). Is one Secure Attachment Enough? Infant Cortisol Reactivity and the Security of Infant-Mother and Infant-Father Attachments at the End of the First Year. *Attachment & Human Development, 21*(5), 426–444. https://doi.org/10.1080/14616734.2019.1582595

Lamb, M. E. (1977). The Development of Mother-Infant and Father-Infant Attachments in the Second Year of Life. *Developmental Psychology, 13*, 639–649.

Liddle, H. A., & Schwartz, S. J. (2002). Attachment and Family Therapy: Clinical Utility of Adolescent-Family Attachment Research. *Family Process, 41*(3), 455–476.

Lindsay & Totsika. (2017). The Effectiveness of Universal Parenting Programmes: The CANparent Trial. *BioMed Central Psychology, 5*(35), 1–11. https://doi.org/10.1186/s40359-017-0204-1

Lorenz, K. (1935). The Companion to the Bird's World. *Auk, 54*, 245–273.

Lyons-Ruth, K., Choi-Kain, L., Pechtel, P., Bertha, E., & Gunderson, J. (2011). Perceived Parental Protection and Cortisol Responses among Young Females with Borderline Personality Disorder and Controls. *Psychiatry Research, 189(3*, 426–432. https://doi.org/10.1016/j.psychres.2011.07.038

Main, M., & Goldwyn, R. (1987). Adult Attachment Interview Rating and Classification System, Unpublished manuscript, University of California, Berkeley.

Main, M., & Hesse, E. (1990). Parents' Unresolved Traumatic Experiences are Related to Disorganised Attachment Status. Is Frightened and/or Frightening Parental Behaviour the Linking Mechanism? In M. T. Greenberg, D. Cicchetti, & E. M. Cummings (Eds.), *Attachment in the Pre-School Years*. University of Chicago Press.

Meeus, W., Oosterwegel, A., & Vollebergh, W. (2002). Parental and Peer Attachment and Identity Development in Adolescence. Journal of Adolescence, 25, 93–106. https://doi.org/10.1006/jado.2001.0451, http://www.idealibrary.com

Moccia, L., Janiri, D., Pepe, M., Dattolie, L., Molinaro, M., De Martin, V., Chieffo, D., Janini, L., & Fiorillo, A. (2020). Affective Temperament, Attachment Style, and the Psychological Impact of the COVID-19 Outbreak: An Early Report on the Italian General Population. *Brain Behaviour and Immunity, 87*, 75–79. https://doi.org/10.1016/j.bbi.2020.04.048

Mooya, H., Sichimbaa, F., & Bakermans-Kranenburgh. (2016). Infant–mother and Infant–sibling Attachment in Zambia. *Attachment & Human Development, 18*(6), 618–635. https://doi.org/10.1080/14616734.2016.1235216

NICHD Study of Early Child Care NICHD. (1997). The Effects of Infant Child Care on Infant-Mother Attachment Security: Results of the NICHD Study of Early Child Care NICHD Early Child Care Research Network. NICHD Early Child Care Research Network. *Child Development, 68*(5), 860–879. https://doi.org/10.1111/j.1467-8624.1997.tb01967.x

Pace, C. S., Di Folco, S., & Guerriero, V. (2017). Late-adoptions in Adolescence: Can Attachment and Emotion Regulation Influence Behaviour Problems? A Controlled Study Using a Moderation Approach. *Clinical Psychology and Psychotherapy, 25*(2), 250–262. https://doi.org/10.1002/cpp.2158

Padilla-Walker, L. M., & Nelson, L. J. (2012). Black Hawk Down? : Establishing Helicopter Parenting as a Distinct Construct from Other Forms of Parental Control During Emerging Adulthood. *Journal of Adolescence, 35*, 1177–1190. https://doi.org/10.1016/j.adolescence.2012.03.007

Patterson, M. W., Cheung, A. K., Mann, F. D., Tucker-Drob, E. M., & Harden, K. P. (2017). Multivariate Analysis of Genetic and Environmental Influences on Parenting in Adolescence. *Journal of Family Psychology, 31*(5), 532–541. https://doi.org/10.1037/fam0000298

Pratt, M., Zeev-Wolf, M., Goldstein, A., & Feldman, R. (2019). Exposure to Early and Persistent Maternal Depression Impairs the Neural basis of Attachment in Preadolescence. *Progress in Neuro-Psychopharmacology and Biological Psychiatry, 93*, 21–30. https://doi.org/10.1016/j.pnpbp.2019.03.005

Robertson, J., & Robertson, J. (1967–1973). *Film Series, Young Children in Brief Separation*. Tavistock.

Rose, J., McGuire-Snieckus, R., Gilbert, L., & McInnes, K. (2019). Attachment Aware Schools: the Impact of a Targeted and Collaborative Intervention. *International Journal of Personal, Social and Emotional Development, 37*, 162–184. https://doi.org/10.1080/02643944.2019.1625429

Rutter, M. (1972). *Maternal Deprivation Reassessed*. Penguin.

Schaffer, H. R. (1996). *Social Development*. Blackwell.

Schaffer, H. R. (2004). *Introducing Child Psychology*. Blackwell.

Schaffer, H. R., & Emerson, P. E. (1964). The Development of Social Attachments in Infancy. *Monographs of the Society for Research in Child Psychology, 29* (Whole No. 3.)

Smetana, J. G. (2017). Current Research on Parenting Styles, Dimensions, and Beliefs. *Current Opinion in Psychology, 15*, 19–25. https://doi.org/10.1016/j.copsyc.2017.02.012

Sorkhabi, N. (2005). Applicability of Baumrind's Parent Typology to Collective Cultures: Analysis of Cultural Explanations of Parent Socialization Effect. *International Journal of Behavioral Development, 29*(6), 552–563. https://doi.org/10.1080/01650250500172640

Sorkhabi, N., & Mandara, J. (2013). Are the Effects of Baumrind's Parenting Styles Culturally Specific or Culturally Equivalent? In R. E. Larzelere, A. S. Morris, & A. W. Harrist (Eds.), *Authoritative Parenting: Synthesizing Nurturance and Discipline for Optimal Child Development* (pp. 113–135). American Psychological Association. https://doi.org/10.1037/13948-006

Steele, H., Steele, M., Croft, C., & Fonagy, P. (1999). Infant-Mother Attachment at One Year Predicts Children's Understanding of Mixed Emotions at Six Years. *Social Development, 8*(2), 161–178. https://doi.org/10.1111/1467-9507.00089

Steele, M., Steele, H., & Beebe, B. (2017). Applying an Attachment and Microanalytic Lens to "Embodied Mentalization": Commentary on "Mentalizing Homeostasis: The Social Origins of Interoceptive Inference" by Fotopoulou and Tsakiris. *Neuropsychoanalysis, 19*(1), 59–66. https://doi.org/10.1080/15294145.2017.1295218

Stepp, S. D. (2001). Development of Borderline Personality Disorder in Adolescence and Young Adulthood: Introduction to the Special Section Stephanie D. Stepp. *Journal of Abnormal Child Psychology, 40*, 1–5. https://doi.org/10.1007/s10802-011-9594-3

Stern, D. (1977). *The First Relationship: Infant and Mother.* Fontana.

Sutton, T. A. (2019). Review of Attachment Theory: Familial Predictors, Continuity and Change, and Intrapersonal and Relational Outcomes. *Marriage & Family Review, 55*(1), 1–22. https://doi.org/10.1080/01494929.2018.145800

Tizard, B. (1977). *Adoption: A Second Chance.* Open Books.

Usher, K., Navjot Bhullar, N., Durkin, J., Gyamfi, N., & Jackson, D. (2020). *International Journal of Mental Health Nursing, 29*, 549–552. https://doi.org/10.1111/inm.12735

Walter, I., Landers, S., Quehenberger, J., Carlson, E., & Brisch, K. H. (2019). The Efficacy of the Attachment-based SAFE Prevention Program: A Randomized Control Trial including Mothers and Fathers. *Attachment & Human Development, 21*(5), 510–531. https://doi.org/10.1080/14616734.2019.1582599

Wilkinson, R. B., & Walford, W. A. (2001). Attachment and Personality in the Psychological Health of Adolescents. *Personality and Individual Differences, 31*, 473–484.

Zeegers, M. A. J., Colonnesi, C., Stams, G. J. J. M., & Meins, E. (2017). Mind matters: A Three-Level Meta-Analysis on Parental Mentalization and Sensitivity as Predictors of Infant–Parent Attachment. *Psychological Bulletin, 143*, 1245–1272. https://doi.org/10.1037/bul0000114

Sociability, Self-identity, and Self-esteem

5

An individual's self-concept and level of self-esteem are influenced by their biology and culturally specific experiences. Children and adolescents are required to 'fit in' and conform to current, cultural expectations of age-related behaviour. Those developing or behaving in ways incompatible with such expectations may face public criticism and be rejected by their peers. However, differences in physical abilities, cognitive development, early attachment relationships, socio-economic status, gender, and ethnicity can mean that it is difficult for some children and adolescents to comply with the complex age-related behaviour judged appropriate within Western society. Being considered 'different' can be stressful and contribute to poor physical and psychological health. Therefore, a psychosocial approach needs to be taken to understand and help reduce such experiences which can have a powerful effect on the self-concept and level of self-esteem developed during childhood and adolescence.

5.1 Influence of Temperament and Attachment on Sociability

5.1.1 Temperament, Age, and Sociability

As mentioned within the previous chapter, an individual's inherited temperament can be identified during infancy by noting their biological, emotional, and physiological reactions to their environment. Such knowledge is useful in predicting a child's future ability to socialise successfully with others. Social interactions provide important opportunities for the child to gain a sense of being a separate 'self'. The child's sense of self-esteem is then seen as a reflection of the positive and negative ways that others have reacted during such interactions. It is, therefore, useful to start by considering the biological mechanisms thought to be responsible for initiating this process.

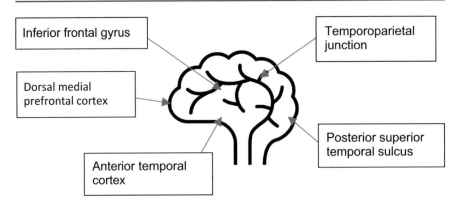

Fig. 5.1 Areas of the brain involved in social cognition according to Kilford et al. (2016)

The biological basis of perceiving and reacting to other humans (social perception) is thought to be linked to specific aspects of visual processing within the brain which influence other areas associated with cognition and emotions during social interactions. Such interactions require the ability to recognise faces and join with others in paying attention to specific stimuli (Guyer et al., 2014). Such abilities develop in early infancy and eventually enable the child to make inferences and recognise the emotional states of others. Such awareness is necessary to guide future responses to others and negotiate complex social situations. The complex, highly integrated nature of the brain regions responsible for social processing includes the dorsal medial prefrontal cortex, temporoparietal junction, posterior superior temporal sulcus, anterior temporal cortex, and interior frontal gyrus (see Fig. 5.1).

Kilford et al. (2016) suggest that, despite the current debatable nature of the specific contributions of these areas, they influence social cognition in ways outlined in Table 5.1.

Individual differences in this complex processing can mean that some infants exhibit 'behavioural inhibition' which involves a tendency to withdraw from social situations that continues into late adolescence and early adulthood. Behavioural inhibition has been linked, in some cases, to pathological disorders such as social anxiety disorder (SAD) which may even lay latent until children and adolescents face stressful social situations. Such children may fear meeting new peers. Unfortunately, their inability to act appropriately establishes a reinforcing cycle of rejection, avoidance, and self-criticism. Rates of social anxiety disorder increase as children approach adolescence. According to Kilford et al. (2016), this is because cognitive and social changes during this period can create unusual activity and connectivity within the reward-related circuits of adolescents' brains. This causes them to feel intensely emotional about peer friendships and their ability to form intimate relationships. Those adolescents identified as experiencing behavioural inhibition are more vulnerable to the effects of peer rejection, which increases the risk of depression, anxiety, risk taking, substance use, and suicidality.

Table 5.1 Specific role of brain areas involved with social cognitions according to Kilford et al. (2016)

Region	Involvement with social cognition
Dorsal medial prefrontal cortex and temporoparietal junction	Reflecting on mental states
Posterior superior temporal sulcus	Identifying faces and biologically based motion
Anterior temporal cortex	Application of social knowledge
Inferior frontal gyrus	Appreciate the meaning of others' emotions and actions

However, Guyer et al. (2014) point out that certain experiences can help reduce the creation of such a cycle. They describe the success of early interventions, such as experiencing being cared for by others in addition to their mothers, can help reduce later anxious behaviours in young children identified with behavioural inhibition. Also, it appears that as adolescents prepare to cope with the increased complexities of adult life their brains develop a heightened neural plasticity during this period, making them particularly amenable to change through social experiences. Kilford et al. (2016) point out the benefits of understanding such neurological changes within this period and applying strategies informed by interventionist studies. For example, reducing the potential positive rewards gained from gang membership and crime. There is a need to gain greater understanding of how developments in social perception within childhood and adolescence interact dynamically with the changing cultural demands during different life stages.

Biological changes within the autonomic nervous system created by experiences within early attachment relationships between children and their caregivers have also been found to impact on social development. For example, Stern and Cassidy (2018) explain how interactions between dopamine-system genes, parenting, and attachment can influence children's prosocial behaviour. They also refer to the role played by the hypothalamic–pituitary–adrenocortical (HPA) axis and oxytocin system in controlling levels of empathy and sensitive caregiving necessary for secure attachments. Insecure attachments can create physiological changes such as vasodilation/constriction, reduced heart rate, and inflammation. It appears that attachment-related experiences become 'biologically embedded' and when of a negative nature can be associated with social impairments in children and adolescents.

Animal studies have demonstrated the need for social cooperation for the survival of some species. As an evolutionary-based theory, attachment theory offers a useful framework for understanding the importance of caring for others and the resulting social behaviour in humans. Attachment influences the development of internal working models through which children learn to regulate emotions necessary for the foundation of future good peer relationships and social competence (Stern & Cassidy, 2018).

5.1.2 Development of Self-concept

The ability to achieve the social competence expected within the society into which children are born impacts upon their self-concept. As discussed above, the ability to meet such social expectations depends initially upon a biologically inherited preparedness for social interactions which differs between individual children. Early emotional expressions of smiling, crying, and proximity seeking create early social signals and promote bonding with parents and other caretakers. Readers who work with very young children will easily appreciate the enormous power of an infant's smile. It is impossible as a caretaker not to feel a warm glow once your own gaze has been captured by those appealing eyes and the infant's look of pure pleasure when smiled at in return. Similarly, it is impossible not to feel uncomfortable when hearing an infant cry, but also appreciate the physically and emotionally rewarding experience of having soothed it back to sleep.

Such signalling occurs cross-culturally and even blind babies smile at gentle touch or noise. The early communication system established through conveying primitive emotions, including recognised facial expressions, becomes modified and more complex through a child's experiences. This bi-directional process means that from early life children influence their environment and the resulting responses from their environment influence children's future actions (Schaffer, 2003).

A sense of an individual 'self' emerges as the child becomes more aware of their own 'self-awareness', their separateness from others, and ability to create an effect on their environment. Cooley (1902) used the term 'looking glass self' to explain this process and how it involves children internalising the reactions of others towards them. Children's 'self-concept' is therefore a reflection of the way caregivers and others have reacted towards them. However, G.H. Mead (1934) points out that a sense of self includes two elements, the 'perceiving process' and what is 'perceived'. He describes the 'self' as involving an 'I', (existential self), which is the process of perceiving, as well as a 'me' (categorical self), which includes aspects of the self that are perceived through interactions with the environment. It is difficult to know what is involved in the 'I' (existential) element of the 'self' as this very awareness or 'consciousness' is not easy to study objectively. However, through social interactions, this awareness does allow infants to gradually identify qualities they possess such as, age, sex, preferences, and similarities and differences between themselves and others. These qualities provide the basis of who a child thinks they are which forms the 'me' ('categorical' self).

Infants' developing awareness of their separateness from others becomes apparent through the separation anxiety they express. This becomes particularly visible from about nine months of age and reaches a peak when they are about eighteen months to two years old. Expressing distress when their caregiver is out of sight suggests that an infant's cognitive development is such that they now have a sense of 'person permanence'; that is they recognise that their caregiver is absent but will return. This demonstrates the development of imagination and an increased ability to remember past experiences. Infants now have developed an ability to store and retrieve information as they are not only able to recognise that their caregiver exists and may disappear but that they will re-appear in response to its own signals of distress. Infants, therefore, also begin to recognise their own 'sense of agency' in relation to affecting the behaviour of others. This builds upon their earlier, emerging ability to change their environment, when, for example, purposefully moving their hand to create noise and movement in the rattles strung across their pushchair. The 'me' and related sense of 'agency' created by a developing sense of self is, therefore, an integrated reflection of responses of others to them and their own actions.

An enlightening study was carried out by Lewis and Brookes-Gunn (1979) to investigate how early young children recognised themselves as separate individuals. They arranged for mothers to place a spot of red rouge on their infants' noses and monitored each child's reactions at seeing their reflection in a mirror. They found that before the age of fifteen months infants merely continued to react to their reflection as an object of interest. However, between 5% and 25% of infants aged between fifteen and eighteen months and 75% of one-year-old infants touched their own noses, suggesting they associated the dot seen in the mirror as on their own face. Interestingly, Lewis and Brookes-Gunn's (1979) found that when red spots of rouge were placed on their mother's nose infants connected the reflection with her much earlier than associating their own reflection with themselves.

By the time they are two years old, securely attached children will use their attachment figure as a safe-base whilst attempting independent exploration and demands. Many caregivers term this period as the 'terrible twos' and find their child's wilful behaviour challenging. However, such determination reflects children's healthy, awareness of self-agency and secure knowledge of support whilst they explore their environment (Kagan, 1981). Infants' ability to monitor their own actions through their emerging sense of self is enhanced through developing language. Infants gradually demonstrate their ability for joint attention and conscious communication, initially through ritualised gestures involving pointing to objects. This is usually accompanied by adults' verbal responses, using simplified language ('motherese'). Interestingly, children soon use the terms 'I' and 'me' correctly which is surprising given that adults will refer to themselves as 'I' and 'me' whilst addressing the infant as 'you'.

By three years of age children's mastering of language enables them to make more complex comparison between themselves and others. Around four to five years of age they begin to appreciate that there are private aspects of the self, not visible to others, such as thoughts and actions carried out alone. These contrast to public aspects of the self which are visible as carried out in the presence of others. By eleven years the child has built up quite a complex sense of the type of person they think they are, based on stored memories of past experiences. In adolescence the self-concept becomes even more complex as it includes more abstract qualities such as ideas, hopes, and how successfully they meet others' expectations.

Adolescents begin to develop a more socially integrated self-identity but also become so acutely self-aware that they are particularly sensitive to being judged by others. They may feel that they are being constantly observed, even when this is not the case. Kilford et al. (2016) refer to the 'New Look Theory' to explain such oversensitivity during this period as due to two interrelated processes. These involve adolescents feeling vulnerable as they attempt to develop an identity separate from that of their parents. They often feel so self-conscious that they overestimate the severity of the way they are being judged by some 'imaginary audience'. Kilford et al. (2016) also point out that, although such self-consciousness peaks in adolescence, it can persist, to some extent, into early adulthood.

It is important that during childhood and adolescence, the development of a concept of 'self' takes place within a trusting relationship, involving secure attachments. For example, early negative responses from others can influence a child's view of their world and confidence in their own ability to act appropriately. Should their affectionate embrace be rejected by their carer, they may feel unworthy and unsure about how to display their emotions. Cognitive and social development are interdependent and secure attachments are important for facilitating both (Schaffer, 2003).

5.2   The Role of Empathy and Theory of Mind in Sociability

5.2.1   Empathy and Awareness of the Needs of Others

Empathy is thought to be a relatively stable human trait involving emotional identification through an ability to share the feelings of another person and understand these from their point of view. Empathetic understanding appears to stem from an inherited neurobiological preparedness and impacts on an individual's ability to develop social relationships. This is enhanced by early secure attachments which promote emotional self-regulation and the development of a conscience. The internal working model developed in childhood and modified during adolescence is shaped by exposure to caregivers' emotion-focussed language and expressions of concern for others (Stern & Cassidy, 2018).

By four years of age a child's capacity for empathy becomes particularly evident as they can now connect images, beliefs, and actions and distinguish between pretence and reality. They have now developed enough self-awareness to form a 'theory of mind' which means that they can now appreciate that others may think differently to themselves. For example, in their study, Perner et al. (1987) found that on seeing a 'smartie' tube filled with pencils, children of this age would have no hesitation in explaining that others given the tube would still expect to find 'smarties' inside. Baron-Cohen (2001) believes that the ability to form a theory of mind entails areas of the brain including the amygdala, orbito-frontal cortex, and medial frontal cortex.

To demonstrate that young children hold a 'theory of mind' Baron-Cohen et al. (1985) developed the 'Sally-Anne' test. This entails acting out a scenario using dolls named Sally and Anne who each have a basket. After ensuring that children knew the names of the dolls, Baron-Cohen et al. (1985) moved the dolls in ways to show Sally placing a marble in her basket and leaving the scene. Anne was then moved in ways to show that she was taking the marble and hiding it in her own basket. When the Sally doll 'returned' the children were asked where she would think her marble would be. Children pointing to Sally's basket demonstrated their ability to know that Sally had a false belief. They were aware that, given Sally had not seen the marble being moved, she would have expected it still to be in her own basket. To check that the children really understood what had transpired they were asked to show where the marble really was and then, where it was originally.

Schaffer (2003) describes how children who have numerous siblings have been found to develop a theory of mind earlier than others. This suggests that environmental influences also impact on the rate that children develop a 'theory of mind'.

5.2.2 Problems with Understanding Others in Childhood and Adolescence

Social and cultural environments as well as biological changes all impact on the development of a 'theory of mind' throughout childhood and during adolescence. The ability to recognise and successfully read facial expressions plays a dominant role in understanding the feelings and intentions of others. Kilford et al. (2016) point to a biological preparedness for such ability. They refer to newborn infants' ability to detect human faces and how core-face processing is evident by the time a child is about seven years old with related brain systems continuing to develop during adolescence. Such development culminates in the use of specific cognitive strategies in adulthood, through having greater experience of others' mental states, including their beliefs, desires, and intentions.

Adolescence is, therefore, a period in which great changes occur within areas of the brain responsible for social perception. The pruning and increase of myelin sheathing of neural connections during this period suggest that areas of the brain concerned with such higher order, social cognitive function need time to mature. Kilford et al. (2016) found that awareness of the perspectives of others, so important for successful social functioning, is particularly cognitively demanding during adolescence. They describe how during adolescence more regions of the brain are used for social functioning than in adulthood.

The capacity to feel compassion also becomes evident during adolescence. Preckel et al. (2017) explain that increased cognitive development means that in addition to the ability to empathise, compassion provides the motivation to help alleviate suffering. They see compassion as helping to regulate emotions and reduce potential distress caused by empathetic 'overload'. Such processes enable adolescents to engage in increasingly complex social situations.

The complex process of sociability becomes particularly apparent when considering children and adolescents with a learning disability. For example, those diagnosed with autism have been thought to lack a 'theory of mind' and appear to have little or no idea that others may not think or feel like them (Baron-Cohen, 2001). Similarly, Maoz et al. (2017) report that children diagnosed with attention deficit and hyperactivity disorder (ADHD) show impaired empathy and 'theory of mind' but, that, this improves if such children are given the stimulant methylphenidate. Gvirts et al. (2021) also found that children with ADHD lack an ability to consciously synchronise their behaviour successfully with others during social interactions and have difficulty anticipating the intentions and movements of others which require a 'theory of mind'.

However, despite much research supporting the development of a 'theory of mind' the tests for possessing this have been seen, by some, as questionable. For example, Quesque and Rossetti (2020) reviewed current methods of assessing 'theory of mind' and report that the majority are not assessing the ability to represent another's mental state, or in some cases, any kind of mental state. Also, Gernsbacher and Yergeau (2019) caution against claiming that autistic people lack a 'theory of mind' as they feel that it is an impossible concept to identify and measure. They point out that it can lead to stigma and cause emotional harm for those given such a diagnosis as it suggests an impaired understanding of themselves and others, which questions their autonomy and credibility.

5.2.3   Cognitive Control Over Prosocial and Antisocial Behaviour

Increased cognitive functioning enables improved social perception with greater ability to consider the views and intentions of others. Understanding the need for fairness is evident from when children are about seven to eight years of age. They also develop a greater appreciation of the role of trust and cooperation by the time they are nine years old (Kilford et al., 2016). The understanding of intentions of others within social interactions continues to develop gradually during adolescence but is not fully developed until adulthood.

However, deficits in social perception during adolescents can result in antisocial behaviour. Kilford et al. (2016) suggest that this is because of an imbalance between brain systems responsible for gaining rewards and avoiding discomfort which can lead to greater risk taking. Heightened reward sensitivity can increase the potential for such risky behaviour as substance abuse, unsafe sex, crime, and dangerous driving. However, Kilford et al. (2016) point out that the role of cognitive control during this period of life is complex. Although in some situations it appears that areas of the brain responsible for cognitive control are not as well developed as those areas responsible for pleasure seeking, in other situations it can be more influential than it is later in adulthood. They believe social cognition to be a highly complex process which involves the development and interplay of overlapping and interdependent brain regions and networks.

The important influence of peer relationships during adolescence has become increasingly recognised, but again this is complex. For example, Kilford et al. (2016) describe how peer's positive and negative feedback has been found to be helpful for late adolescent males but detrimental to the performance of tasks carried out by female adolescents. However, when compared to adults, adolescents' risk-taking actions were found to be influenced more by peers and social context. There is a need for adolescents to experience good adult as well as peer relationships as both have been found to have a potentially positive effect in different contexts. For example, Kilford et al. (2016) report that adolescents were less likely to engage in risk-taking behaviour in the presence of their mother than when alone and exhibit more pro-social behaviour when receiving peer feedback.

5.3   Socialisation, Sociability, and Self-esteem

It is important to take account of the context in which relationships develop as this can not only influence children's ability to 'read' others but also impact on their self-esteem. Self-esteem has been defined as the subjective evaluation a person makes of their own worthiness and is a relatively stable trait impacting on wellbeing and relationships (Orth & Robins, 2014; Orth et al., 2018). By two years of age infants seek the approval of others when they are engaged in activities. They develop a sense of worthiness and competence through the response they receive. Past studies have suggested that self-esteem decreases during middle childhood (about four to eight years) as by this age cognitive development means that children are more aware of their private and public 'selves', make social comparisons, and distinguish between their 'ideal' and 'real' selves. This can result in the ability to feel pride and shame. However, Orth et al. (2018) found that, despite increased self-awareness sensitising children to potential negative views of themselves, their overall self-esteem increases during this period. They suggest that this may be the result of other gains they have made in personal autonomy and a general sense of increased mastery of their world.

Orth et al. (2018) also report that in contrast to past reports of a decline in self-esteem during the transition from childhood to adolescence, current research indicates that, on average, self-esteem remains constant for those aged about eleven to fifteen years of age. They suggest that adolescence may not be quite the time of 'storm and stress' generally expected within Western society. However, individual differences will mean that some adolescents may experience a decline in their self-esteem due to changes in puberty, mood swings, and the impact of their social environment. To appreciate the ways that the social environment influences the development of self-esteem it is important to understand the different ways in which it is influenced by the responses of significant others.

5.3.1   The Influence of the Family on Concepts of Self and Self-esteem

Although genetic inheritance plays some part in a child's potential self-esteem, personal qualities valued by wider society are passed on (directly and indirectly) through the child's family and become a basis of self-judgement and their self-esteem. Rogers' (1961) humanistic theory suggests that self-esteem is heavily influenced by the extent to which basic human needs of acceptance and love are given. He saw low self-esteem resulting from caregivers demanding that the child be the person they wished them to be, rather than accept who they really were. This creates the feeling in the child of a gap between the 'ideal self', desired by others, and 'real self' the child feels that they are. A wide gap can create an individual who is constantly striving to be something better than they think they really are and lead to depression.

Box 5.1 David's story

David had returned to school to study and re-sit the General Certificate in Education Examinations (GCSEs) due to the poor results he had achieved previously. He was not an easy student to teach or popular with his classmates due to his constant boasting, irritating comments, and practical jokes. During a 'parents' evening' his parents were found to be very demanding and to consistently criticise their son for the poor GCSE grades he had achieved. They insisted that he would work harder this year and gain better grades so that he could go on to university as this was what they planned for his future.

Despite studying hard, the results from David's re-sit GCSE examinations were little better than the original grades. David decided to enrol at the local college to train as an electrician. When met again at the college, David was much happier, more confident, and was well thought of by his work placement supervisors. He had even gained a girlfriend.

The example offered in Box 5.1 experienced by the first author when teaching in a school and local college (name changed for anonymity) helps to illustrate Rogers' theory.

The response of caregivers to developmental changes within childhood is, therefore, highly influential on children's self-esteem. As seen in the previous chapter, parenting responses can be permissive, authoritarian, neglectful, and authoritative. The impact of parenting styles appears to be complex, but elements of authoritative parenting appear to help in fostering a high sense of self-esteem in children. For example, Coopersmith (1967) found high self-esteem in boys whose parents were strict but interested. However, the level and timing of parental strictness along with the child's gender are important as Gittins and Hunt (2019) report little benefit from strict parental control during late childhood and early adolescence and that it can even lead to greater levels of self-criticism in girls. Perez-Gramaje et al. (2019) emphasise the importance of caregivers' warm attitudes in developing high self-esteem. They found the lowest self-esteem and highest levels of aggression in adolescents raised by neglectful or strict authoritarian parents. However, Pinquart and Gerke (2019) suggest that more evidence from longitudinal studies is needed as children's behaviour may also impact on parenting styles. There are also many other features of family life which also impact on the self-esteem of children and adolescents which are addressed in further chapters of this book.

5.3.2 Self-identity, Class, Ethnicity, and Gender Socialisation

A secure sense of self and self-worth is heavily influenced by the ability of children and adolescents to adapt to, and balance the different age-related, social roles which are demanded by the society into which they are born. These roles vary between cultures. For example, within Western society individuality is prized in contrast to societies, such as China, where social competence is measured more in terms of the ability to recognise and put the needs of their group first. An ability to adapt to social roles is also influenced by factors such as age, class, gender, and ethnicity.

A highly influential feature of family life impacting on children's emerging self-identity and related self-esteem is the attitude of parents to the way that their social class is perceived and responded to within society. Easterbrook et al. (2020) define social class in terms of income, education, and employment position. They found this to influence an individual's self-identity as much as their ethnic origin or gender and influence the choice of political affiliation as well as marriage partner. Parents will quickly and accurately use class to assess their own social status, as well as that of others. Parents' perception of the class to which they belong has a powerful effect on the self-concept and self-esteem of all family members. The self-identities of those from lower class backgrounds are more dependent upon their position within their family and community, whereas the self-identities of those from higher class backgrounds are based more on their personal achievements. Easterbrook et al. (2020) explain that the rise in economic inequality and decrease in social mobility within the UK have meant that since the 1980s positive attitudes to traditional working-class values have changed. They point out that despite the deputy leader of the Labour Party at the time, John Prescott, claiming that everyone was now middle class, this was not the case. Huge inequalities still exist and the increased tendency to measure social status on individual achievement, autonomy, and high income further marginalises many lower class families.

Whilst social inequalities appear to threaten current working-class solidarity, they have been found to strengthen group boundaries within ethnic minority populations (Easterbrook et al., 2020) which can positively influence the self-esteem of children and adolescents. However, within the UK, children and adolescents from many ethnic minority groups are likely to suffer a low standard of living and experience authoritarian parenting. This along with a greater vulnerability to prejudice and discrimination (discussed further in Chap. 8) can have a negative impact on children's and adolescents' self-concept and self-esteem.

Preferences for some ethnic groups over others, possibly based on perceived inequalities of wealth, have been demonstrated in some children as young as pre-school age. For example, Godfrey et al. (2017) report that white American children recognised and preferred their group due to it having a higher status than groups including children from different ethnic backgrounds. However, they point out that Afro-American children, from what were considered lower status groups, did not display such preferences. Also, cultural stereotypes based on skin colour are easily recognised by middle childhood and children around ten years old are aware of explicit and implicit discriminatory behaviour (Benner et al., 2018). A greater sense of ethnic identity is evident during early adolescence and by late adolescence this includes an increased awareness of racism and privilege within wider society. Godfrey et al. (2017) point to a decline in self-esteem amongst adolescents from minority ethnic groups who accept the hierarchical nature of Western society as they increasingly feel marginalised. Experiencing discrimination based on ethnicity can also impact on adolescents' mental health and create risky health behaviours (Benner et al., 2018).

However, it must be noted that despite continuing inequalities, prejudice, and discrimination, the self-esteem of Afro-Americans was radically improved due to the civil rights movement in America during the 1960s. The positive impact of this movement on the way children and adolescents of colour were encouraged to see themselves and feel pride in their group heritage cannot be underestimated.

It has been traditionally thought that those adolescents from multiracial backgrounds will be more vulnerable to the negative effects of discrimination and subsequently have lower self-esteem than those who have parents from the same ethnic group. However, Shih et al. (2019) found that currently having a multiracial identity was associated with a more positive self-esteem. They attribute this to strategies adopted by such adolescents, to deal with potential stereotypes and stigma. These have been found to involve protective measures, consciously and unconsciously, which include selecting the appropriate aspects of their multiracial identity to match different social situations and placing less emphasis on the importance of race. Shih et al. (2019) point out that this enables such adolescents to actively create positive identities. They add that such strategies can also be adopted by those from single racial groups such as when Afro-American adolescents move between predominantly Caucasian American or Afro-American social groups.

In addition to class and ethnicity, gender also impacts on the self-concept and self-esteem of children and adolescents. Although labels of male and female are based on a child's physical sexual characteristics at birth, the process of acquiring a gender identity is influenced by not only biology, but also the ability to conform to expectations of gender-related behaviour held by the society into which the child is born. Successful adaptation to the gender role they have been ascribed has a profound effect on the child's future self-concept and self-esteem.

It appears that gender development results from a complex interaction between socialisation and biology, including sex hormones. Early studies, such as those by Maccoby and Jacklin (1974), identified some potentially inherited gender differences in that, on average, boys show a stronger tendency towards aggression and do well in tasks demanding spatial abilities and maths, whilst girls are better at verbal tasks. Although it is difficult to identify such skills before considerable socialisation has taken place, later studies have found some support for such differences. Interestingly, Nagy et al. (2007) tested the responses of very young babies and found that girls demonstrated more accurate imitative abilities. Schaffer (2003) also points out that by the time boys are a year old their behaviour is more exploratory and involves many 'touching' interventions. Also, Eriksson et al. (2012) refer to the many studies which suggest that girls develop verbal skills earlier than boys. These skills involve early communicative gestures, combining words and acquiring a vocabulary. They found cross-cultural support for these differences and suggest that such abilities may facilitate interactions within social situations, which then create further differences between boys and girls in their later socio-emotional and cognitive development.

However, there appear to be no gender differences in the nurturing responses of boys and girls. Also, as the differences which have been identified occur within as well as between the sexes, there are, obviously, some boys who, for example, excel in verbal tasks and girls who are excellent at maths. Schaffer (2003) explains how cultural expectations can account for some differences. For example, although within Western culture strong mathematical ability is generally more prevalent in males, in China and Japan, where girls are praised for such abilities, they equally excel in the subject.

Nevertheless, some evidence for innate gender differences exists in the gendered type of toys children choose, even before they have had the opportunity to learn gender-based behaviour. It is possible that the potential for boys to be drawn to 'masculine' toys such as cars, trains, and guns is based on their predisposition to be active and exploratory. In contrast girls' choice of 'feminine' play, such as dressing up, using the 'home corner' and 'cooking' may be because this facilitates communication and social interaction. It appears that children's self-selected play is in tune with some gender differentiated pathways which overlap between the sexes and become magnified depending upon social experience. It is likely that the family acts as the initial socialising force and, that, later also peer pressure becomes influential.

Social learning theory and social cognitive theory offer useful ways of explaining gender socialisation, given that they stress the importance of observation, imitation, and role models. Cognitive theory points out how the internal working model, suggested by attachment theory, facilitates development of gender-based schemas (networks of mental representations organised in terms of gendered experience) which are used to understand and comply with the gender with which the child identifies (Schaffer, 2003). Work by Kohlberg (1981) and others later suggests that children observe, memorise, and associate with gender-specific behaviour in stages. Pre-school children soon display a knowledge of their own gender and from six years are said to have achieved 'gender constancy' in that they know that this will not change. Halim et al. (2013) point out that although individual differences exist in gender-related behaviour, the gender identified remains stable.

Children are active learners, using gender stereotypes in their decision making and behaviour. This is possible through gender schemas developed within their 'internal working model', which provides a framework to help children understand their world. Children then process new information in line with the internalised gender expectations of their specific culture. This bidirectional process means that, through interacting with others, children develop a social network, which Goble et al. (2012) liken to a kind of feedback loop in which both social experience and cognitive process are informed by each other. Gender can, therefore, be seen to have a powerful effect on children in terms of direct and indirect pathways.

Gender is particularly influential on social interactions. For example, it is used as a basis for acknowledging 'within-group similarity' and 'between-group differences' and provides a collective identity. It can also be seen how children soon learn the complexity of social situations and how to adapt their behaviour accordingly. For example, Goble et al. (2012) found that although pre-school children usually choose same-sex playmates and gender-typed activities, they adapt their play to more neutral activities if playing with an opposite sex-playmate. Interestingly, being observed by adults impacted upon gender type play. For example, boys played significantly more in obviously feminine activities when interacting with teachers.

Although social cognitive learning theory and cognitive theory help to explain how gender identity is formed through internal processing of social experience, Halpern and Perry-Jenkins (2016) think that a feminist perspective is also needed to fully understand the role of social and contextual factors, including power, class, and ethnicity, on such development. Feminist theory emphasises the way societies are consistently organised in terms of gender segregation and power which is passed on implicitly and explicitly through the family, peers, school, and media, as well as types of toys available and how these are marketed.

Maccoby et al. (1987) identified how several forces, including dominance based on gender and gender labelling, combined to create gender segregation. Although, diverse family forms and more shared parenting are currently developing within Western culture, Halpern and Perry-Jenkins (2016) feel that differences in social class still impact on gender role development. They point out how the way family life and related household labour is different between working-class and middle-class parents. They explain how the potentially more traditional gender role models offered by working-class, low-income mothers will include low-paid employment and responsibility for most of the housework. In contrast children of middle-class, professional parents will possibly witness more shared, equitable parental duties within the home and socially aware, educated mothers. Halpern and Perry-Jenkins (2016) point out that working-class parents may not choose such traditional gender divisions of labour but are often forced to do so due to financial restrictions. They explain how, through taking a feminist approach, it is possible to see how early gender socialisation of children is influenced by social inequalities

Fathers appear to be highly influential on children's gender identity, particularly sons, despite changes within Western culture, with single-sex, same-sex parenting and father involvement in childcare more common. However, children from such families have been found to be less likely to stereotype on grounds of gender. In response to concerns that explanations of gender role development may be biased given the past dominance of studies from European countries Halpern and Perry-Jenkins (2016) studied families from a range of diverse nationalities. They found that even though expectations of gender roles may vary across cultural contexts, parents in all cases were a powerful force in reinforcing socially approved gender-related behaviour and discouraging that which is not considered 'normal'.

The complex impact of gender socialisation becomes particularly evident during late childhood and adolescence. The rapid physical and emotional changes which take place during this period have a profound effect on an individual. For example, Coopersmith (1967) found that developing early or late in comparison to peers impacted upon levels of self-confidence. Late developing boys were found to lack confidence, whilst 'early developers' had high levels of confidence which continued into adulthood. In contrast, girls were less confident if late or early developers but rather gained confidence if felt they were average and therefore 'normal'.

Interestingly, when Blum et al. (2017) investigated adolescents' views of gender roles from across fifteen continents, including the UK and USA, they identified common experiences. Gender differences were perceived as powerfully influenced by schools, parents, media, and peers. Even in countries where the vulnerability of boys was acknowledged, girls were felt to need more protection. This was particularly the case during puberty as girls were thought to be most sexually desirable and boys feared as potential predators. Many girls, irrespective of country, lived more restricted lives than boys and under sanctions of punishment, social isolation, and 'gossip'. Adolescents expressed concern that having earlier played together made the later gender segregation difficult, but despite this, boys were less keen to continue friendships with girls. Adolescents from the different countries also expressed awareness of gender nonconforming peers who dressed and behaved in ways associated with their opposite sex, and how this was met with sanctions.

Kane (2006) found that parents were not as concerned with gender nonconformity among their young daughters but held more complex views in relation to sons. Kane says that many parents from different racial and class backgrounds accept some tendencies thought atypical for boys, but this was balanced by efforts to help sons conform to societal views of masculinity. Even lesbian mothers and gay fathers were concerned about the treatment sons may receive if not able to live up to traditional concepts of male gender.

Currently within Western society there is a movement by some groups to broaden the definitions of gender to include more than just masculinity and femininity. Shumer et al. (2016) explain that an individual's internal sense of gender can include being a boy or girl, man or woman, non-binary understanding of own gender, or agender (having no gender). Olson-Kennedy et al. (2016) describe how some gender nonconforming adolescents are thought to suffer gender dysphoria, given that they experience a conflict between the sex they were identified as at birth and an internal sense of being the opposite gender. However, they report that those adolescents who choose to adopt the physical attributes of their opposite gender (transgender) form a high-risk group in terms of psychosocial adjustment including depression, suicide, illicit drug use, and HIV infection.

The force of societal views on conforming to traditional gender roles becomes starkly clear as a high number of transgender individuals are victimised, and suicide is more prevalent amongst such adolescents who have suffered verbal and physical abuse. Class appears to make transgender individuals even more vulnerable, as rates of suicide have been found to be higher amongst those who are young, unemployed, poor, and less educated (Shumer et al., 2016).

However, there is growing concern about the numbers of children requesting treatment to adopt their opposite gender prior to puberty. This is possibly due to increased awareness of such possibilities conveyed through the media and internet. The diagnostic criterion for gender dysphoria in children and adolescents is that they have experienced, for at least six months, a marked difference between the gender to which they have been assigned and that which they feel to be, and that this is causing impaired functioning as well as significant distress. Some children and adolescents diagnosed with this condition are reported to have greater emotional and behavioural problems and even autism. Although a Dutch study demonstrated post-treatment improvement for such individuals, Shumer et al. (2016) report that most transgender people do not have gender dysphoria, and the majority of young children who are gender non-conforming do not continue to identify as transgender during adolescence.

Although the American Psychological Association has developed developmentally and culturally sensitive guidelines for psychologists working with transgender individuals, the uncertainty of gender dysphoria persisting into adolescence or adulthood when diagnosed in young children has meant that this has become a controversial issue. Within the UK, there has been a recent high court ruling against the use of puberty-blocking drugs for such children (reported by The Guardian, 06.12.2020). This was in relation to a case brought by a young adolescent who had been given such drugs much earlier by a gender identity development service as part of treatment for gender dysphoria.

The court ruled that the service had misinterpreted the law on child consent when prescribing puberty-blocking drugs for children as young as ten years old. Concern was raised about the use of such drugs as an experimental treatment for gender dysphoria as so little is known about this condition. Moreover, such drugs are invariably followed by cross-sex hormones, which have long-term effects on sexual function and fertility. The court also pointed out that gender dysphoria may resolve itself by teenage years but, taking puberty blockers may serve to support the condition. Accordingly, the court ruled that in such cases it was unlikely that children could offer informed consent.

This case highlighted concerns about pressure placed on children and adolescents to consider alternative genders through poorly informed data and misinformation presented in the media and in online material. An emerging trend of bias towards transgender may be developing as it was reported that the staff, from the clinic referred to in this case, who raised concerns were silenced by claims that they were transphobic.

Moreover, it is possible that the sensitivity of this topic is such that it may be responsible for the 'silencing' of debate in some current academic communities. Conflicting views have been expressed about the rights of those men who 'feel' they are the opposite gender so identify as female and thus gain entry to female spaces. For example, recently a university professor, who raised concerns about such rights, was accused of transphobia (see Adams, 2021; Hayton 2020). This issue appears to raise wider, ethical, and political concerns around free speech which need to be considered through taking a biopsychosocial approach.

In 2002, Martin et al. warned of the dangers of highlighting gender too forcefully, as this can increase gender stereotyping and negative discrimination, reducing the diversity of behaviour choices available to children. They pointed out how gender socialisation is likely to be influenced by various interrelated factors including prenatal biological influences, media portrayals, peer, and parental attitudes. Interestingly, recent studies have found additional gender differences in the use of digital technology and self-concept. For example, Jackson et al. (2010) found that videogames, played more by boys than girls regardless of race, negatively influence self-esteem whilst the use of the internet, popular with girls, has a positive effect. Also, Jackson et al. (2010) identified gender differences in the way girls and boys measured self-esteem. It appeared that girls took account of academic and behavioural success whilst boys were more concerned with successful physical appearance and athletic ability. However, ethnicity was also found to influence self-concept as, in their study, African Americans demonstrated lower self-concepts than Caucasian Americans in terms of satisfaction with their own behaviour.

Jackson et al. (2010) also found confirmation that children and adolescents from higher income households had higher levels of self-concept and self-esteem than those from low-income families. The work of Pickett and Wilkinson (2010) demonstrates how, in more unequal societies, such as the USA and UK, inequalities in terms of income, ethnicity, and gender impact on the health of children and adolescents. They argue that increased inequality creates greater social distances and intensifies stigma and shame associated with being of low social status. Blum et al. (2017) found that adolescents across cultures expressed a desire for more gender equality which De Looze et al. (2018) point out will benefit boys as well as girls. The 'spirit level' argument used by Wilkinson and Pickett (2010) suggests that greater income, race, and gender equality in all societies will improve the wellbeing of all children and adolescents.

Summary

- The ability to be sociable requires an ability to fit in with cultural expectations of 'normal' behaviour. A biological preparedness enables children to gain experiences and form an internal working model of their world, through using attachment figures. A sense of separateness from others and concept of self emerge through awareness that people and things may disappear and regularly reappear as well as responses received from others. Communication, including language, facilitates the sense of a self-concept and private and public aspects of the self. Cognitive and social development are interdependent.

- Becoming sociable involves the ability to recognise and adapt to the needs of others through the development of empathy. Empathy requires an ability to possess a 'theory of mind' which means appreciating differing points of view held by others. Experiences with significant others are thought to influence the development of empathy but a biological basis for a lack of a 'theory of mind' has been linked to learning disabilities such as ADHD and autism. However, currently within Western society there are some who challenge the testing for a 'theory of mind' and question the diagnosis of this type of learning disability.

- Self-esteem represents the level of self-worth children and adolescents develop from awareness of the reaction of others such as family and peers. Early or late biological development when approaching adolescence, gender, ethnicity, and class all have the potential to impact on self-esteem. There is an increased acceptance of more varied gender identities within current Western society yet growing concern about medical methods and acceptance of 'gender realignment' for children and adolescents.

Case Study Questions

Read the family case study on page 265 and consider the following:

- What would be taken into consideration if Liam was tested for ADHD?
- Why might Gemma, Liam, and Ben be expected to take on different responsibilities when contributing to their family life?
- How could the self-esteem of each child be influenced by their age and having parents from different ethnic origins?

Reflective Questions

- The current 'I am worth it!' attitude within Western culture is thought to promote individualism rather than collectivism. How easy or desirable is it for all in children and adolescents to develop such an attitude?
- To what extent can ethnic and gender equality be seen to have been achieved within Western society?
- How might issues of class, race, and gender impact on an individual's experiences across their lifespan?

References

Adams, R. (2021, October 28). Sussex Professor Resigns after Transgender Rights Row. *The Guardian.*

Baron-Cohen, S. (2001). Theory of Mind in Normal Development and Autism. *Prisme, 34,* 174–183.

Baron-Cohen, S., Leslie, A. M., & Frith, U. (1985). Does the Autistic Child have a 'Theory of Mind'? *Cognition, 21,* 37–46.

Benner, A. D., Wang, Y., Shen, Y., Boyle, A. E., Polk, R., & Chen, Y.-P. (2018). Racial/Ethnic Discrimination and Well-Being during Adolescence: A Meta-Analytic Review. *American Psychologist, 73*(7), 855–883. https://doi.org/10.1037/amp0000204

Blum, R. W., Mmari, K., & Moreau, C. (2017). It Begins at 10: How Gender Expectations Shape Early Adolescence Around the World. *Journal of Adolescent Health, 61* (2017), S3eS4. 1054-139X/ 2017 Society for Adolescent Health and Medicine. Open Access Article. https://doi.org/10.1016/j.jadohealth.2017.07.009

Cooley, C. H. (1902). *Human Nature and Social Order.* Charles Scribner.

Coopersmith, S. (1967). *The Antecedents of Self-Esteem.* Freeman.

De Looze, M. E., Huijts, T., Stevens, G. W. J. M., Torsheim, T., & Vollebergh, W. A. M. (2018). The Happiest Kids on Earth: Gender Equality and Adolescent Life Satisfaction in Europe and North America. *Journal of Youth and Adolescence, 47,* 1073–1085. https://doi.org/10.1007/s10964-017-0756-7

Easterbrook, M., Kuppens, T., & Manstead, A. (2020). Socioeconomic Status and the Structure of the Self-Concept. *British Journal of Social Psychology, 59*(1), 66–86. https://doi.org/10.1111/bjso.12334

Eriksson, M., Marschik, P. B., Tulviste, T., Almgren, M., Pereira, M. P., Wehberg, S., Marjanovic-Umek, L., Gayraud, F., Kovacevic, M., & Gallego, C. (2012). Differences between Girls and Boys in emerging Language Skills: Evidence from 10 language communities. *British Journal of Developmental Psychology, 30,* 326–343. https://doi.org/10.1111/j.2044-835X.2011.02042.x

Gernsbacher, M. A., & Yergeau, M. (2019). Empirical Failures of the Claim that Autistic People Lack a Theory of Mind. *Archives of Scientific Psychology, 7*, 102–118. https://doi.org/10.1037/arc000006

Gittins, C. B., & Hunt, C. (2019). Parental Behavioural Control in Adolescence: How Does it affect Self-Esteem and Self-Criticism? *Journal of Adolescence, 73*, 26–35. https://doi.org/10.1016/j.adolescence

Goble, P., Martin, C. L., Hanish, L. D., & Fabes, R. A. (2012). Children's Gender-Typed Activity Choices across Preschool Social Contexts. *Sex Roles, 67*, 435–451. https://doi.org/10.1007/s11199-012-0176-9

Godfrey, E. B., Santos, C. E., & Burson, E. (2017). For Better or Worse? System-Justifying Beliefs in Sixth-Grade Predict Trajectories of Self-Esteem and Behavior Across Early Adolescence. *Child Development, 90*(1), 180–195. https://doi.org/10.1111/cdev.12854

Guardian High Court's Ruling on Puberty-blocking Drugs for Children. (2020, December 6).

Guyer, A. E., Benson, B., Choate, V. R., Bar-Haim, Y., Perez-Edgar, K., Jarcho, J. M., Pine, D. S., Ernst, M., Fox, N. A., & Nelson, E. E. (2014). Lasting Associations between Early-Childhood Temperament and Late-Adolescent Reward-Circuitry Response to Peer Feedback. *Development and Psychopathology, 26*, 229–243. https://doi.org/10.1017/S0954579413000941

Gvirts Poblovski, H. Z., Levi, D., Yozevitch, R., Sherman, M., Hagay, Y., & Dahan, A. (2021). Impairments of Interpersonal Synchrony evident in Attention Deficit Hyperactivity Disorder (ADHD). *Acta Psychologica, 212*, 103210. On Line. https://doi.org/10.1016/j.actpsy,2020.103210

Halim, M. L., Ruble, D. N., Tamis-LeMonda, C. S., & Shrout, P. (2013). Rigidity in Gender-Typed Behaviors in Early Childhood: A Longitudinal Study of Ethnic Minority Children. *Child Development, 84*(4), 1269–1284. https://doi.org/10.1111/cdev.12057

Halpern, H. P., & Perry-Jenkins, M. (2016). Parents' Gender Ideology and Gendered Behavior as Predictors of Children's Gender-Role Attitudes: A Longitudinal Exploration. *Sex Roles, 74*(11), 527–542. https://doi.org/10.1007/s11199-015-0539-0

Hayton, D. (2020, June 29). The Silencing of Graham Linehan. *The Spectator*.

Jackson, L. A., von Eye, A., Fitzgerald, H. E., Zhao, Y., & Witt, E. A. (2010). Self-Concept, Self-Esteem, Gender, Race and Information Technology Use. *Computers in Human Behavior, 26*, 323–328. https://doi.org/10.1016/j.chb.2009.11.001

Kagan, J. (1981). *The Second Year: The Emergence of Self-Awareness*. Harvard University Press.

Kane, E. W. (2006). 'No Way My Boys are Going to be like That!' Parents' Responses to Children's Gender Nonconformity. *Gender & Society, 20*(2), 149–176. https://doi.org/10.1177/0891243205284276

Kilford, E. E., Garrett, E., & Blakemore, S.-J. (2016). The Development of Social Cognition in Adolescence: An Integrated Perspective. *Neuroscience & Behavioural Reviews, 70*, 106–120. https://doi.org/10.1016/j.neubiorev.2016.08.016

Kohlberg, L. (1981). *Essays on Moral Development* (Vol. 1). Harper and Row.

Lewis, M., & Brookes-Gunn, J. (1979). *Social Cognition and the Acquisition of Self*. Plenum.

Maccoby, E. E., & Jacklin, C. N. (1974). *The Psychology of Sex differences*. Stanford University Press.

Maccoby, E. E., & Jacklin, C. N., & Nagy, C. (1987). Gender Segregation in Childhood. *Part of Advances in Child Development and Behavior, 20*, 239–287. New York, NY: Elsevier.

Maoz, H., Gvirts, H. Z., Sheffer, M., & Bloch, Y. (2017). Theory of Mind and Empathy in Children with ADHD. *Journal of Attention Disorder, 23*, 11. https://doi.org/10.1177/1087054717710766

Martin, C. L., Ruble, D. N., & Szkrybalo, J. (2002). Cognitive Theories of Early Gender Development. *Psychological Bulletin Copyright 2002 by the American Psychological Association, 128*(6), 903–933. https://doi.org/10.1037//0033-2909.128.6.903

Mead, G. H. (1934). *Mind. Self and Society*. Chicago.

Nagy, E., Kompagne, H., Orvos, H., & Pal, A. (2007). *Gender-Related Differences in Neonatal Imitation.*, *16*(3), 267–276. https://doi.org/10.1002/icd.497

Olson-Kennedy, J., Cohen-Kettenis, P. T., Kreukels, B. P. C., Meyer-Bahlburg, H. F. L., Garofalo, R., Meyer, W., & Rosenthal, S. M. (2016). Research Priorities for Gender Nonconforming/ Transgender Youth: Gender Identity Development and Biopsychosocial Outcomes. *Current Opinion in Endocrinol Diabetes Obesity, 23*(2), 172–179. https://doi.org/10.1097/ MED.0000000000000236

Orth, R., Erol, R. J., & Luciano, E. C. (2018). Development of Self Esteem from age 4 to 94 years: A Meta-Analysis of Longitudinal Studies, American Psychological Society. *Psychological Bulletin, 144*(10), 1045–1080. https://doi.org/10.1037/bul0000161

Orth, U., & Robins, R. W. (2014). The Development of Self-Esteem. *Current Directions in Psychological Science., 23*(5), 381–387. https://doi.org/10.1177/0963721414547414

Perez-Gramaje, A. F., Garcia, O. F., Reyes, M., Serra, E., & Garcia, F. (2019). Parenting Styles and Aggressive Adolescents: Relationships with Self-esteem and Personal Maladjustment. *The European Journal of Psychology Applied to Legal Context, 12*(1). 2020. Pages 1–10. https:// doi.org/10.5093/ejpalc2020a1

Perner, J., Leekham, S. R., & Wimmer, H. (1987). Three-Year-olds' Difficulty with False Belief: The Case for a Conceptual Deficit. *British Journal of Developmental Psychology, 5*(2), 125–137. https://doi.org/10.1111/j.2044-835X.1987.tb01048.x

Pickett, K. E., & Wilkinson, R. G. (2010). Inequality: an Under Acknowledged Source of Mental Illness and Distress. *The British Journal of Psychiatry, 197*, 426–428. https://doi.org/10.1192/ bjp.bp.109.072066

Pinquart, M., & Gerke, D. C. (2019). Associations of Parenting Styles with Self-Esteem in Children and Adolescents: A Meta-Analysis. *Journal of Child and Family Studies, 28*, 2017–2035. https://doi.org/10.1007/s10826-019-01417-5

Preckel, K., Kanske, P., & Singer, T. (2017). On the interaction of Social Affect and Cognition: Empathy, Compassion and Theory of Mind. *Current Opinion in Behavioral Sciences, 19*, 1–6. www.sciencedirect.com

Quesque, F., & Rossetti, Y. (2020). What Do Theory-of-Mind Tasks Actually Measure? Theory and Practice. *Perspectives on Psychological Science, 15*(2), 1–13. https://doi. org/10.1177/1745691619896607

Rogers, C. R. (1961). *On Becoming a Person.* Houghton Mifflin.

Schaffer, H. R. (2003). *Social Development.* Blackwell.

Shih, M., Wilton, L. S., Does, S., Goodale, B. M., & Sanchez, D. T. (2019). Multiple Racial Identities as Sources of Psychological Resilience. Social and Personality. *Compass, e12469*, 1–13. https://doi.org/10.1111/spc3.12469

Shumer, D. E., Nokoff, N. J., & Spack, N. P. (2016). Advances in the Care of Transgender Children and Adolescents. *Advances in Pediatrics, 63*(1), 79–102. https://doi.org/10.1016/j. yapd.2016.04.018

Stern, J. A., & Cassidy, J. (2018). Empathy from Infancy to Adolescence: An Attachment Perspective on the Development of Individual Differences. *Developmental Review, 47*, 1–22. https://doi.org/10.1016/j.dr.2017.09.002

Wilkinson, R. G., & Pickett, K. E. (2010). *The Spirit Level: Why Equality is Better for Everyone.* Penguin.

Play, Learning, and Developmental Wellbeing

6

A key feature of childhood is the child's free capacity to experience their environment and engage with others through play. As adults we also recognise that there are numerous learning and developmental benefits of play. However, we must not lose sight of how children are innately driven to engage in play because it leads them to joyful or enriching experiences. In addition, the understanding and skills gained from play also help children gain more mastery and control over their world. This chapter considers firstly what we mean by learning and its impact on wellbeing. We then explore the varied definitions and types of play and how play in its different guises can influence and support learning and developmental wellbeing in children and adolescents. Cultural differences and challenges to play in contemporary society are also discussed.

6.1 Learning and its Impact on Wellbeing

Wellbeing is achieved when we have developed sufficient skills necessary to exist comfortably within a given environment. Within Western society it is expected that learning requires academic achievement and the development of skills useful in contributing to a country's economy and ability to compete with other countries. However, play provides much broader skills for living than just those focussed on within educational institutions. Several theories underpin current attempts to help children develop such skills. These theories include the works of Piaget and Vygotsky who revolutionised the Western education system and expectations of what children need to learn and how they can best do this. This also includes the development and usefulness of different types of play. Indeed, cognitive theory has changed how children and adolescents are now perceived as active participants in their learning.

Piaget's (1896–1980) and Vygotsky's (1896–1934) work highlight how the schemas we have developed through experiences are then drawn upon to enable us to encode and interpret our future experiences. This notion suggests the flexibility of the brain to adapt and learn. Piaget suggested a child's senses or actions (he termed operations) are mentally encoded by neural connections. These connections (schemas) adapt once new information is gleaned (assimilation) and increase considerably when experiences are very different so new, related schemas are created (accommodation). Piaget suggested this was a continuous process in child development.

Although, stages are used to explain Piaget's theory of children's cognitive development, this does not mean that they develop in discrete stages as such, but rather that within certain age groups it is possible to identify specific abilities which increase over time.

Different 'Stages' of Cognitive Development Suggested by Piaget's Theories

▶   Between 0–2 years (Sensori Motor Stage) infants' reflexes allow information to be processed such that they develop a schema of their own body and increased motor control, recognise that people and objects exist even when not seen (object permanence), can memorise and copy actions (deferred imitation), and begin to engage in make-believe play.

Between 2–7 years (Pre-Operational Stage) although much cognitive development has taken place the dominance of visual perception means children still have problems in abstract tasks. For example, if required to describe a scene from different perspectives, (decentring) or recognising that the amount of liquid is the same whether in a tall thin glass or a short, wide glass (conservation). However, when offered tasks within social contexts children can display awareness of different perspectives.

Between 7–11 years (Concrete Operational Stage) children can carry out abstract and logical tasks if they are given concrete examples.

From about 11 years (Formal Operational Stage) older children and adolescents display logical reasoning, systematic planning, and can form hypothesis due to the increased complexity of schemas formed through their past experiences.

Vygotsky's theory of cognitive development is compatible with the work of Piaget, to a great extent, however, he emphasised the role of socio-cultural influences on cognitive development. He was also heavily influenced by Marxist philosophy which purports that 'historical changes in society and material life produce changes in human nature' (see Blake & Pope, 2008, p. 60) and stressed how social interaction facilitates the development of mental functions. Further discussion and detail of these theories are provided in Chap. 3.

Vygotsky, like Piaget, advocated active, hands-on methods to facilitate learning, but he saw negotiation and interaction with others as necessary to develop cognitive abilities. He saw non-verbal communication as playing an important role in this process but also how the use of language enabled the learner to successfully integrate their experiences within their unique set of thought processes. Vygotsky suggested three types of speech exist: social, private, and internal. He saw that social language was used to give information to children by those older and more experienced. This form of communication is translated by the child into their private language to help them process what has been said and apply what is learned to similar situations. Internal or inner speech was then thought to occur as the child carries out a silent, abbreviated form of dialogue which forms the essence of conscious mental activity. Vygotsky was, therefore, suggesting that thinking equals social speech which has been transformed into private speech and become internalised (Blake & Pope, 2008).

6.2 Definitions and Types of Play

Play involves a broad array of behaviours, influenced and interpreted differently by time, culture, and contexts. As such, many researchers have tried to define play, including Erikson (1963), Bruner (1972), and Vygotsky (1978).

▶ **Definitions of Play**

Erikson (1963, p. 212)

'When man plays, he must intermingle with things and people in a similarly uninvolved and light fashion. He must do something which he has chosen to do without being compelled by urgent interests or impelled by strong passion. He must feel entertained and free of any fear or hope of serious consequences. He is on vacation from social and economic reality—or as is most emphasised: he does not work'.

Bruner (1972, **p. 693**)

'Play appears to serve several centrally important functions. First, it is a means of minimising the consequences of one's actions and of learning, therefore … [it is] … a less risky situation. … Second, play provides an excellent opportunity to try combinations of behaviour that would, under functional pressure, never be tried'.

Vygotsky (1978, **p. 102**)

Argues that imaginative play is the key to child development as: 'Play creates a zone of proximal development in the child. In play, the child always behaves beyond their average age, above their daily behaviour; in play it is as though they were a head taller than himself. As in the focus of a magnifying glass, play contains all developmental tendencies in a condensed form and is itself a major source of development'.

These three seminal authors define and conceptualise play from developmental psychology perspectives. They each consider the increasing maturity of children to be related to the complexity of their play (Fromberg & Bergen, 2015). In addition,

Table 6.1 Characteristics and benefits of object and symbolic play

Play	Characteristics	Key benefits
Object play	Begins from early sensorimotor explorations; infants use their mouths to explore objects and as children develop and become more mobile, they use symbolic objects for communication, language, and abstract thought. For example, playing while talking on the telephone with a piece of fruit	Object play allows the child's imagination to flourish and their motor and problem-solving skills to develop
Symbolic play—Language	Infants and toddlers' experiment with language sounds, mouthing sounds, engaging in the repetition of words, projecting their sounds, exploring rhyme, and alliteration	Children's knowledge of nursery rhymes and how often they engage in word play predict children's phonological awareness
Symbolic play—Musical play	Young children will engage in much physical activity whilst playfully dancing and singing	The 'musicality' of early parent and infant interactions establishes early communicative abilities. Prosocial behaviour (helping each other and co-operating) improves more rapidly in children participating in musical play. Children who engage in informal musical activities are more sensitive to slight changes in sounds, suggesting advanced auditory development
Symbolic play—Drawing and writing	As suggested by Vygotsky (1978) young children will engage in mark-making and there are strong links between early drawing and writing	Like language and musical play, play with mark-making and drawing is seen in children across cultures, and is widely accepted as a way in which children, before they are literate, record their experiences and ideas

Piaget (1952) considered play as the construction of knowledge within the individual child by interacting with objects including toys. Alternatively, Vygotsky (1978) perceived play as a means for social interaction and considered that children learn about themselves through being sociable and interacting with others.

To show how play functions as a source of enjoyment for children and adolescents and to learn and develop, it is helpful to appreciate some of the commonly recognised types of play, their characteristics, and key benefits for children and adolescents outlined in Tables 6.1, 6.2, and 6.3.

6.3 Play and Child Development

There are many benefits that result from play, including development in several domains. Where the child experiences childhood adversity, the role of play can hold even greater importance. The shared joy and attunement that parents can experience together with children through play can lower the bodily stress response of the

Table 6.2   Characteristics and benefits of social or pretend play

Play	Characteristics	Key benefits
Social or pretend play (alone or with others)	Young children experiment with social roles via play. Infants smile and are vocal in response to others and will practice turn taking. Older children will create games with rules assigning relationships between players and guidelines. This creativity can be aided by 'dress up' and 'make believe'. Play of this type is categorised as child lead or self-directed as opposed to that guided or lead by adults. Although guided play can maintain child agency, it is the adult who designs the activity or play-related goals. Board games with rules and goals would also fit into this category	Play with other children enables negotiation of 'rules' and cooperation. Self-directed play allows children to explore their world and discover their interests. Games that transcend generations such as 'Head, Shoulders, Knees, and Toes' improve executive functioning skills as children learn to control their bodily reactions. Guided play links to Vygotsky's work and his notion of the zone of proximal development. Where children are unable to master skills on their own, they can master them in the context of a safe, stable, and nurturing relationship with an adult

Table 6.3   Characteristics and benefits of physical play

Play	Characteristics	Key benefits
Physical and rough and tumble play	This type of play progresses from pat-a-cake type games between parent and infant to achieving foundational motor skills in toddlers to free rough and tumble play in older children. In rough and tumble play, children will mimic play fighting and other social dominances (bull dog or tig). Within this context, children differentiate real aggression from play fighting. Children however learn to appreciate socially acceptable norms, and perfect their athletic and behavioural dominance skills	Learning to cooperate and negotiate promotes critical social skills. Children's playful negotiations through physical play build empathetic and prosocial behaviour. In addition, imaginary play facilitates a Theory-of-Mind (TOM) framework (understanding the perceptions of others). Through physical play children experience both winning and losing without feeling upset, because, for example, it was their turn to lose
Outdoor play	Over recent years we have seen the dwindling away of outside spaces for children and find children are playing more within the home environment	There are associations between obesity and low levels of physical activity in children and adolescents. Outdoor play including walking, running, climbing, and stretching is exercise that develops physical strength and co-ordination. Contact with nature in the outdoors is also associated with wider wellbeing benefits and reducing levels of stress

child. Hence, play may be an effective and protective resilience factor that influences the biopsychosocial outcomes that can result from childhood adverse events and related toxic stress. It is useful to understand however that this depends on the type of play activity and parents' role in this. For example, if parents try to determine the type and content of make-believe play too much it can minimise the pleasure of being in control that children can get from play. It is the one area of their (mainly adult controlled) lives where they can be in complete control. It is therefore important that parents let the child lead this type of play.

6.3.1 Language Development

The act of play is influential in learning language and communication skills (Weisberg et al., 2013). Significant correlations have been observed between symbolic play or pretend play, and language. Studies identify how developmental aspects of play are linked with early communication and language as well as pre-operational and sensorimotor periods of cognitive development (Mohan et al., 2021; Piaget, 1952). Indeed, the development of language and symbolic play appear to have similar developmental sequencing (Lillard et al., 2013). As children grow older, they move on from the infant babble and sound making to learning they can experiment with words and manipulate their use, meaning, and grammar. Through words, children also practice rhythm, sound, and form. Whilst playing, children will draw on their language skills to enhance their social interaction with others. Through different interactions they apply different tones and sounds to regulate speech and their developing vocabulary (Mohan et al., 2021).

Bruner (1983) sees that prior to language development children's learning about their world is mostly through their physical senses and visual images. Learning to use the symbols which make up a language enables them to develop much more complex forms of thinking. Bruner's theory of how language develops reflects Vygotsky's concept of scaffolding and the importance of social interactions. He points out how early interactions, particularly when playful, between babies and parents provide a structure for language. Turn taking activities are engaged in with parents initially articulating their own role and the baby's response. Language development is, therefore, aided by non-verbal cues and the social setting in which it takes place. Learning gained from past, social interactions is represented in a symbolic form through rule-governed sounds (or gestures for those who cannot hear) and communicated to others. Emotional bonds developed between parents and their young children mean that they are finely tuned into each other's non-verbal cues and these, along with corresponding physical interactions, thus, provide a framework for language to develop.

6.3.2 Socio-Eemotional and Physical Development

Children develop their own elaborate cognitive and behavioural scripts for interaction and practice operating within the flexible rules of their self-created world via play. However, as children's skills develop, they move more towards abstract thought, and their play-oriented challenges shift them from the flexibility of pre-schoolers' play to the athletic and competitive activities of middle childhood characterised by rules. It is in these middle years of childhood where the scaffolding of 'prosocial behaviour' is a distinct need as within current Western society, bullying (and cyberbullying) incidents peak from now into early adolescence. Bullying and cyberbullying can account for many different behaviours and can occur anywhere, including online, at school or at home. Classic features include being called names, teased, or humiliated; posting, commenting on or liking nasty photos, videos, or posts about individuals online; being pushed, hit, or hurt; having money and other belongings stolen; spreading rumours or starting group chats about individuals; being ignored, purposely side-lined/isolated or made to feel like you're not wanted; being threatened, intimidated, or sent nasty messages; being trolled or having commenting on your posts or pictures saying nasty things; someone revealing an individual's personal details without permission and where you are targeted over and over again in an online game (Childline, 2021).

Play is an excellent vehicle for helping children with their emotional development and coping skills. Through the vehicle of play, children can explore their anxieties, frustrations, trauma, and events they have found upsetting in the real world. Play can help children find new ways of dealing with their emotions and their reality. As children play, they explore the properties of things and extract information about their environments. They imitate, re-create, and rehearse roles that help them understand and solve problems related to everyday living. They form relationships, share, cooperate, master their feelings, extend the range of their experience, test ideas, and form associations between things, events, and concepts. Another major emotional benefit of play is that it gives children numerous opportunities to feel good about themselves. Because there is no right or wrong way to pretend play, children have multiple experiences in play, which positively influences their concepts of self. (This is not so simple in relation to playing with rules.)

Goldstein and Lerner (2018) investigated the influence of pretend play on emotional control in young children. Three groups of children, each receiving different activities over the course of twenty-four sessions, were studied. The activities involved guided dramatic pretend play games, guided block play, and story time. The children who were involved in pretend play games over the course of twenty-four sessions had lower *personal distress across two measures of emotional control* compared to the children who participated in the other two groups (p. 8). It was also discovered that involvement in pretend play games was related to increased levels of positive social behaviours.

Cognitive self-regulation involves the ability to plan, regulate task behaviour, and sustain attention, while emotional self-regulation involves the ability to understand one's own emotions, control the expression emotions, and resolve conflict with others (Slot et al., 2017). Slot et al. (2017, p. 16) state, 'Pretend play requires children to coordinate their goals, negotiate plans, monitor their play and the children they play with as the play progresses, and adapt their actions accordingly. Hence, complex pretend play requires metacognitive regulation strategies and persistence'. *Therefore*, pretend play settings provide an opportunity for children to develop their ability to communicate and regulate their emotions in a socially acceptable manner. Unstructured free play provides opportunities for children to develop problem-solving skills and emotional intelligence, while pretend play offers children the avenue to take risks and learn skills from pretending to be someone or something they are not.

Through play, children can exert their energies, creating movement and physical expression, through physical play activity. It is through these types of play activities that children can increase their physical motor development, drawing on the mechanisms of their large muscles. Other types of play activities, such as cutting, eating, writing, painting, and dressing, provide for their fine motor development, or refinement of the skills that require the use of smaller muscles. Through play, children can improve their coordination abilities and perfect their fine motor skills. With increasing physical maturity large and fine muscle movements become more integrated (Pagnano-Richardson & Henninger, 2008).

6.4   Play and Learning

Research has consistently shown that the different domains of development we have highlighted are interrelated, development in one area can influence development in another. In addition, neuroscience highlights how learning is dynamic and cannot easily be separated into independent mental processes. At a policy and practice level, over recent decades adults have insisted that children learn academic skills at increasingly young ages. As stated in prior chapters, this is to ensure that children can become part of a productive future workforce. For example, reception classes in the UK and USA have shifted curricula towards more literacy and numeracy content, direct instruction, and assessment, over creative and child-led activities (Bassok et al., 2016).

International evidence is mounting, however, on the importance of learning through play and child-centred practices. This movement is being encouraged by the success of interventions such as ReachUp. This home visiting programme evolved from a Jamaican study (Gertler et al., 2014) and has provided positive outcomes for children living in low socioeconomic (SES) contexts. The intervention involves community health care workers attending the homes of new mothers for one hour per week, teaching them parenting skills, encouraging play and related interaction with their children. Those children studied have shown they could reach the same level of cognitive development, mental health, and social behaviour as children with more privileged backgrounds. Associated research has identified how child-centred preschool activities provide a more stable foundation for learning in later years than can be achieved by an earlier academic focus (Weisberg et al., 2013).

6.4.1   Educational Play-Centred Programmes

Several educational programmes offer further encouragement for child-centred curricula. For example, the Montessori curriculum is a programme of education that encourages the importance of children actively directing their own experiences. This method has evidenced numerous positive results on academic, social, and behavioural measures (Lillard, 2016). The American Montessori Society (as cited in Bagnoli, 2021) details the five main components of Montessori Education including trained Montessori educators, a multi-aged classroom, using Montessori materials, child-directed work, and uninterrupted work periods. The AMS website reads:

> Within the community of a multi-aged classroom—designed to create natural opportunities for independence, citizenship, and accountability—children embrace multi-sensory learning and passionate inquiry. Individual students follow their own curiosity at their own pace, taking the time they need to fully understand each concept and meet individualised learning goals. (American Montessori Society, 2021, para. 2, as cited in Bagnoli, 2021)

Lillard et al. (2013) compared Montessori education with other forms of playful learning, suggesting similarities and key differences. Montessori education differs mostly in how unstructured and pretend play are not supported. For example, the programme contains specific learning materials that are provided to children through sequenced lessons and are used by instruction. One classic Montessori material is labelled the Brown Stair; it includes ten blocks, each one larger than the former and the activity is to arrange the blocks sequentially. Children, for example, would not be allowed to use these blocks as building blocks for free play (Lillard et al., 2013). Alternatively, a play-based curriculum or activity would support children to use the blocks with their free will, encouraging the child to use their imagination and creativity. Torrence (2001, p. 8) argues, 'Despite this surge of interest in play from the scientific community, there exists a shared belief among many in the Montessori community that children's pretend-play is trivial and rather inconsequential'.

Maria Montessori founder of Montessori education stated play is 'developmentally irrelevant' and traditional Montessorians uphold this understanding. According to Lillard et al. (2013), Montessori educationalists revoke pretend play for several reasons:

1. Maria Montessori was an empirical researcher. She had tested out providing toys in classroom spaces but had found that children instead use the materials she had designed (Lillard et al., 2013).
2. Montessori also believed it to be inappropriate to encourage fantasies in children; she feared children would believe them and then this would result in internal conflict. The child would be left confused as to what is real and what is fantasy (Lillard et al., 2013).
3. Although Montessori placed importance on imagination, she believed that *truth underpins all great acts of imagination and, thus, that children should be told the truth* (Lillard et al., 2013, p. 173).

It is worth mentioning that such fears of children being overpowered by fantasy have been shown to have little evidence to support them. For example, Schaffer (2004) reports that children can easily move from fantasy to reality and have mechanisms to ensure fantasy does not take over. He cites an observed example of two boys playing a pretend game in preschool which involved a ghost eating up the tools of the broken-down fire engine that they were pretending to mend. During the game one boy reminds the other that they are only pretending and later the other boy reassures him that there are no such things as ghosts whilst pretending to call for the ghostbusters to come and help.

Within many early childhood programmes, play is integral and used to help children to explore their thoughts. In traditional Montessori classrooms play is not an integral feature, in fact it is discouraged. This can put progressive Montessori educators at conflict with the philosophy that the child's mind is best developed through the senses and real-life experiences, which is what the collection of carefully designed materials provides, against how Montessori educators find themselves naturally wanting to 'follow the child', another tenet of the Montessori approach, and where following the child can often result in pretend play. Torrence (2001, p. 8) shared her experience as a Montessori teacher in her journal article Montessori and Play: Theory vs. Practice:

> My own interest in play developed through observation in my 3–6 classroom. Despite my best efforts at the practice of redirecting children toward a carefully prepared, reality-based curriculum, and despite their obvious interest in and enjoyment of same, I frequently observed children's spontaneous and persistent interest in pretend-play. I had the nagging and uncomfortable feeling that a rich layer of hidden meaning quite important to the children lay just beyond the scope of my vision.

Another programme worthy of mention here is the Abecedarian Approach (Ramey et al., 2012). This is also an early childhood education programme that targets both infants and young children from low socioeconomic status families. The aim of the intervention was to determine if providing children with enriched learning experiences, embedded in stable, nurturing, and responsive relationships with caregivers, could buffer against the adverse effects of poverty. A longitudinal study compared two groups of children (intervention n = 57, control n = 54). Both groups involved family support, food, supportive social services, and health care throughout the child's first five years. Those in the intervention group also attended a full-day preschool programme. The programme included activities designed to be highly engaging and fun for children. Learning was observed over the course of each day from engagement with the routines, physical play, and exploration. Findings identified that the children receiving the Abecedarian Approach intervention had improved outcomes on measures of academic and social competencies. They achieved higher education levels, and were more likely to have full-time, higher paying jobs than the control group in their later years. It is clear that more research is needed as there remains a lack of joined up thinking when we consider the importance of play for learning and consistent gaps between the evidence base, policies, and actual practices (Thornton et al., 2016).

It is also worth mentioning the role play had in the original Sure Start programmes in the UK and how despite their value the government have reduced the whole programme for financial reasons. Simons (2021, p. 374), a clinical research fellow and speciality registrar in rehabilitation medicine, recently in the *British Medical Journal* stated:

I was lucky enough to have my children during the period the centres were available and cannot praise the scheme highly enough. They gave me a reason to get out of the house, walk for an hour, and spend time with my children and other people. ... The staff in the centres modelled how to play, make healthy snacks, and care for young children, while offering advice, training, support, and the loan of equipment. I would predict that the centres, and the peer support resulting from them, also improved the long term physical and mental health outcomes of parents and, in turn, their ability to work. Better educational outcomes for the children who attended were also expected as fewer would have undetected communication problems or delayed abilities. The centres were inclusive and introduced families that would not have interacted otherwise, creating communities, and improving wellbeing.

It is further argued that schemes such as Sure Start which focus on child wellbeing and the positive influence of play on learning and on child and family wellbeing are of much greater benefit to communities than interventions that then 'take pathologies and retrospectively try to prevent them'.

6.5 Cultural and Societal Challenges to Play

Cultural universals have been noted in children's play, such as preferences for same gendered or aged play companions. Cross-cultural similarities may also exist in terms of certain features of play such as the sociality of play (dyadic or group play) and imagination (e.g. pretending to feed doll or friends). In addition, the deep structure of certain play forms (e.g. pretend play) seems to be preserved cross-culturally. Differences across cultural communities however are evident in the context where play occurs (i.e. when children are permitted to play), the type and availability of play company (e.g. parent or peers), and the use of toys and outdoor play areas (Gaskins, 2013).

Although there are shared characteristics of play behaviour across cultures, there are also some cultural variations in activities. It is important that we consider cultural values and variations and how they impact children's play to explore implications for cultural identity and self-esteem. The current evidence base suggests that appreciating the inter-relationship between play and culture is more important than considering the impact of wider sociocultural influences such as the impact of social class on child outcomes (Whitebread & Basilio, 2013).

6.5.1 Play Spaces

Studies have been undertaken to examine children's play across physical settings, such as rural versus urban settings. Findings from parental survey responses of one of the larger studies (n=830) on the topic do not identify variance between children's play experiences in urban and rural settings in the United States (Clements, 2004). A study conducted in the UK employing interviews and observations of over 400 children aged 5 to 12 (Smith & Barker, 2001) residing in three rural areas of

England and Wales revealed that geographical isolation, fear over lack of local supervision, and lack of mobility limited play opportunities. The rise of children's technology use (e.g. digital tablets) (Hofferth, 2010) has also been proposed to explain the decline of play in rural areas. Barriers to play in urban areas, however, include limited green spaces, increased street traffic, and poor urban planning (e.g. lack of play facilities in public places) (Veitch et al., 2006).

As gatekeepers to play experiences, parents and the parenting role are important considerations in understanding children's use of rural and urban space for play purposes (Aziz & Said, 2012). In urban areas, safety is a major concern for parents, and their safety-related beliefs may determine the number of opportunities they afford to their children for active play outdoors.

6.5.2 Parental Beliefs

In general, research suggests that parental beliefs about the role of play in learning and developmental wellbeing vary across demographics and relate to both community practices and economic circumstances (Smith et al., 2015). In communities geared to preparing children for schooling, activities such as play or didactic lessons may be prevalent, while in other communities where schooling is not as important, economic activities (e.g. running errands, buying bread) may predominate.

Research findings have also indicated that there is cultural variance in perceptions of play. In middle-class Western cultures, parents generally posit a connection between children's play and various domains of development, such as cognitive, language, and intrapersonal domains (e.g., Colliver, 2016). DiBianca Fasoli (2014) found ethnic differences between Latino and European-American parents in terms of how they believed children learned in a museum setting. Euro-American parents most commonly (85%) attributed learning to the child's self-directed and independent engagement in activities, whereas Latino parents were less likely to give such responses (33%) and instead referenced learning as engagement and interaction with parents (54%) and peers (30%).

Parents' perceptions of play are an important area of investigation as they are thought to structure cognitive and social activities for children. Positive parenting perceptions of play may increase the amount of childhood playtime (Lillard, 2011). They may also serve to shape parent-child interactions in play. Several studies have demonstrated that the endorsement of the significance of certain play forms for child development determines the extent to which parents will provide support and participate in this form of play (e.g. Manz & Bracaliello, 2016). It is important to note that the actual means of parental support in play vary considerably and appropriately across cultures and economic backgrounds (Lancy, 2007). Empirical studies have revealed that parental involvement may be atypical in some non-Western cultures. In fact, in certain cultures (e.g. Latino), siblings and peers may replace parents as playmates and even interact with their younger siblings as a mature parent might.

Several explanations exist for the absence of parent-child play. One salient consideration is the economic structure of the community, which may cause workload constraints. Another relates to parental beliefs, particularly the belief that parent-child interactions interfere with children's inborn character and sense of autonomy and that play occurs naturally, without intervention. Lancy (2007) argued that parent-child play may be far from universal even among Western parenting groups. Studies indicating that mother-child play is largely absent in lower class households provide support for this claim. A recent study (Smith et al., 2015) sheds light on the potential effects of intergenerational poverty on parental beliefs regarding their role in children's play. The researchers interviewed an ethnically diverse group of Australian mothers and found that the mothers did not see themselves as suitable play partners for their children despite having observed various positive benefits of parent-child play. Play was perceived as the work of children, not necessitating the involvement of parents. Parents nonetheless valued play for developmental purposes. The findings align with Lancy's (2007) assertion that mother-child play seems to be a product of a distinct middle-class cultural milieu in which parents have relatively high levels of schooling. It is important to note that additional studies are warranted to fully understand the dynamics of parent-child play, given the focus appears to be restricted (e.g. to either parenting groups in undeveloped countries with little formal education or those in developed countries with high levels of education).

Roopnarine and Davidson (2015, p. 237) asserted in their literature review that 'parent-child play as a medium for upward educational mobility may be gaining appeal and traction in newly developed and developing economies.' Their assertion is based on studies using field observations and estimates obtained through interviews and self-reports. For example, Bornstein and Putnick (2012) demonstrated in their large-scale study of 127,000 families in 28 developing countries that parents worldwide spend considerable time playing and engaging with their children. In fact, the researchers found that across all countries, taking children outdoors and playing were the most predominant activities. In middle-class societies, research has demonstrated that parents tend to value play and correspondingly consider themselves appropriate play partners. They may involve themselves in children's play directly (e.g. teaching) or indirectly (e.g. providing time, space, resources). Through effectively interacting with children, parents have the potential to promote problem-solving skills, build imagination, develop language, and social competence. Parent-child interactions, whether social (e.g., turn-taking) or didactic (teaching), can result in important benefits for the child. Benefits may be apparent in the social domain. For example, mother-child play in the early years has been found to build a foundation for peer competence (e.g. social connectedness) in the school years which may demonstrate that a child's ability to engage with peers in a task requiring sustained interaction and joint attention has its roots in successful, early mother-child interactions. There may be also important cognitive benefits (e.g. representational thinking, problem-solving skills) related to mother-child play. Several studies have demonstrated that mother-child play is more complex, sophisticated, frequent, and sustained than solitary play.

The meanings attached to beliefs about play as well as involvement in play activities are not arbitrary. Rather, meanings are driven by community goals for children's development with apparent differences in value systems. According to Lancy (2007), the common theme which motivates mothers in modern middle-class societies to engage in high levels of mother–child play and verbal interaction relate to their childrearing goals of educational success and eventual participation in the information economy. Conversely, in societies where social class is equated with destiny and children are not seen as having such futures, mothers may not spend time playing with their children.

6.5.3 Modern-Day Challenges

For many families, there are limits placed on children's play time not least due to curricula focussed on achievement, after-school academic enrichment programmes, increased homework, concerns about test performance, and college acceptance pressures. The stressful effects of this contemporary approach to learning could result in the later development of anxiety and depression and a lack of creativity. Parents also feel increasing pressure to do the best for their children and can be carried along with the increasing norm of registering their children to attend multiple 'enrichment opportunities'. This good intention however can then leave children with little free time, time for free play, conversation, and mealtimes with families. Schools have also increasingly limited creative arts and physical education over the years to make room for them to prepare children for examinations in academic subjects. Unsafe local neighbourhoods and playgrounds have also led to nature-deficit disorder for many children. A national survey of 8950 preschool children and parents found that only 51% of children went outside to walk or play once per day with either parent (Tandon et al., 2012).

Today many parents feel they need to supplement their children's learning with technology, to keep them apace with the competition for future job prospects. However, there are studies that contradict the perceived benefits of increased formal learning. Researchers have compared pre-schoolers playing with blocks independently and creatively with pre-schoolers who are encouraged to watch Baby Einstein tapes. These US-based videos aim to expose infants to engaging patterns, puppets, animals, and toys, accompanied by classical music and traditional rhymes in ways to demonstrate kindness and compassion. The findings highlight how children playing with blocks independently developed better language and cognitive skills than their peers watching the educational videos. This is not to say that there are no benefits to children watching and playing with different media and more so if accompanied by peers or parents. But media cannot take the place of the benefits of play, which include developmental wellbeing and learning benefits (Rich, 2019). This also supports Vygotsky's view of the need for interaction with others to achieve learning.

Despite research that reveals an association between television watching and a sedentary lifestyle and greater risks of obesity, the typical pre-schooler watches

4.5 hours of television per day. This not only means risks to children's physical health but also the benefits of social interactions. It displaces conversation with parents and the practice of joint attention (focus by the parent and child on a common object) as well as physical activity. It is also acknowledged that easy access to electronic media purposefully designed to be attractive and engaging can be difficult for parents to compete with (Rich, 2019).

The importance of play, particularly during middle childhood, requires specific attention as much of the play literature attends to the needs and experiences of infants and young children. Little attention is given to the play of those in middle childhood and its benefits. Goldstein and Winner (2011), however, provided preliminary evidence that the engagement of 8- to 11-year-olds in role play, pretence, and acting classes predicted theory of mind skills, which is consistent with findings regarding younger children. Howard et al. (2017) also revealed the importance of listening to children when studying play in middle childhood, suggesting that play is essential for 7- to 11-year-olds. Indeed, children's perceptions of play at this age highlight the benefits of play for social competence. This notion is congruent with Erikson's (1963) view that there is a relationship or association between play and socio-emotional development in middle childhood.

6.5.4 Reduced Child-Driven Play

Although we are aware of the benefits of play for children, time for free play has reduced over the years at home and at school. This trend within schools has even affected reception-aged children, to make room for more academic time (Pellegrini, 2009). Our academic knowledge of cognitive psychology and particularly around the storage and retrieval of information suggests that the lack of play can impact on children's memory. We know that children's cognitive capacity is enhanced when there are clear changes in activity and cognitive effort. Even a physical education class will be structured, and rule bound, and will not provide the benefits of a free play break. Reduced time for free play physical activity could also be adding to the gendered difference in academic abilities; sedentary styles of learning have been shown to be more difficult for boys to experience (Gurian et al., 2009).

Some children are given less time for free exploratory play as they are hurried to adapt into adult roles and prepare for their future at earlier ages. Organised activities do have developmental benefits for children, but less is understood about how children can become 'overscheduled' to their developmental detriment or emotional distress.

Breaks can also allow parents and children to engage in valuable interaction. Without guidance, parents are left to negotiate how many activities are appropriate and be in fear of their children being left behind academically. Studies have suggested that parents can be made to feel inadequate in their parenting if they do not participate in the academic enriched lifestyle. There is also evidence that childhood and adolescent depression is on the rise through the college years (Ginsburg, 2007). Although there are certainly many factors involved and current research has as yet failed to find a direct link between the early pressure-filled intense preparation for a high-achieving adulthood and these mental health concerns, it is important that we consider the possibility of such a linkage. We can be certain that when families still promote play time and family time this can be protective against the negative impacts of the current highly scheduled childhood within Western society. It would also be inappropriate to suggest that an array of extracurricular academic activities is inappropriate for all children. In fact, many children, particularly those in poverty, should receive more enrichment activities. However, it is important to recognise the benefits of balance and downtime.

The increased pressures of adolescence, however, do leave some young people struggling with their transition to college years and independence. Many students' health services and counselling centres on college campuses have not been able to keep pace with the increased need for mental health services, and surveys have substantiated this need by reporting an increase in depression and anxiety among college students. Several studies have linked feelings of anxiety and depression with that of perfectionism and an overly critical self-evaluation. Other studies have linked this perfectionism with highly critical parents who instil pressures to excel (Soenens & Vansteenkiste, 2005). Longitudinal studies are required to assess the possibility of a direct link between intense preparation for adulthood during childhood and this rise in mental health needs. There certainly are other causes, but some experts believe today's pressured lifestyle is an important contributor.

6.6   Impact of COVID-19

Children are not at the forefront of our current pandemic; however, the wide-ranging effects of the coronavirus could lead to long-lasting consequences. For example, the effects of physical distancing measures and movement restrictions on children's wellbeing represent an obvious cause for concern. We already know from information based in China that children's and adolescents' lifestyle behaviours, such as outdoor play and their sedentary behaviours, may have been drastically impacted due to prolonged school closures and home confinement during the COVID-19 pandemic (Liu et al., 2020). Play is an essential part of children and adolescent's physical and social development. The closure of public spaces and the introduction and persistence of social distancing measures have meant many children have struggled to socialise and play outdoors. This loss has been accompanied by fear, where children have learnt that to break the rules and engage in social activities is dangerous for them.

Children's play in situations of crisis has received minimal academic attention and so there are significant gaps in our knowledge base. To date, we have little research evidence to know all the impacts of COVID-19 on children because of social distancing, lack of opportunities for outdoor play, and opportunities to socialise. However, an analysis of seventeen relevant European and America studies by Kourti et al. (2021) has revealed a reduction in outdoor play in most countries, except in Ireland where it was found to have increased. There was an overall increase in indoor play and use of video games during this period. It appeared that children of older parents and those working from home engaged in less physical play. Children have continued to use their imagination during this period, and interestingly, often include references to COVID-19 within their pretend play. Greater interaction between family members was found, with an increase in the time that children and parents played games together which appeared to strengthen emotional bonds and improve children's mood.

Future studies will help us to navigate through the impact of this unique phenomenon whereby we have been able to continue play within the family, with parents, and siblings, in isolation or online. Perhaps the impact of a lack of peer contact and movement restrictions will be most notable on the developmental milestones and wellbeing of those in their adolescent years when transitioning to college and university life. They have no doubt to some extent missed out on experimental behaviours (and learning from them) and have been unable to become independent from family supervision due to movement restrictions.

6.7 Solutions

Play is so important to optimal child development that it has been recognised by the United Nations High Commission for Human Rights, as a right of every child (Assembly, 1989). This birth right is challenged in many countries by forces including child labour and exploitation practices, and war. Within Western societies there still are limited resources available for children living in poverty and experiencing neighbourhood violence. In addition, we now have the impact of COVID-19 to consider and the impacts on those who are left anxious due to the over scheduling of their lives and over focus on academic attainment. Child advocates need to be mindful of the protective and developmental benefits of play and the fact that children receive much joy and happiness from engagement in playful activities.

6.7.1 The Therapeutic Use of Play

It is useful to consider what is known about how play can be used to help children resolve emotional difficulties. For example, Kourti et al. (2021) point out how playing outdoors not only offers children a sense of connection with nature but also boosts their immune system and regulates their sleep patterns. Play can also be used as a coping mechanism for dealing with difficult situations as a distraction or safe way to confront and come to terms with problems. This can help in reducing anxiety and depression (Schaffer, 2004).

Undirected and directed play is often used as a therapeutic tool in helping children understand difficult experiences in a concrete way. This was demonstrated by the ground-breaking studies carried out by James and Joyce Robertson (1971) who used play as one of their methods to help children they fostered cope with separation from their mothers who were in hospital having another baby. Joyce Robertson would engage the children in playing with dolls which she used to represent herself and her husband as well as the child and his/her parents and the new baby. Identifying themselves and the adults in their lives with the dolls and their interactions within play enabled the children to understand what was happening in their lives and be more prepared for the changes to come.

Whilst the idea of using play to help children understand and come to terms with difficulties in their lives may seem obvious to those currently responsible for caring for children, at the time the Robertsons were carrying out their work this was not the case. The success they achieved in reducing the distress normally exhibited by children in this situation was particularly evident when the reactions of their fostered children were compared to James Robertson's film of the harrowing, distress, and later problematic behaviour exhibited by John, an infant placed in a residential nursery until his mother could leave hospital (see Beardsworth & Stevenson, 1976).

James Robertson's earlier work also included filming the distress that young children experienced during periods of hospitalisation. Whilst medical professionals initially rejected his findings, they later acknowledged the emotional damage children were suffering and changes were made which have radically changed how children are now cared for in hospitals and other institutions. As a result of the acceptance of this work carried out by Robertson the Platt Report was published in 1959, which included recommendations that children be allowed unrestricted visiting and be cared for in dedicated children's wards providing facilities for play (see Lindsay, 2009). It must be said, however, that despite those providing care being fully aware on the need for such changes, it took many years for these recommendations to be fully implemented. Thankfully, it is now common practice within healthcare to use play to help young children cope better with hospitalisation as well as teaching them how to cope with their illness and treatment, for example, giving teddy an injection.

Play therapy is used extensively by those working with children experiencing adverse life events. The varied ways in which it is approached reflect the different psychological theories described in Chap. 3. For example, as suggested within psychodynamic theory, it offers a useful diagnostic tool to tap the child's unconscious and help him/her articulate feelings which cannot be expressed verbally; those taking a cognitive approach explain it as enabling deeper understanding of children restricted by the dominance of concrete thought at such a young age, and play therapists informed by humanistic theories stress the importance of viewing the child as having the potential for growth, maturity, and self-healing (Lin & Bratton, 2015). Also, principles within Behaviourist theory underpin many ways that play therapy is used to reduce problem behaviour in young children.

The cross-cultural value of play therapy is pointed out by Lin and Bratton (2015). They describe how it is a useful way for mental health professionals to communicate with children whose language is different from that of the culture in which they now live. Also, the usefulness of play therapy within schools is described by Ray et al. (2015) as they are one of the easiest places to contact and offer more children mental health support. They suggest that this should involve trained specialists, using age-related toys and the ability to develop trusting relationships with the children. When applying this in their own study, Ray et al. (2015) found that children in the treatment group improved by 0.20 standard deviations over their control group and concluded that play therapy is of real value in elementary schools. They admit that more research is needed to assess the long-term implications of play therapy in schools, but report that research to date suggests that it has the potential to reduce difficult behaviour and improve learning ability, self-esteem, and wellbeing.

6.7.2 Supporting Parents

In an age of conflicting messages and pressures for parents to scaffold their children's academic achievements, it is important that professionals and advocates are also in a position, to help support families and caregivers to help children to engage in activities that will act as protective strategies for children to become resilient and to reduce their anxieties. These could include:

- Helping parents and caregivers to understand that free play is a healthy and needed feature of childhood.
- Emphasising that although parents can certainly monitor play for safety, a large proportion of play should be child driven rather than adult directed.
- Supporting and praising parents who share unscheduled free time with their children and who spend time in engaging in play, letting them know about the array of developmental and wellbeing benefits that these actions can result in for their children.
- Reminding parents of their importance in their child's development and wellbeing and how listening and sharing time with their children can lead to their children transitioning into successful and happy young adults.
- Advocating for more development of 'safe spaces' in under resourced neighbourhoods perhaps by opening school, library, or community facilities to be used by children and their parents after school hours and on weekends.
- Explaining how it is good to allow children to explore many different interests whilst trying to maintain a balance and refraining from expecting excellence in each discipline.

It feels insufficient to just suggest that children learn and develop through play, we need to better understand what play activities can promote what types of learning and development and how. Studies suggest that where children are asked to reflect on their play experiences, they can articulate their own learning. This method may stop the delineation of play and learning and allow play to become more dominant in children's lives, within and outside of the school setting, given the current cultural obsession with academic achievement in Western society. A more sophisticated understanding of play and how children can report benefits to learning and their happiness can only influence the improvement of pedagogical practices that aim to enhance children's developmental wellbeing (Theobald, 2019).

Summary

- Play is a feature of childhood across all cultures, with wide ranging developmental, learning, and wellbeing benefits. However, current societal demands are combining to impact on the environments and time made available for children to play. It remains important that children are encouraged to play, and that child carers and education policy makers are made aware of how play provides multiple learning opportunities for children and can boost their learning capacity.
- Play can also buffer the effects of stressful living conditions and provide children with joyful experiences and promote good family relationships. Further research is needed however to explore how play can best accommodate individual children's needs and compliment schedules that include academic enrichment.
- Children's play opportunities are increasingly shifting to include more virtual play opportunities, even for young children. Chapter 11 further addresses the importance and implications of play, extending the discussion to virtual settings.

Case Study Questions

Read the family case study on page 265 and consider the following:

- What family circumstances may have limited Lily's opportunities to play with her children?
- How might play therapy be used to help control Liam's difficult behaviour?
- In what ways may Chrissy be benefitting from the play opportunities offered when she attends nursery?

Reflective Questions

- To what extent should educational institutions use play as a means of helping young children learn?
- How might culture, class, and gender impact on children's ability to play?
- Is current new technology reducing the opportunity for children and adolescents to learn, think, and play?

References

American Montessori Society Website. https://amshq.org/Educators/Membership/Montessori-Life. Cited in: Bagnoli, D. C. (2021). Montessori by Design: School Spaces that Stay True to the Montessori Method. *Montessori Life: A Publication of the American Montessori Society, 33*(1), 26–34.

Assembly, U. G. (1989). Convention on the Rights of the Child. *United Nations, Treaty Series, 1577*(3), 1–23.

Aziz, N. F., & Said, I. (2012). The Trends and Influential Factors of Children's Use of Outdoor Environments: A Revliew. *Procedia-Social and Behavioral Sciences, 38*, 204–212.

Bagnoli, D. C. (2021). Montessori by Design: School Spaces That Stay True to the Montessori Method. *Montessori Life: A Publication of the American Montessori Society, 33*(1), 26–34.

Bassok, D., Latham, S., & Rorem, A. (2016). Is Kindergarten the New First Grade? *AERA Open, 2*(1), 2332858415616358.

Beardsworth, T., & Stevenson, O. (1976). The Effect on a Young Child of Brief Separation from his Mother: Five Films by the Robertsons. *The British Journal of Social Work, 6*(3), 393–401. Published by: Oxford University Press Stable https://www.jstor.org/stable/23693942

Blake, B., & Pope, T. (2008). Developmental Psychology: Incorporating Piaget's and Vygotsky's Theories in Classrooms. *Journal of Cross-Disciplinary Perspectives in Education, 1*(1), 59–67.

Bornstein, M. H., & Putnick, D. L. (2012). Cognitive and Socioemotional Care: Giving in Developing Countries. *Child Development, 83*, 46–61.

Bruner, J. S. (1972). Nature and Uses of Immaturity. *American psychologist, 27*(8), 687.

Bruner, J. S. (1983). *Child's Talk*. Oxford University Press.

Childline. (2021). https://www.childline.org.uk

Clements, R. (2004). An Investigation of the Status of Outdoor Play. *Contemporary Issues in Early Childhood, 5*(1), 68–80.

Colliver, Y. (2016). Mothers' Perspectives on Learning Through Play in the Home. *Australasian Journal of Early Childhood, 41*(1), 4–12.

DiBianca Fasoli, A. (2014). To Play or Not to Play: Diverse Motives for Latino and Euro-American Parent–Child Play in a Children's Museum. *Infant and Child Development, 23*(6), 605–621.

Erikson, E. (1963). *Childhood and Society*. Norton.

Fromberg, D. P., & Bergen, D. (2015). Play as Ritual in Health Care Settings Laura Gaynard. In *Play from Birth to Twelve* (pp. 361–372). Routledge.

Gaskins, S. (2013). Pretend Play as Culturally Constructed Activity. *The Oxford Handbook of the Development of Imagination*, 224–247.

Gertler, P., Heckman, J., Pinto, R., Zanolini, A., Vermeersch, C., Walker, S., Chang, S. M., & Grantham-McGregor, S. (2014). Labor Market Returns to an Early Childhood Stimulation Intervention in Jamaica. *Science, 344*(6187), 998–1001.

Ginsburg, K. R., & Committee on Communications, & Committee on Psychosocial Aspects of Child and Family Health. (2007). The Importance of Play in Promoting Healthy Child Development and Maintaining Strong Parent-Child Bonds. *Pediatrics, 119*(1), 182–191.

Goldstein, T. R., & Lerner, M. D. (2018). Dramatic Pretend Play Games Uniquely Improve Emotional Control in Young Children. *Developmental science, 21*(4), e12603.

Goldstein, T. R., & Winner, E. (2011). Engagement in Role Play, Pretense, and Acting Classes Predict Advanced Theory of Mind Skill in Middle Childhood. *Imagination, Cognition and Personality, 30*(3), 249–258.

Gurian, M., Stevens, K., & Daniels, P. (2009). *Successful Single-Sex Classrooms: A Practical Guide to Teaching Boys & Girls Separately*. John Wiley & Sons.

Hofferth, S. L. (2010). Home Media and Children's Achievement and Behavior. *Child development, 81*(5), 1598–1619.

Howard, J., Miles, G. E., Rees-Davies, L., & Bertenshaw, E. J. (2017). Play in Middle Childhood: Everyday Play Behaviour and Associated Emotions. *Children & Society, 31*(5), 378–389.

James Robertson & Joyce Robertson (1971) Young Children in Brief Separation, The Psychoanalytic Study of the Child, 26:1, 264–315, https://doi.org/10.1080/00797308.1971.11822274.

Kourti, A., Stavridou, A., Panagouli, E., Psaltopoulou, T., Tsolia, M., Sergentanis, T. N., & Tsitsika, A. (2021). Play Behaviors in Children During the COVID-19 Pandemic: A Review of the Literature. *Children, 8*, 706. https://doi.org/10.3390/children8080706

Lancy, D. F. (2007). Accounting for Variability in Mother–Child Play. *American Anthropologist, 109*(2), 273–284.

Lillard, A. S. (2011). Mother-Child Fantasy. play.psycnet.apa.org.

Lillard, A. S. (2016). *Montessori: The Science Behind the Genius*. Oxford University Press.

Lillard, A. S., Lerner, M. D., Hopkins, E. J., Dore, R. A., Smith, E. D., & Palmquist, C. M. (2013). The Impact of Pretend Play on Children's Development: A Review of the Evidence. *Psychological Bulletin, 139*(1), 1.

Lin, Y. W., & Bratton, S. C. (2015). A Met-Analytic Review of Child-Centered Play Therapy Approaches. *Journal of Counseling & Development, 93*, 45–56. https://doi.org/10.1002/j.1556-6676.2015.00180.x

Lindsay, M. (2009, March). Comments on the Article "Changing Attitudes Towards the Care of Children in Hospital: A New Assessment of the Influence of the Work of Bowlby and Robertson in the UK, 1940–1970" by Frank C.P. *van der Horst and Rene van der Veer (Attachment and Human Development, 11*(2), 119–142), *Attachment & Human Development, 11*(6), 563–567. https://doi.org/10.1080/14616730903282506

Liu, W., Zhang, Q. I., Chen, J., Xiang, R., Song, H., Shu, S., Chen, L., Liang, L., Zhou, J., You, L., Wu, P., Zhang, B., Lu, Y., Xia, L., Huang, L., Yang, Y., Liu, F., Semple, M. G., Cowling, B. J., ... Yu, H. (2020). Detection of Covid-19 in Children in Early January 2020 in Wuhan. *China. New England Journal of Medicine, 382*(14), 1370–1371.

Manz, P. H., & Bracaliello, C. B. (2016). Expanding Home Visiting Outcomes: Collaborative Measurement of Parental Play Beliefs and Examination of Their Association With Parents' Involvement in Toddler's Learning. *Early Childhood Research Quarterly, 36*, 157–167.

Mohan, M., Bajaj, G., Deshpande, A., Anil, M. A., & Bhat, J. S. (2021). Child, Parent, and Play– An Insight Into These Dimensions Among Children with and without Receptive Expressive Language Disorder Using Video-Based Analysis. *Psychology Research and Behavior Management, 14*, 971.

Pagnano-Richardson, K., & Henninger, M. L. (2008). A Model for Developing and Assessing Tactical Decision-Making Competency in Game Play. *Journal of Physical Education, Recreation & Dance, 79*(3), 24–29.

Pellegrini, A. D. (2009). Research and Policy on Children's Play. *Child Development Perspectives, 3*(2), 131–136.

Piaget, J. (1952). Play, Dreams and Imitation In Childhood.

Ramey, C. T., Sparling, J. J., & Ramey, S. L. (2012). *Abecedarian. The Ideas, the Approach and the Findings*. Sociometrics.

Ray, D.C., Armstrong, S.A., Balkin, R.S., & Kimberly, J.M. (2015). Child Centered Play Therapy in the Schools: Review and Meta-Analysis. *Psychology in Schools, 52*(2), 102–124. https://onlinelibrary.wiley.com/doi/epdf/10.1002/pits.21798

Rich, E. (2019). Making Gender and Motherhood Through Pedagogies of Digital Health and Fitness Consumption:'Soon It Made Us More Active as a Family'. In *Digital Dilemmas* (pp. 205–223). Palgrave Macmillan.

Robertson, J., & Robertson, J. (1971). Young Children in Brief Separation. *The Psychoanalytic Study of the Child, 26*(1), 264–315, https://doi.org/10.1080/00797308.1971.11822274

Roopnarine, J. L., & Davidson, K. L. (2015). Parent-Child Play Across Cultures: Advancing Play Research. *American Journal of Play, 7*(2), 228–253.

Schaffer, H. R. (2004). *Introducing Child Psychology*. Blackwell.

Simons, G.N. (2021) Sure Start Children's Centres Did So Much More Than Prevent Paediatric Admissions. *BMJ, 374*, n2303. Retrieved September 21, 2021, from https://doi.org/10.1136/bmj.n2303

Slot, P. L., Mulder, H., Verhagen, J., & Leseman, P. P. (2017). Preschoolers' Cognitive and Emotional Self-Regulation in Pretend Play: Relations with Executive Functions and Quality of Play. *Infant and Child Development, 26*(6), e2038.

Smith, F., & Barker, J. (2001). Commodifying the Countryside: The Impact of Out-of-School Care on Rural Landscapes of Children's Play. *Area, 33*(2), 169–176.

Smith, L., Gardner, B., Aggio, D., & Hamer, M. (2015). Association Between Participation in Outdoor Play and Sport at 10 Years Old with Physical Activity in Adulthood. *Preventive Medicine, 74*, 31–35.

Soenens, B., & Vansteenkiste, M. (2005). Antecedents and Outcomes of Self-Determination in 3 Life Domains: The Role of Parents' and Teachers' Autonomy Support. *Journal of Youth and Adolescence, 34*(6), 589–604.

Tandon, P. S., Zhou, C., & Christakis, D. A. (2012). Frequency of Parent-Supervised Outdoor Play of US Preschool-Aged Children. *Archives of Pediatrics & Adolescent Medicine, 166*(8), 707–712.

Theobald, M. (2019). UN Convention on the Rights of the Child:"Where Are We at in Recognising Children's Rights in Early Childhood, Three Decades on…?". *International Journal of Early Childhood, 51*(3), 251–257.

Thornton, R. L., Glover, C. M., Cené, C. W., Glik, D. C., Henderson, J. A., & Williams, D. R. (2016). Evaluating Strategies for Reducing Health Disparities by Addressing the Social Determinants of Health. *Health Affairs, 35*(8), 1416–1423.

Torrence, M. (2001). Montessori and Play: Theory vs. Practice. *Montessori Life—A Publication of the American Montessori Society, 13*(3), 8–11.

Veitch, J., Bagley, S., Ball, K., & Salmon, J. (2006). Where Do Children Usually Play? A Qualitative Study of Parents' Perceptions of Influences on Children's Active Free-Play. *Health & Place, 12*(4), 383–393.

Vygotsky, L. S. (1978). Socio-Cultural Theory. *Mind in society, 6*, 52–58.

Weisberg, D. S., Hirsh-Pasek, K., & Golinkoff, R. M. (2013). Guided Play: Where Curricular Goals Meet a Playful Pedagogy. *Mind, Brain, and Education, 7*(2), 104–112.

Whitebread, D., & Basilio, M. (2013). *Play, Culture and Creativity. Cultures of Creativity*. The LEGO Foundation.

Ambiguity Within Family Life

7

Given that families are such a powerful force in shaping the early experiences of children and adolescents, it is useful to consider how this impacts on their wellbeing. However, the concept of 'family' proves difficult to define, as those who are considered as part of a family can vary between cultures and historical periods. Despite this, most people recognise the essential features of what is usually considered 'family' to include a group of people, providing emotional, social, and economic support for each other, often related by blood, and living in the same household. Attachment theory explains how strong emotional bonds usually develop between family members which ensure the protection necessary for children's survival. That others are prepared to put, at the very least, their children's survival needs above their own places the child in a state of moral obligation which becomes cemented over time and influences family loyalties. Although, in Western society, parents are held responsible for their children's care, governments have increasingly intervened, imposing legal expectations and limitations on parental behaviour. Although it is not possible to do full justice to sociological explanations for such increased state intervention into family life, an attempt is made within this chapter to explain how families both reflect and contribute to the wider social system in which they exist.

7.1 Function of Families

7.1.1 Families as Social Systems

As relatively small units, families are suitable for meeting the needs of individual members and protect them against adverse events, such as economic hardship, neighbourhood violence, and parental divorce. Routines developed within individual families offer stability and consistency necessary in early child development and positive family functioning promotes better mental health in adolescence (Balistreri & Alvira-Hammond, 2016).

© The Author(s), under exclusive license to Springer Nature Switzerland AG 2022
J. M. Waite-Jones, A. M. Rodriguez, *Psychosocial Approaches to Child and Adolescent Health and Wellbeing*, https://doi.org/10.1007/978-3-030-99354-2_7

Although each family unit is unique, they are all influenced by the wider social systems in which they exist. For example, industrialisation, new forms of work, decrease in mortality rates, and increased life expectancy have impacted heavily on family life. Within the UK, the current view, of family life as a refuge, providing safety and protection, reflects images promoted within the British Victorian era. It is no accident that traditional celebrations depicted on British Christmas cards are often set during this historical period. Nevertheless, just as the snow usually accompanying such scenes is rarely seen here at Christmas, the harmonious family scenes depicted do not necessarily reflect reality.

The idea of the ideal family type, emerging from the Victorian era, was accepted by functionalist sociologists within the 1950s and 1960s as good for society. Such theorists saw the function of families was to socialise members, regulate sexual relationships, clarify inheritance, and transmit social status. These functionalist views were expressed by Parsons (1951) who believed that, in helping to meet members' emotional and material need, families ensured a stable society. He saw family roles and responsibilities highly gendered, with fathers as 'breadwinners' and mothers as carers. However, interactionist theorists, such as Berger (1963), disagreed and pointed out that the nature of family life is determined by social conditions and attitudes. Within Western society, these ensure that children internalise dominant values of achievement, individualism, and anti-collectivism. Goulden (2019) particularly criticises Parson's idea of 'family' as promoting inequality and ignoring variations within family life created by race, class, gender, and poverty.

Feminists also reject the idea of the ideal family type suggested by Parsons and point out how its highly gendered roles create a power imbalance detrimental to women. For example, assigning males as family wage earners suggests that they have a higher value than females and reduce women's bargaining power within family disputes and social situations. This view also sees Parsons' ideal family as serving capitalist production as the husband's power over his wife acts as a buffer against frustrations created by work. Such power imbalance also has the potential to lead to domestic violence. Bochel et al. (2005) point out that the functionalist view of the family is not only 'masculinist' but also ethnocentric. They demonstrate this by referring back to the Beveridge report (1942, p. 53), which established the foundations for the current welfare state. Here, it is clearly stated that 'housewives' have a vital role to play in raising children who will promote the value of the British race and British ideals.

Evidence of an acceptance of Parsons' explanation for the function of the family is also evident within later government policy and rhetoric used by politicians. For example, in 1988, Margaret Thatcher claimed that:

The family is the building block of society. It's a nursery, a school, a hospital a leisure place, a place of refuge and a place of rest. It encompasses the whole of society. It fashions beliefs. It's the preparation for the rest of our lives and women run it. (cited by Bochel et al., 2005, p. 518)

Women are clearly seen here to be responsible for the extent to which family life contributes to the good of society. To ensure a stable family life, women were expected to see their role of homemaker as a full-time career. It is highly ironic that such a statement should have been made by a woman, who, herself, worked outside the home and would have paid others to carry out her 'housewifely' and mothering duties. Later prime ministers also held families responsible for ensuring a stable, prosperous society. For example, Tony Blair (1997–2007) blamed a 'break down' in family life as responsible for national social problems, and David Cameron (2010–2016) maintained that Britain was now 'broken' due to the large number of troubled families and increasing chaotic nature of family life.

Although current UK government policies have started to reflect greater acceptance of different family forms, 'problem families', based on their inability to fit in with existing ideas about family life, continue to be identified, targeted, and brought 'into line' by agencies such as social services. Nevertheless, Punch et al. (2013), adopting a more interactionist stance, insist that, despite strong pressure on families to conform to expectations within wider society, family members are not totally powerless as they possess 'agency'. By this, they mean that families are also shaped by the choices made by different family members which then contribute to wider changes within their environment. Such a view illustrates well the need to take psychosocial approach when considering family life.

7.1.2 Family, Images, Ideals, and Reality

The view of a traditional, harmonious family, suggested by Parsons, tends to glorify the past and has become an idealised concept. The family is seen as private and trusting, offering safety, security, and warmth, set apart from the troubled 'outside' world. However, seeing families as self-sufficient units, relatively free from social pressures, can polarise family and society. For example, Punch et al. (2013) point out how, at the start of twenty-first century, the UK government identified both family life and paid employment as responsible for moral, strong communities but ignored how security within family life depends on the availability of employment and a living wage. Also, expectations of a unified family experience assume that all family members have common interests and ignore potential tensions due to power relations, work patterns, and emotional pressures.

Parsons' view of the ideal family also reflects assumptions of a past predominance of extended families with different generations sharing households, being replaced by a smaller nuclear family, consisting only of parents and children. Such smaller family units were thought to have developed in response to industrialisation, given that they offered a flexible workforce which could move locations in response to new employment opportunities. In fact, previous high mortality rates amongst the very young, old, pregnant females and those in dangerous occupations meant many families were not extended, but rather varied due to second and third marriages. Moreover, Goulden (2019) explains that, far from the nuclear family being most common, increased forms of communication and easy travel have meant that many families are currently enmeshed within extended kinship networks.

In the past marriage had moral, political, and economic implications and was entered into for pragmatic reasons given that it legally sanctioned relationships required for childrearing and property inheritance. Due to high mortality rates the time parents spent together could be relatively short in comparison to current Western society, where many parental partnerships are expected to be lengthy and based on romantic ties. High mortality rates, economic pressures, and religious disapproval meant that in the past, divorce was uncommon; however, legal changes have contributed to its relatively recent increase within the UK. For example, the impact of the Equal Pay Act (1970) cannot be underestimated. Previously, women were paid less than two thirds of the wage received by men doing the same work and, thus, not in a position to support their children alone if trapped in unhappy and possibly abusive marriages. In addition, the Divorce Reform Act (1969) meant divorce became quicker and less expensive. This, along with the rapid decline in the power of major religious institutions, has contributed to higher rates of divorce and resulted in less public censure.

The media has proved a powerful force in promoting the ideal family as usually nuclear, white, and middle class. Kelly and Emery (2003) point out that within the media, as well as health and care services, divorce has previously been linked to behavioural and emotional problems in children and adolescents. Families headed by married couples have been assumed to provide the necessary nurturing environments for children. However, Kelly and Emery (2003) found that even though, two-parent families have the potential to offer a secure environment, some are not able to do so, whilst most children who experience parental divorce are emotionally well-adjusted.

Currently, more diverse family structures and types are being acknowledged and portrayed in advertisements, programmes, and policies. This should prove beneficial as Gittins (1993) insists that, trying to live up to a sense of an 'ideal' family, can leave family members feeling inadequate, disappointed, and guilty. Nevertheless, for those in power, promoting such an ideal can be highly useful as it allows those families who are unwilling or unable to aspire to such an ideal to be blamed for the erosion of moral values. It, therefore, provides a powerful rhetoric which increases psychological pressure on individuals to conform and reduces the opportunity to recognise inequalities which require changes at a much broader, structural level in society.

7.1.3   Family Paradox

Family life is influenced by the conditions of the time in which it exists. Prior to industrialisation family life was relatively public, given that families formed integral components of a joint community life. Industrialisation not only separated work from home but also created a wider gap between private and public spheres within family life. Increased pressure from having to work lengthy hours away from home in intolerable conditions yet needing to conform to the 'idealised' family for fear of public shame, placed many families in a paradoxical position. Consequently, responses to tensions between family members were hidden from public view.

The increasingly private nature of family life can be explained in terms of Goffman's (1959) concept of 'backstage area'. Goffman believed that, as individuals wish to control how they are perceived by others, they put on particular 'performances' to achieve a desired reaction. Families operate in a similar way by monitoring members' behaviour in public so that it appears compatible with the idealised view of family life, whilst concealing family disputes. Therefore, in private, family members may act in 'backstage' ways that they would not wish others to see. This means that although, individuals may have their own 'backstage' view of their own family, they can only judge other families in terms of their particular 'front stage' performances.

Over the years, growing awareness of disturbingly large numbers of domestic violence incidents suggests a dark side may exist in the increasingly private nature of family life. Parsons' functionalist approach explained how the nuclear family benefits both family and societal functioning. Vogel and Bell (1960) also used this functionalist approach to explain that families' (as identifiable units) continued contributions to the good of society may be at the expense of the wellbeing of some individual family members. They refer to the historical use of scapegoating which helped to release collective tensions within communities. Vogel and Bell (1960) suggest that, in a similar way, scapegoating a particular family member can relieve family tensions and allow families to continue as productive units. They fully realised that scapegoating may lead to emotional and/or physical abuse but, thought this may be necessary for the whole family to continue functioning and contributing to society. This highlights the disturbing way that the functionalist approach, which initially may seem very positive and rational, can include the notion that the suffering of a powerless individual is acceptable if it is for the good of the many.

Although also subscribing to functionalism, the social anthropologist Leach (1910–1989) disagreed with Parsons' view of the ideal nuclear family form, seeing kinship as much broader, more fluid, and operating pragmatically. Leach believed that the narrow, private nature of the nuclear family puts members under intolerable pressure to live up to impossible ideals (see Kuper, 1986). The powerful force of emotional pressures within nuclear families was also recognised by psychiatrists Laing and Esterson (1979), who identified this as the cause of much mental illness.

The feminist movements have been particularly responsible for raising awareness of how the family home can be a dangerous place to live. For example, they have exposed the high number of women murdered by male partners. It is now accepted that the physical chastisement of wives by husbands, previously supported in the past by both law and religion, is unacceptable and illegal. However, despite successes made by feminists in achieving some legal changes to prevent domestic violence and child abuse, much more still needs to be done. Carpenter and Stacks (2009) explain how intimate partner violence (IPV) often first occurs whilst women are pregnant and that the devastatingly high number of children under twelve known to have witnessed IPV is grossly under-representative. They add that such children, particularly when under the age of three years, are also likely to experience abuse and neglect. Indeed, by 2020 it was shockingly estimated that 2.3 million children in the UK were living in vulnerable family backgrounds, with 829,000 'invisible to the system', and an additional 761,000 known to the system but with 'unclear' support (Children's Commissioner, 2020 cited by Thembekile Levine et al., 2020). It is not surprising that White (2011) states that, although it is assumed that family life is a safe way of raising children, some families cannot provide the necessary security and alternative forms of care are needed, including substitute families or institutions if necessary.

It is possible that the apparent increase of domestic violence may be partly explained by current expectations of a family fulfilment which is not always possible to achieve. The ideal family image now includes romantically attached parents, seeking self-fulfilment, both within and outside family life in contrast to past family ideals of duty, responsibility, work, and self-denial. Partners may outgrow their potentially much lengthier monogamous relationship if it no longer permits continual self-development. Greater use of birth control and alternative ways of creating a family within current Western society have meant smaller numbers of children and helped to enhance their status. This may also have influenced the increasingly romanticised view of parenthood as intrinsically fulfilling. The emotional investment required to offer the ideal, intensive parenting full of quality time spent interacting with children believed critical to their development can prove exhausting. Also, in comparison to the ideal family, the reality of the many mundane elements of family life can result in feelings of disillusionment and disappointment.

7.2   Family Structures

7.2.1   Diversity of Family Lives

The formation of families is primarily determined by economic opportunities, legal policies, public attitudes, and family members who actively shape their families in response to their social environments (Smetana, 2017). Given the diverse ways that members provide the essential features of family life including, caring, stability, responsibilities, and obligations means that reference should be made to 'families' rather than 'the family'. Indeed, within sociology, attempts to replace the term with concepts such as 'households' and 'intimacy' have failed to fully capture the powerful appeal and common understanding of 'family life'.

Alternatives to family structures have been attempted, such as those practiced within Israelian Kibbutz when first established in 1909. Initially, all adults worked outside the home and children were placed in residential nurseries, only visiting their parents for short periods each day and at weekends. Interestingly, it was found that only very rarely did children raised in full-time, non-biologically based groups marry during adulthood. Eventually, the power of emotional ties between parents and children, which had been underestimated, was acknowledged and families were permitted to reside together.

Currently within Western society, reduced birth rate, better health, longer life, home ownership, and geographical mobility mean that a 'bean pole' family structure is emerging including parents and children closely linked with grandparents and great-grandparents. The multigenerational nature of such families provides mutual support, based on emotional ties, relationships, and companionship. Such a structure can include co-habiting, re-constituted, modified, and blended existing families as well as single parent-led households and gay- and lesbian-led families which include adopted or fostered, non-biological members. Interestingly though, families mostly include married couples which Punch et al. (2013) see as demonstrating the continued preference for a public demonstration of commitment.

7.2.2   Roles and Relationships Within Families

To appreciate the impact of the rising number of alternative family structures on children and adolescents, it is useful to consider what has been learned about the changing nature of roles and relationships within traditional forms of family life. For example, historically wives and children were legally the property of fathers and it is only relatively recently that changes in legislation and social attitudes have allowed mothers to be given custody of their children.

Despite the limited legal status of women, it has always been assumed that they should take on caretaking duties, particularly in relation to young children. Such role expectations have meant that mothers have usually remained at the centre of extended family networks in which they are more likely to continue caring for others. They have tended to maintain greater contact with their own family, drawing their husbands and children into this unit. Since industrialisation, work outside the home has added to the pressure on mothers as principal homemakers. Although this has lessened, to some extent, through current greater equality between mothers and fathers within the home, mothers are still more likely to take a lead role in childcare, experience career disruption, work part-time, do more housework, and offer greater emotional labour. Forbes et al. (2020) found that current working mothers feel that their experience of motherhood is very different to the expected 'ideal', as it involves juggling priorities, feeling physically and emotionally overloaded, and having to constantly ignore their own needs.

There seems very little difference between the ability of mothers and fathers to care for their children. Some differences reported by Steele (2002) suggest that mothers may provide a consistent, comforting role which helps children to develop a unique, inner emotional world, whilst a father's role is more likely to be based on the care that they had experienced and influence their child's future peer relationships. Support for this can be found by Psouni (2019) who found some fathers' expectations of caregiving to be influenced by past rejection by their own father. However overall, it appears that both mothers and fathers share a similar capacity to respond sensitively to their children's needs and emotional states (Psouni, 2019).

Whilst attachment theory has been vital in highlighting the importance of early child–parent relationships, sadly it initially relegated fathers to providers of social, emotional, and economic support for mothers and sometimes allowed mothers to become mediators for the father and child relationship. Male-led households were, then, automatically seen as a social problem. However, Burman (2008) points out that the rise of feminism, varied work patterns, and diversity in family forms, as well as, to some extent, a male liberation movement within the 1990s, have led to recognition of the important caretaking contributions of fathers within families.

Recent changes in legislation, flexible working patterns, and social attitudes have offered opportunities for fathers to play a more integral caring role within families. For example, within the UK, financial help is offered through paid maternity leave (initially first established in 1986 with the latest amendment to date, in 2017), paternity leave (established in 2002), and the possibility of shared parental leave (established in 2014). Although most mothers still take on the primary caretaking role, Andersen (2018) found that increased participation from fathers offered financial benefits and greater gender equality. Moreover, Pettsa and Knoester (2018) report that longer periods of leave offer fathers the opportunity to be more engaged in daily childcare duties which strengthens their commitment to their infant's development and early years of life.

Interestingly, taking a feminist perspective, Burman (2008) identifies an ambiguity with greater male involvement in children's care. She points out that, whilst it may be liberating for women and enable closer relationships between fathers and their children, it can also mean that males may be taking over the one area of life where women previously (if only relatively recently) held more power and control. She points out how the involvement of women into male-dominated work outside the home has not progressed at the same rate.

Nevertheless, it is impossible for any research to measure, quantify, and compare the strength of the emotional rewards of parenthood for both fathers and mothers. Despite inequalities, personal sacrifices, and relentless hard work, it is still the case that most parents would easily sacrifice their own lives to protect their young ones. A haunting example can be offered from a recent newspaper article which described how the father of a family fatally trapped in their car which had been swept away in a swollen river struggled to hand out the baby to be saved by a person trying to help them.

Past family research has tended to concentrate on interactions between parent and child with less attention given to the role of sibling relationships. Siblings can form the longest lasting family relationship and provide support for each other in older age. They are endowed with a shared biological inheritance as well as experiencing the same family culture, if slightly differently. Siblings provide additional attachment figures, reinforce family routines, and, also vicariously, share some of their experiences outside family life. All this, and the intimate shared knowledge and emotional intensity of their relationship, means that siblings have the potential to significantly impact on one another's development and wellbeing.

The emotionally charged nature of sibling relationships fosters learning and imaginative play but also means that they are acutely aware of differential treatment from parents. Dunn (2002) reports that first-born children may display more problematic behaviour after the birth of a new baby as mothers demand more of them.

Despite all the best parental endeavours to spend more time with the older child, eventually the care demanded by the baby increases until by mid-childhood, the younger child has the most attention. Although having to compete for parents' attention, siblings provide important mutual support and act as role models. It has even been found that having an older sibling can help younger siblings to develop a theory of mind earlier than those children who do not have siblings (White & Hughes, 2018). Also, levels of harmony within sibling relationships often reflect the level of satisfaction within their parents' relationship.

Pike et al. (2009) investigated sibling relationships and found that although there were slight indications that birth order, spacing between siblings, and gender (sisters usually being closer than brothers) may have some influence on their relationships, overall, this was negligible. They also stress that family structure was only minimally influential as, in contrast to popular expectations, they found no difference between sibling relationships within single mother-led families and those from two-parent families. Biological inheritance cannot be ignored, as Pike et al. (2009) finally conclude that sibling relationships are influenced as much by their individual characteristics as their family environment.

Increase in home ownership, more mothers working outside the home, and the potential for longer active, healthy lives within the UK have meant that grandparents are playing an even larger part within family life. However, there are important variations in grandparent support depending on ethnicity and education (Margolis & Wright, 2017). Grandparents can influence family life explicitly by offering financial help and advice based on their own family experience but, also implicitly through expectations and emotionally supporting family members. For example, they can act as a buffer during times of stress, such as illness, unemployment, divorce, and bereavement. The role of grandparents can often act in similar ways to a pressure cooker valve, in that parents and grandchildren can use them to relieve family tensions through confidentially 'offloading' their frustrations. Grandchildren can also gain companionship from grandparents who help teach them not only pro-social behaviour, self-regulation, and independence but also how to enjoy life (Giraudeau et al., 2020). However, grandparents have limited legal rights to their grandchildren and may lose contact with them if their parents divorce.

Interestingly, Brown et al. (2021) describe the impact of grandchildren on the relationship between married grandparents. They report that within the USA the divorce between couples aged about fifty years was less likely to happen after grandchildren were born. They explain that the deeply emotional nature of grandparenthood revitalises marriage and reduces the likelihood of divorce. However, such effects were not found within stepfamilies. These findings demonstrate the complex, bi-directional, intergenerational nature of the emotional links within the web of the larger family network.

7.2.3   Impact of New Family Forms

Grandparents and other extended family members can play an important role in offering support and a sense of stability for grandchildren during family separation (Rabindrakumar et al., 2018). Within the UK greater diversity in family structures including single parent, step/blended families as well as single-sex parent families can mean that children and adolescents now often experience a 'chain of relationships' extending across multiple households (Smart et al., 2001). For example, Rabindrakumar et al. (2018) report that, currently, not only are one in four families headed by a single parent, but over a six-year period, one in three children experience such a family form as it often proves to be a transitional period, after which parents marry or cohabit with new partners. Nevertheless, Rabindrakumar et al. (2018) found that in terms of self-reported life satisfaction, quality of peer relationships, and positive views of family life, children who had experienced single-parent family life scored as highly or higher than those who had always lived in two-parent families.

Nevertheless, single-parent families have been portrayed as problematic, particularly within politics and the media (Kushner, 2009), and linked to reduced academic achievement and greater emotional difficulties in children and adolescents. Flouri (2010) suggests that such negative consequences could be explained in terms of genetics, with parents passing on a biological propensity for problematic behaviour. She also explains how it could also be that the problematic behaviour of the child causes family disruption leading to parental separation and divorce. Nevertheless, Flouri (2010) acknowledges that it is possible that the stressful family environment prior to divorce is responsible for any later, problematic behaviour in children. She adds that children from single-mother-led households appear to fare better than those from father-led households, but in both cases, adverse effects are modified by the number and timing of parents' partnership transitions, the age of the child, and economic conditions created by family disruptions.

The impact of single-parent family life on children can, therefore, be seen to be very complex. Flouri (2010) suggests the need to take account of parenting styles as well as child and parent psychopathology. Other influential factors have been found to be involvement of the non-residential parent, financial support, level of conflict following divorce, quality of parenting, and potential joint custody. Also, in some cases, parental separation and divorce can prove beneficial, such as when children and adolescents are raised by parents who display a high level of conflict within their relationship, and particularly in families experiencing domestic violence.

Divorce and single parenthood can often mean reduced family income with poverty acting as both a cause and effect of problems for such families. A sub-culture of poverty has been identified with specific norms and values, including a sense of fatalism and helplessness. It inhibits participation outside family life and any attempts to change situations. Families experiencing poverty are often blamed for many social problems and, as on state benefit, face greater public interventions than those who are financially self-sufficient. Interestingly, a new form of 'semi-detached' family is emerging, which Punch et al. (2013) refer to as 'living apart but together', given that parents are emotionally close but reside in separate households. They suggest that potential reasons for creating this kind of family include previous commitments to caring for relatives, career constraints, or previous lack of success in living together. However, a further reason could be that economic forces determine this family form as, if both parents are claiming state benefit, they may be entitled to more money if classed as separate individuals, with one heading a one-parent family.

An increasing number of children become members of stepfamilies when their parents bring a new partner into the family unit. If the new partner also has children, this may mean the creation of a new and more complex 'blended' family. Having to create new family ways of behaving may feel frustrating and confusing, especially for children whose non-custodial parent is not supportive (Perry & Fraser, 2020). Also, stepparents may find it challenging to establish a warm relationship with step-children and it can be difficult for a biological parent to adjust to co-parenting when they have previously operated as a single parent (Repond et al., 2018). Even so, Punch et al. (2013) found that initial tensions due to previous relationships and loyalties reduce over time and family life becomes more traditional. Even though there may be potential problems when parents attempt to 'cement' their relationship by producing a common offspring within step/blended families, over time, this can increase family satisfaction. It seems that for step/blended families to succeed, members must be open about previous family histories (Sanner et al., 2020), and achieve a level of cohesion and stability that is the same or greater than they experienced within their previous family life (Perry & Fraser, 2020).

Changing attitudes, adoption, and methods of technically assisted reproduction have created other family structures such as those with same-sex parents. Although, it is still possible that children and adolescents from such newly emerging types of family may face stress and stigma, Farr (2016) found that by middle-childhood, children from families headed by lesbian or gay parents were as emotionally and socially adjusted as those by heterosexual parents. Also, Parke (2020) found that gay fathers were as deeply attached to their children as heterosexual fathers were. They also found highly equitable relationships between lesbian parents who were willing to share childcare and household responsibilities. It appears that acceptance from extended families, friends, neighbours, and others within their community is important for such families, and that many same sex parents attempt to ensure that their children have opposite sex role models available.

When parents are of the same sex it can create added complexities for step/blended families. Even so, Gold (2017) suggests that although such families may lack the traditional formal social template of family life, this can free them in terms of how they carry out family roles. They found children from such families to be no different to those from nuclear families in terms of psychological development, gender identity, sexual orientation, self-esteem, or social competence. However, older children may come into the family with established views and fear peer pressure and stigma.

A further newly emerging family form is that including transgender parenting. Hafford-Letchfield et al. (2019) suggest that such parents face even greater prejudice and less support than those who are of the same sex. Stotzer et al. (2014) report a higher percentage of transgender women and those who 'transition' later in life to have children, but no evidence that such children were affected in terms of their gender identity, sexual orientation, or developmental milestones. However, Sullis (2015) suggests that relationships between same sex couples may provide a less stable family life than opposite sex couples. Given the relatively new emergence of such families, he stresses the need for further research on the long-term effects on their children's wellbeing.

Another, newly emerging family form, also worth considering, is that including gender variant children. Gray et al. (2016, p. 123) define such children as having a 'subjective sense of gender identity and/or preferences regarding clothing, activities, and/or playmates that are different from what is culturally normative for their biological sex'. They describe complex attitudes towards such children that are interwoven within social systems, including extended family and schools. Gray et al. (2016) found that the reaction of some parents was to try to protect their child from social stigma whilst others strove to achieve greater tolerance within existing social systems. As, again this is such a new family form, more research is needed into the impact of these early experiences on the wellbeing of children and adolescents.

It is difficult to tease out whether it is the type of family or the impact of stress from being different to the majority of families within a society which may threaten the wellbeing of children and adolescents. LeBlanc (2015) explains how stress is experienced through internalising negative attitudes towards minority groups, which can also include those identified by ethnic origin. Within the UK, family structures vary between families from different ethnic origins. For example, many Afro-Caribbean families live in single female-headed households which exist within a wider matriarchal kinship network, whilst those from India, Pakistan, and Bangladesh may live in extended family households. Children may be expected to contribute to the family income, for example Chinese families running takeaways may expect this through family loyalty, based on Confucian principals (Wyness, 2012). Also, transnational families may have prior commitments and ties to their wider family network which spans national borders. Family practices, such as arranged marriages, within some ethnic minority groups may not be compatible with those expected within the UK.

It is, therefore, necessary to consider cultural and subcultural expectations when seeking to assess the impact of family structure on the wellbeing of children and adolescents from ethnic minority families. This is becoming increasingly important, as Rees et al. (2017) report a significant rise in the number of ethnic minority groups within the UK and predict a greater number of diverse family forms in the future. However, when considering the impact of any minority group it is also useful to bear in mind that, as Smart et al. pointed out in 2001, children view their families positively, and as 'typical', despite differences in how they are organised, as they balance the fluidity in family boundaries and hierarchy of family roles with differing cultural expectations.

7.3   Responding to Family Needs in Practice

There is a need for professionals responsible for children and adolescents, particularly those experiencing adversity such as abuse and neglect, to be aware of the diversity of family forms and function within Western society. Often, family breakdown is used to explain many social ills by treating the family as building blocks of society rather than a product of social conditions. This ignores the structural reasons for some forms of family diversity and suggests the powerful hold that the 'ideal nuclear family' still has on public opinion. Such blame suggests that a return to traditional family forms could solve social and economic problems and allow the public and the governments to escape social responsibilities. The impact of wider social forces on social inequalities experienced by families is captured by the model proposed by Dahlgren and Whitehead (1993). This illustrates how families are influenced by social and community networks; living and working conditions; and general socio-economic, cultural, and environmental conditions.

Although it is beyond the scope of this text to address ways of reducing social inequalities created by such wider social structures, it is possible to discuss ways those working with children and adolescents can help alleviate their influence on family dynamics. Such an undertaking is complex, given that each family is unique, and some form of theoretical base is required from which to assess and identify individual family dynamics, including appreciating subcultural values and beliefs and how these relate to those currently held within wider Western society. Saltiel (2013) concludes that a theoretical framework is necessary as a starting point in understanding the complexity of relationships within families. This could help to avoid potential errors of judgement being made by practitioners left to tease out family practices, which may threaten child and adolescent safety. Saltiel (2013) stresses that such a framework should involve assessing individual family practices and who are considered as 'family' by children and adolescents. This may include carers not related by kinship and outside what would conventionally be considered their 'typical family'.

7.3.1   Family Theories as Frameworks for Child and Adolescent Care

Although Dahlgren and Whitehead (1993) outline how the personal is embedded in wider social connectedness, there is also a need to recognise the power of individual values and beliefs. Parents and other caregivers may pass on social norms but, they also influence children's emotional learning, implicitly and explicitly. To understand how family members react to stressful, socially created events, such as unemployment and poverty, it is useful to take account of family structure, roles, communication, power relationships, and boundaries which create their unique family life (Schaffer, 2004).

Family systems theory, which sees each family operating as a system with each component influencing other components, is currently used as a base for many policies and practices within health and social care. The family group is considered greater than the 'sum of its parts' and its aim is to promote family survival by meeting the basic physical and psychological needs of members. The concepts underlying family systems theory originate from a therapeutic approach initiated by Bowen (1913–1990) which also recognises the need to take a multigenerational approach and examine how rules and customs learned by parents within their original families become repeated within their new family (see Haefner, 2014). The aim is to provide members with an understanding of their situation and help them find more positive ways of interacting. A similar approach is adopted within structural therapy, which particularly emphasises how problems are often caused by a family's inability to adapt to changes. This may be because of limitations on family interactions due to the rigidity of family role boundaries, or that family members are unable to develop a sense of autonomy as their roles are so enmeshed.

Brief strategic family therapy (see Carr, 2016) includes a strategic communication approach (see Voelkl & Colburn, 1984), which focusses on ways in which family rules are communicated verbally and non-verbally. Ambiguous interactions, particularly when non-verbal and verbal messages do not match, create a disorganised system and potential problematic responses, for example, if a parent stiffens at their child's touch, whilst simultaneously saying how much they love them. Members insisting on having the last word display greater power and dominate the whole family. Severe, lasting family disequilibrium is possible if relationships between some members are continually competitive and include mutual distrust with other members having to compromise their sense of self. To try and improve functioning within such families, all members as well as other important figures such as teachers, extended family, and friends are involved in meetings.

Whilst useful within family policies and practice, the limitations of family systems theories are also recognised as individual psychological factors may be neglected. Feminist theory suggests a need for greater awareness of the context in which such families exist and more consideration of gender, class, ethnicity, and wider social role expectations. It becomes clear that family systems theory is most useful when embedded within a wider biopsychosocial approach, such as that suggested by Bronfenbrenner (1979) which sees the bidirectional influences of an individual, their family, community, and social systems.

7.3.2 Family-based Policies and Initiatives

Recognition of the need to consider the whole family when attempting to improve the wellbeing of children and adolescents has become evident within government policies. For example, in 1998 the Sure Start initiative was established by the UK Labour government. It was a response to high rates of child poverty and child and adolescent mental health problems, resulting from policies of the Thatcher government in the 1980s and 1990s (Rutter, 2006). The government intended to fund this intervention programme for ten years, after which it would become the responsibility of local authorities, who could apply for grants. All children under four years of age were included within Sure Start, which aimed to establish partnerships between health services, social services, education, private and voluntary sectors, and parents. Types of services were tailored to identify community needs including home visits for families, quality childcare experience, primary and community healthcare, and specific support for families with children who had special needs.

In 2001 an attempt was made to evaluate the success of Sure Start, but difficulties arose due to the lack of consistency in types of services provided within different areas. Rutter (2006) suggests that the reticence for a more systematic evaluation may also have been politically motivated to avoid the initiative being viewed as a failure. However, some progress was detected such as less families claiming benefit, more adults in work, less crime, less school absence, and improved academic grades. Although no improvement in general child health was observed, less child accidents were reported. In 2005 the programme was transformed into children's centres under local authority control from which positive outcomes have been reported, including better health, greater use of services, and social behaviour of children (Melhuish et al., 2010).

Interestingly, an attempt was made to conduct a randomised controlled evaluation of a form of Sure Start provision in Wales. This included the Incredible Years Parent Training programme and was found to be particularly successful (Rutter, 2006). The programme involved trained supervised facilitators, equipped with necessary resources, setting homework, and making weekly checks with parents (Letarte et al., 2010). Although Sure Start provision is no longer offered in its original form, such programmes have continued to be offered by various organisations within different settings.

Other UK government, family-based policies have been particularly concerned with safeguarding, that is, actively protecting vulnerable family members from neglect and abuse. Many of these follow the safeguarding initiatives implemented in New Zealand, Australia, and the USA. In 2008, the UK Cabinet Office established specific policies and practice initiatives based on the concept of 'Think Family'. These were developed from the Children Act 1989 and controlled safeguarding measures implemented by local authorities, courts, parents, and other agencies in the UK, to enable greater professional engagement with families (Morris, 2012).

Initiatives were particularly aimed at creating long-term changes in families with multiple needs, from which a specific group were identified as proving costly due to their entrenched problems. Such families were deemed as resisting current forms of support, including preventative programmes, and in need of specifically focussed interventions (Morris, 2012). Early intervention was suggested to enable such families to improve, and services were to be joined up. The aim was to harness family resources, through family group conferences and kinship care, and use appropriate services for families with an 'inherited dysfunctionality'. However, Morris (2013) identifies contradictions between some policies as, for example, they could mean that the same extended family is identified as problematic but, also a resource for kinship care of a child unable to live with their parents.

Nevertheless, later legislation such as the Child and Families Act (2014) also acknowledges the importance of protecting children through supporting the whole family. In addition, the Child and Family Relations Act (2015) recognises the current diversity of some family forms.

7.3.3 Family-Centred Health and Social Care and Joined-Up Services

A family-centred approach is now accepted as a theoretical and practical framework to guide decision making within child health and social care services. This is generally taken to mean that when offering care and service delivery to a child or adolescent, it is in their best interest to also appreciate needs within the extended network of relationships in which they are embedded. Due to increased costs and new thinking on how best to deliver care, the provision within health and social care also aims to foster empowerment and self-help. This requires collaborative decision making between professionals, parents, and, depending on age and ability, the child or adolescent. The aim is to encourage families to participate in their care and decision making at a level they choose, and with a mutual sense of respect between them and professionals. Key features within family and professional interactions are meant to include negotiation based on respect for the knowledge, values, beliefs, and cultural backgrounds of family members. This approach is aimed at helping family members to develop the confidence and abilities necessary once initial care provision is reduced.

However, providing family-centred care to improve the lives of ill, disabled, or disadvantaged children and adolescents can be problematic. Uniacke et al. (2018) point out how tensions may exist between the needs of the child or adolescent, and those of the family who may be required to make considerable sacrifices in the type of care or changes they need to make. They also see that although meant to be equal, the views of professionals and parents may dominate over those of the child or adolescent which undermines their fundamental right to promote their own wellbeing (United Nations, 1989).

A lack of consensus as to what collaborative practice involves also makes it difficult to assess just how this is implemented within service delivery. Unless sensitively delivered, families may suffer a lack of information or, conversely, 'information overload'. Families and professionals may differ in their expectations of appropriate strategies, which can have a financial, social, and emotional impact on family members who may feel pressured into taking on a caring role. Also, in the case of a chronically ill or disabled child, family carers must quickly learn skills that healthcare professionals have taken years to master.

Professionals offering family-centred care face difficult dilemmas, such as when there are conflicting concerns about the ability of certain families to make safe care and protection plans. Morris (2012) explains how, if family members are required to make decisions which are beyond their capacity their reaction may be to use avoidance tactics. Also, seeking wider kinship care for children and adolescents can prove problematic when the child or adolescent's wider kinship network is also considered as unstable, and distrustful of professional interventions (Saltiel, 2013).

Concerns have also been raised about who is specifically considered as family, when providing family-centred care. Morris (2013) suggests that often this just means focussing on parents or even mothers, with a continued dominance of the idea of a traditional family form. Indeed, the extended family network may include significant others who may not be related, live near, or be connected by blood. Tensions between old and new expectations of who should be considered as family create difficulties in responding to family diversity when working within rigid family policies (Morris, 2013).

True equality in partnerships between professionals and families is problematic due to an inherent power imbalance. For example, professionals can determine what is discussed within family conferences and meetings which often take place after their professional opinion has been determined. Also, some situations exist which offer families little choice (Morris, 2013). Families are also automatically placed in a less powerful position given that they are dependent on the skills and knowledge of professionals, embedded in established processes of which family members are not familiar. It also must be noted that, professionals are placed in an ambivalent position, in that whilst trying to create an equal partnership with families, they also have a duty to act on their professional knowledge and experience. They also must take professional responsibility for decisions which may require confidentiality and ultimate accountability to their own professional bodies.

The inherent power imbalance between professionals and families can mean that family members reluctantly acquiesce to the dictates of professionals or be perceived in ways that undermine their confidence and leave them feeling unsupported (Reeder & Morris, 2021). However, tensions between the positions of families and professionals can at least be eased by mutual recognition of the constraints on both their positions and striving to establish relationships based on mutual respect. The need to establish good relationships between families and professionals cannot be understated, as Morris (2013) explains that families recognise and value attempts to understand their specific experience of family life and as a result will engage more in family services.

Interestingly, Rutter (2006) found that within the provision of Sure Start, nurses were particularly successful in establishing such relationships with families. They were reported by families to understand their different needs, be good record keepers, and provide tailored support. It could be that because of the type of intimate, often invasive, physical care required within nursing, nurses must develop ways of quickly establishing trusting relationships. Also, possibly the necessary 'breaking of body boundaries' experienced by those receiving such nursing care creates a readiness to trust and confide.

As families often feel overwhelmed by the different types of services they may be required to engage with, which often requires constant repetition of the same information about their needs, there is a move to offer services in a 'joined up' way. However, Roets et al. (2016) believe that such moves are also based on market-based principles and policies. They point out that, unintended consequences of such initiatives can mean that those most constantly in contact with families are reduced to 'signposting' them to increasingly specialised services. Roets et al. (2016) see such initiatives as reducing the opportunity for professionals, such as social workers, to develop close and trusting relationships which can help avoid the need for more specialist services. Overall, although highly valued, the success of family-centred practice needs to be more evidence based as it may not be the best way of meeting the needs of all children and adolescents (Shields, 2017).

Summary

- Families are human groupings small enough to meet family members' physical and emotional needs. They socialise offspring through passing on values and beliefs of their specific culture which involves regulating sexual behaviour, reproduction, inheritance, and status. In Western culture, images of an ideal harmonious, nuclear family life are promoted through agencies such as the government and media. However, family life is determined by a family's economic position and includes many mundane features. A paradox exists between the public and private spheres of family life, given that the family is portrayed as a refuge and 'safe-haven' yet can include domestic violence and abuse.
- Due to changes in legislation and public attitudes within Western culture there is increasing diversity in family structures and the roles of family members. More mothers work outside the home and fathers take greater responsibility for childcare whilst the contributions of siblings and grandparents to family life are increasingly recognised. Various family forms now exist, including those headed by a single parent, step/blended families, and families headed by single-sex couples. There is a need to recognise the potential stress experienced by children and adolescents from these and other minority families, including those of different ethnic origins.
- A family systems approach, supporting the whole family, currently underpins child- and adolescent-focussed legislation, policies, and initiatives. This also guides current health and social care provision which aims to promote family empowerment and self-help, along with 'joined up' services. Mutually respectful relationships between professionals and families are required to overcome an inherent imbalance of power.

Case Study Questions

Read the family case study on page 265 and consider the following:

- In what ways does the Wilson family differ from what is considered the 'ideal' family?
- How might the children react to having more contact with Damian and his partner?
- In what ways could the family's social worker help Lily deal with Stuart's constant unwelcome visits as well as Ben's truanting and shoplifting behaviour?

- How well can the new, diverse family forms provide the secure attachments necessary for the wellbeing of children and adolescents?
- How might children and adolescents benefit from fathers' greater engagement in early childcare and general family life?
- In what ways will relationships change within families across different members' lifespan?

References

Andersen, S. H. (2018). Paternity Leave and the Motherhood Penalty: New Causal Evidence. *Journal of Marriage and Family, 80*(1125–1143), 1125. https://doi.org/10.1111/jomf.12507

Balistreri, K. S., & Alvira-Hammond, M. (2016). Adverse Childhood Experiences, Family Functioning and Adolescent Emotional Well-being. *Public Health, 132*, 72–78. https://doi.org/10.1016/j.puhe.2015.10.034

Berger, P. L. (1963). *Invitation to Sociology. A Humanistic Perspective*. Doubleday.

The Beveridge Report – Internet Archive. https://archive.org/details/in.ernet.dli.2015.275849

Bochel, H., Bochel, C., Page, R., & Sykes, R. (2005). *Social Policy, Issues and Developments*. Pearson Educational.

Bronfenbrenner, U. (1979). *The Ecology of Human Development: Experiments by the Nature of Design*. Harvard University Press.

Brown, S. L., Lin, I.-F., & Mellencamp, K. A. (2021). Does the Transition to Grandparenthood Deter Gray Divorce? A Test of the Braking Hypothesis. *Social Forces, 99*(3), 1209–1232. https://doi.org/10.1093/sf/soaa030

Burman, E. (2008). *Deconstructing Developmental Psychology*. Routledge.

Carpenter, G. L., & Stacks, A. M. (2009). Developmental Effects of Exposure to Intimate Partner Violence in Early Childhood: A Review of the Literature. *Children and Youth Services Review, 31*, 831–839. https://doi.org/10.1016/j.childyouth.2009.03.005

Carr, A. (2016). Family Therapy for Adolescents. A Research-Informed Perspective. *Australian and New Zealand Journal of Family Therapy, 37*, 467–479. https://doi.org/10.1002/anzf.1184

Dahlgren, G., & Whitehead, M. (1993). *Tackling Inequalities in Health: What Can We Learn from what has been Tried?* King's Fund. Cited by World Health Organisation. (2012). Health 2020: a European Policy Framework Supporting Action Across Government and Society for Health and Well-being. Copenhagen: WHO. http://www.euro.who.int/en/publications/abstracts/health-2020-a-european-policy-frameworksupporting-action-across-government-and-society-for-health-and-well-being

Dunn, J. (2002). Sibling Relationships. In P. K. Smith & C. H. Hart (Eds.), *Blackwell Handbook of Childhood Social Development* (pp. 223–237). Blackwell.

Farr, R. H. (2016). Does Parental Sexual Orientation Matter? A Longitudinal Follow Up of Adoptive Families with School-Age Children. *Developmental Psychology*. Advance online publication. https://doi.org/10.1037/dev0000228.

Flouri, E. (2010). Fathers' Behaviours and Children's problems. *The Psychologist, The British Psychological Society, 23*(10), 802–805.

Forbes, L. K., Lamar, M. R., & Bornstein, R. (2020). Working Mothers' Experiences in an Intensive Mothering Culture: A Phenomenological Qualitative Study. *Journal of Feminist Family Therapy, 7*(1), 1–25. https://doi.org/10.1080/08952833.2020.1798200

Giraudeau, C., Duflos, M., & Chasseigne, G. (2020). Adolescents' Conceptions of "Good" Grandparents: A Reversal Theory Approach. *Journal of Intergenerational Relationships, 8*(25), 1–18. https://doi.org/10.1080/15350770.2020.1804034

Gittins, D. (1993). *The Family in Question*. Macmillan Press.

Goffman, E. (1959). *The Presentation of Self in Everyday Life*. Penguin Books.

Gold, J. M. (2017). Honoring the Experiences of Gay Stepfamilies: An Unnoticed Population. 126–133, Published Online: January 19. https://doi.org/10.1080/10502556.2016.1268020.

Goulden, M. (2019). 'Delete the Family': Platform Families and the Colonisation of the Smart Home. *Information, Communication and Society*. Published online. Retrieved February 02, 2021, from https://doi.org/10.1080/1369118X.2019.1668454.

Gray, S. A. O., Sweeney, K. K., Randazzo, R., & Levitt, H. M. (2016). "Am I Doing the Right Thing?": Pathways to Parenting a Gender Variant Child. *Family Process, 55*(1), 123–138. https://doi.org/10.1111/famp.12128

Haefner, J. (2014). An Application of Bowen Family Systems Theory. *Issues in Mental Health Nursing, 35*, 835–841. https://doi.org/10.3109/01612840.2014.921257

Hafford-Letchfield, T., Cocker, C., Rutter, D., Tinarwo, M., McCormack, K., & Manning, R. (2019). What Do We Know About Transgender Parenting?: Findings from a Systematic Review. *Health & Social Care in the Community, 27*, 1111–1125. https://doi.org/10.1111/hsc.1275

Kelly, J. B., & Emery, R. E. (2003). Children's Adjustment Following Divorce: Risk and Resilience Perspectives. *Family Relations, 52*(4), 352–362. Retrieved March 18, 2019, from http://www.jstor.org/stable/3700316

Kuper, A. (1986). An Interview with Edmund Leach. *Current Anthropology, 27*(4), 375–382. Published by: The University of Chicago Press on behalf of Wenner-Gren Foundation for Anthropological Research Stable URL: https://www.jstor.org/stable/2743059

Kushner, M. A. (2009). A Review of the Empirical Literature About Child Development and Adjustment Postseparation. *Journal of Divorce & Remarriage, 50*(7), 496–516. https://doi.org/10.1080/10502550902970595

Laing, R. D., & Esterson, A. (1979). *Sanity, Madness, and the Family*. Penguin Books.

LeBlanc, A. J., Frost, D. M., & Wight, R. G. (2015). Minority Stress and Stress Proliferation Among Same-Sex and Other Marginalized Couples. *Marriage and Family, 77*(1), 40–59. https://doi.org/10.1111/jomf.12160

Letarte, M. J., Normandeau, S., & Allard, J. (2010). Effectiveness of a Parent Training Program "Incredible Years" in a Child Protection Services. *Child Abuse and Neglect, 34*, 253–261. https://doi.org/10.1016/j.chiabu.2009.06.003

Margolis, R., & Wright, L. (2017). Healthy Grandparenthood: How Long Is It, and How Has It Changed? *Demography, 54*, 2073–2099. https://doi.org/10.1007/s13524-017-0620-0

Melhuish, E., Belsky, J., & Barnes, J. (2010). Evaluation and Value of Sure Start. *Archives of Disease in Childhood, 95*, 159–161. https://doi.org/10.1136/adc.2009.161018

Morris, K. (2012). Thinking Family? The Complexities for Family Engagement in Care and Protection. *British Journal of Social Work, 42*, 906–920. https://doi.org/10.1093/bjsw/bcr116

Morris, K. (2013). Troubled Families: Vulnerable Families' experience of Multiple Service Use. *Child and Family Social Work., 18*, 198–206. https://doi.org/10.1111/j.1365-2206.2011.00822x

Parke, R. D. (2020). Toward a Contextual Perspective on the issue of Gay Fathers and Attachment. *Attachment & Human Development, 22*(1), 129–133. https://doi.org/10.1080/14616734.2019.1589069

Parsons, T. (1951). *The Social System*. Routledge & Keegan Paul.

Perry, C., & Fraser, R. (2020). A Qualitative Analysis of New Norms on Transition Days in Blended Families. *Sociology Mind, 10*, 55–69. https://doi.org/10.4236/sm.2020.102005

Pettsa, R. J., & Knoester, K. (2018). Paternity Leave-Taking and Father Engagement. *Journal of Marriage and Family, 80*(5), 1144–1162. https://doi.org/10.1111/jomf.12494

Pike, A., Kretschmer, T., & Dunn, J. F. (2009). Siblings—Friends or Foes? *The Psychologist, The British Psychological Society, 22*(6), 494–449.

Psouni, E. (2019). The Influence of Attachment Representations and Coparents' Scripted Knowledge of Attachment on Fathers' and Mothers' Caregiving Representations. *Attachment & Human Development, 21*(5), 485–509. https://doi.org/10.1080/14616734.2019.1582598

Punch, S., Marsh, I., Keating, M., & Harden, J. (2013). *Sociology. Making Sense of Society* (5th ed.). Pearson Educational Ltd..

Rabindrakumar, S., Martinex-Perez, Á., Shaw, W., Hughes, N., & Jones, P. M. (2018). *Family Portrait; Single Parent Families and Transitions Over Time*. Sheffield University.

Reeder, J., & Morris, J. (2021). Becoming an Empowered Parent. How do Parents Successfully Take up Their Role as a Collaborative Partner in their Child's Specialist Care? *Journal of Child Health Care., 25*(1), 110–125. https://doi.org/10.1177/1367493520910832

Rees, P. H., Wohland, P., Norman, P., Lomax, N., & Clark, S. D. (2017). Population Projections by Ethnicity: Challenges and Solutions for the United Kingdom. In D. Swanson (Ed.), *The Frontiers of Applied Demography* (Applied Demography Series) (Vol. 9). Springer. https://doi.org/10.1007/978-3-319-43329-5_18

Repond, G., Darwiche, J., El Ghaziri, N., & Antonietti, J.-P. (2018). Coparenting in Stepfamilies: A Cluster Analysis. *Journal of Divorce and Remarriage, 60*(3), 211–233. https://doi.org/10.1080/10502556.2018.1488121

Roets, G., Roose, R., Schiettecat, T., & Vandenbroeck, M. (2016). Reconstructing the Foundations of Joined-Up Working: From Organisational Reform towards a Joint Engagement of Child and Family Services. *British Journal of Social Work, 46*, 306–322. https://doi.org/10.1093/bjsw/bcu121

Rutter, M. (2006). Is Sure-Start an Effective Preventative Intervention? *Child and Adolescent Mental Health, 11*(3), 135–141. https://doi.org/10.1111/j.1475.3588.2006.00402.x

Saltiel, D. (2013). Understanding Complexity in Families' Lives: The Usefulness of 'family practices' as an Aid to Decision Making. *Child and Family Social Work, 18*, 15–24. https://doi.org/10.1111/cfs.12033

Sanner, C., Ganong, L., & Coleman, M. (2020). Shared Children in Stepfamilies: Experiences Living in a Hybrid Family Structure. *Journal of Marriage and Family, 82*(2), 605–621. https://doi.org/10.1111/jomf.12631

Schaffer, H. R. (2004). *Introducing Child Psychology*. Blackwell.

Shields, L. (2017). All is not Well with Family-Centred Care. *Nursing Children and Young People, 29*(4), 14–15. https://doi.org/10.7748/ncyp.29.4.14.s15

Smart, C., Neale, B., & Wade, A. (2001). *The Changing Experience of Childhood: Families and Divorce*. Polity Press.

Smetana, J. G. (2017). Current Research on Parenting Styles, Dimensions, and Beliefs. *Current Opinion in Psychology, 5*, 19–25. https://doi.org/10.1016/j.copsyc.2017.02.012

Steele, H. (2002). State of the Art: Attachment. *The Psychologist, 15*(10), 518–522.

Stotzer, R. L., Herman, J. L., & Hasenbush, A. (2014). *Transgender Parenting: A Review of Existing Research* (pp. 1–27). Williams Institute, University of California. (UCLA). https://escholarship.org/uc/item/3rp0v7qv

Sullis, D. P. (2015). Emotional Problems among Children with Same-Sex Parents: Difference by Definition. *British Journal of Education, Society & Behavioural Science, 7*(2), 99–120. https://doi.org/10.9734/BJESBS/2015/15823

Thembekile Levine, D., Morton, J., & O'Reilly. (2020). Child Safety, Protection, and Safeguarding in the Time of COVID-19 in Great Britain: Proposing a Conceptual Framework. *Child Abuse & Neglect, 110*(2), 1–9. https://doi.org/10.1016/j.chiabu.2020.104668

Uniacke, S., Browne, T. K., & Shields, L. (2018). How should we understand Family-Centred Care? *Journal of Child Health Care., 22*(3), 460–469. https://doi.org/10.1177/1367493517753083

United Nations General Assembly (UN). (1989). https://www.un.org/en/ga/62/plenary/children/bkg.shtml.

Voelkl, G. M., & Colburn, K. (1984). The Clinical Sociologist as Family Therapist: Utilizing the Strategic Communication Approach. *Clinical Sociology Review, 2*(1), Article 11. http://digitalcommons.wayne.edu/csr/vol2/iss1/11

Vogel, E. F., & Bell, N. W. (1960). The Emotionally Disturbed Child as a Family Scapegoat. *Psychoanalytic Review, 47B*(2), 21–42.

White, K. (2011). A Bad Home is Better than a Good Institution. *The Therapeutic Care Journal— Published by The International Centre for Therapeutic Care*.

White, N., & Hughes, C. (2018). *Why Siblings Matter*. Routledge.

Wyness, M. (2012). *Childhood and Society* (2nd ed.). Palgrave Macmillan.

Deviance and Labelling

8

8.1 Defining Deviance

The focus within this chapter is on the biological, psychological, and social processes involved in deviance. Although at first glance, the idea of being deviant may seem simple, when examined closely, it becomes a complex concept. Deviance refers to some form of difference (intended or not) from what is considered 'typical'. It covers a broad area, ranging from breaking laws and social rules to just looking different in some way to what is expected by most people in specific groups or cultures. To understand the impact of 'deviance' on wellbeing in children and adolescents, it is important to consider what is meant by 'typical', as well as the benefits of conforming to 'normality', and the effects of others' reactions when conformity is rejected or not possible.

Understanding the processes involved in judging someone as deviant is important as children and adolescents are more vulnerable to such judgements due to their powerlessness in comparison to adults. For example, being judged and given a negative 'label' during this period can influence the way that others react to them over their lifetime. Also, children and adolescents may absorb and perpetuate prejudice and discriminatory behaviour towards others which they have witnessed in adult behaviour.

8.1.1 Evolutionary Explanations of Conformity and Deviance

Judgements of deviance are made about those who do not conform to the rules of their group. Being accepted as a group member means supressing individual differences and acting in ways that are necessary for the good of the whole group. Rules are developed to promote the safety of the group, although these can also further the interests of those who hold most powerful positions within the group. Pressure to conform to group rules (norms) is applied through threats of punishment and

© The Author(s), under exclusive license to Springer Nature Switzerland AG 2022
J. M. Waite-Jones, A. M. Rodriguez, *Psychosocial Approaches to Child and Adolescent Health and Wellbeing*, https://doi.org/10.1007/978-3-030-99354-2_8

rejection if they are broken. Such group processes are easily visible within societies with a simple structure, but within complex groups such as Western society some of the mechanisms of judgement and control are much more difficult to identify. Bronfenbrenner's (1979) bio-ecological theory is particularly useful in demonstrating the bidirectional forces of biological inheritance, families, community, and ideals of wider society in creating as well as reacting to deviance within Western society. Applying this theory requires examination of the biologically inherited capacities which enable humans to become social animals. Also, the hidden forces that emerge once social groups develop, making them 'greater than the sum of their parts' in terms of power and control, need consideration.

When considered in terms of human evolution, group membership offers individuals security and promotes the survival of the species. Therefore, to survive, humans have developed as social animals. This has meant curbing the inherited capacities for aggression necessary for individual survival and learning to appreciate the needs of others. Such abilities are possible through the development of increasingly sophisticated cognitive and emotional capacities, including empathy, altruism, and a 'theory of mind' which all promote pro-social behaviour. Humans, therefore, possess an inherited ability to achieve a balance between meeting their individual needs, as well as those of others, which is necessary to be accepted as a member of the specific culture into which they are born.

8.1.2   Inherited Pre-dispositions for Pro and Anti-social Behaviour

Although aggression, along with hunger, sex, and flight, has been identified as necessary for human survival (Lorenz, 1966), it needs controlling so that groups can be formed which offer an even greater chance of the human species surviving. Therefore, understanding and, where necessary, limiting potential anti-social uses of aggression are necessary for the survival of any society. Within cultures, an inherited temperament can mean that some individuals have greater propensity towards displaying aggression and limited impulse control. Kotler and McMahon (2005) explain that this can be due to a lack of the anxiety normally felt when fearing punishment, which usually reduces aggressive impulses. This process may also be particularly prevalent during specific developmental stages, such as adolescence. Blakemore and Mills (2014) have demonstrated that at this stage of neurological development areas of the brain responsible for impulse control lag behind those involved in rational decision making. This suggests that adolescents cannot always control impulsive behaviour which they clearly know to be inadvisable. Van Teijlingan and Humphris (2019) point out that, within Western society, although most adolescents manage to successfully negotiate this period, about 20% suffer greater problems with impulse control, have an unrealistic sense of invulnerability, and may be drawn to a youth sub-culture, including anti-social behaviour.

Greater development of inherited emotional capacities for empathy, and cognitive processing, including a 'theory of mind', also helps keep aggressive impulses in check for most people. Empathy involves recognising and (to some extent) vicariously experiencing distress in others with a desire to help alleviate their suffering. Kagan (1981) suggests that children inherit an ability to empathise and desire to help others, but that this can be enhanced or 'bleached out' by the social environment in which the child is raised. Empathy is, therefore, a key building block of prosocial behaviour (Komorosky & O'Neal, 2015) and positively associated with higher levels of social competence in children. Interestingly, a form of empathy appears very early in human development, as demonstrated by the 'contagious crying' exhibited by babies, who start crying in response to hearing the cries of other babies. However, empathy requires the later development of more sophisticated emotional and cognitive abilities including emotion recognition, perspective taking, emotional response, and reparative action (Marshall & Marshall, 2011).

Empathy, therefore, includes an element of cognitive processing which provides a rationalising mechanism, controlling aggressive impulses and providing an ability to develop a 'theory of mind'. As discussed in previous chapters, this allows an awareness of others' beliefs, desires, and needs. Increased cognitive development also enables greater understanding of social rules. Kagan and Snidman (1991) point out that by two years of age, infants have learnt many social rules through experiences within their family, particularly once language is acquired. However, although pro-social rules may be learned, adverse experiences can create distortions in cognitive processing which mean that difficult, ambiguous situations may be interpreted as hostile and responded to aggressively. A vicious cycle can then develop whereby aggression breeds aggression.

Psychopathy can be considered as an extreme example of an inherited inability to follow social rules due to lack of empathy, impaired cognitive development, and restricted 'theory of mind'. Interestingly Kotler and McMahon (2005) found that, although some of those diagnosed as psychopaths did possess a limited 'theory of mind' in sensing that others may hold different beliefs, they were unaware that others could recognise their own false behaviour. Psychopathy involves consistent calculating and unemotional behaviour, as well as an inability to recognise distress in others which normally triggers a violence inhibition mechanism. Kotler and McMahon (2005) explain how children diagnosed as having psychopathic traits focus on rewards brought by aggression but pay little attention to punishment. However, they express concerns about readily applying a diagnosis of psychopathy to children and adolescents as this may not always continue into adulthood. Kotler and McMahon (2005) point out how such a serious diagnosis so early in life would be difficult to lose later and may influence any legal judgements made about any future criminal behaviour.

8.1.3 Social Shaping of Inherited Abilities

Although Kotler and McMahon (2005) found links between parental history of psychopathic traits and their children's diagnosis of psychopathy, they did find a small number of cases where the children's psychopathic traits reduced during adulthood.

This suggests that, at least to some extent, such extreme anti-social behaviour can be enhanced or inhibited by experience. Also, Plomin (2019) acknowledges that, although genetics have an undeniably powerful effect on anti-social behaviour, this can also be influenced by individual experience. Kagan (2018) sees that both cognitive and emotional reactions result from experience as well as inheritance, particularly in relation to the empathy and altruism involved in moral development. He explains that developing a moral code includes awareness of the context in which actions take place including the specific nature of the act, who is the perpetrator and who the recipient, as well as the actual action.

Potential social and anti-social behaviour can, therefore, also be influenced by the environmental conditions in which children and adolescents are raised. For example, anti-social acts may be a result of poverty which creates hardship and the potential for weak attachments, inadequate child supervision, and harsher parenting styles. Also, Schaffer (2003) offers examples of cultural variations in child-rearing practices which reflect differences in the value placed on displays of altruism and aggression. He describes how within the Mundugumor people, aggression is encouraged and little affection evident in parent–child interactions. This contrasts starkly with child rearing within the Philippines where altruism and affection are highly valued. Currently within Western culture good parenting involves encouraging pro-social behaviour. This reflects the extent to which caring for others is valued and the need to reduce anti-social behaviour recognised. However, despite these overt cultural aspirations, on a deeper less obvious level, they are often at odds with the forces of capitalism on which Western culture is based, which aggressively promote competition and individualistic self-gratification.

8.1.4 Function of Attitudes and Prejudice Towards Deviance Within Social Groups

The interaction between inherited human cognitive and emotional capacities and group processes becomes particularly evident when examining the often hidden and intangible pressures social groups exert to ensure conformity. Emotional responses of shame and guilt result from being disapproved of by others. These provide a powerful mechanism for ensuring people conform to what is approved of within social situations and aid the survival of the whole group or culture.

Social approval and disapproval are conveyed through attitudes towards group members and their behaviour, which are expressed explicitly and implicitly. Children learn to adopt attitudes very early in their development through interactions with family members and peers, and later from those within their community and wider society. Attitudes convey who and what is considered as 'deviant' within different cultures and subcultures. However, it seems that holding some form of attitude is difficult to avoid as this process provides an instant cognitive 'sizing up system' to evaluate threat or safety, which aids individual and group survival. Adopting attitudes approved of by specific groups or cultures also ensures being accepted and gaining protection from other members. But the ability to conform to attitudes approved of within groups can impact on an individual's self-identity and self-esteem. Cooley's (1902) 'looking glass' theory suggests that seeing the 'self' through the eyes of others includes awareness of their positive and negative evaluations. Fear of not living up to the expectations of others can create low self-esteem in a person and intensify their need to be critical of others seen as 'deviant' to ensure their own acceptance (Tajfel & Turner, 1986).

The process of attitude formation enables a quick 'sizing up' of new situations when little is known about other people involved. It involves focussing on a particular feature (central trait) of someone and using this to judge them and their behaviour. This feature may then be used to judge and blame a person in difficult situations. Unfortunately, this can involve a 'self-serving' bias which is a psychological mechanism protecting the self-esteem of the person making judgements. This means that a person will judge others in terms of a specific behavioural feature (central trait) but, if they, themselves commit a similar action, they will blame it on the situation. For example, we may judge another person as a 'clumsy' person when they spill their drink at a party. However, we will interpret spilling our own drink, as due to some environmental factors, such as the floor being uneven. Sadly, once an initial negative judgement has been made about a person based on such a feature (central trait), it is very difficult for them to be seen more positively.

Box 8.1 Example of stereotyping

Some time ago, within the UK, a Christmas card was sold by a famous supermarket. This showed a small red-haired child sitting on the knee of Father Christmas and being given a present. The caption below the picture read:

'Father Christmas even loves ginger nuts.'

The Christmas card was removed due to public outcry about the (unintended) prejudicial attitudes that this card conveyed towards people with red hair.

This process of judging someone by specific visible features or behaviour which differ from the majority means stereotyping and expecting other people or groups with those features to be the same. For example, an (unfounded) assumption commonly expressed is that people with red hair have a fiery temper, therefore anyone with red hair is assumed to be hot tempered and treated cautiously. Red hair then becomes a label which links specific different features and behaviour, whilst ignoring aspects that the person shares with all humans. Such prior assumptions can cause distress to those people judged in this way.

It is important to understand such processes as they explain the prejudice which children and adolescents may be exposed to, absorb, and later perpetuate. Prejudice means to have a positive or negative attitude towards a person or group of which little is known. It may, even, merely be based just on what has been previously reported about them. Negative attitudes can mean stigmatising people for their differences and using it to justify discriminatory behaviour by treating them less favourably. This whole process can lead to self-fulfilling prophecies, as being unfairly blamed for being different may make the person more likely to act in this way. For example, being constantly accused of having a fiery temper may irritate red-haired people so much that they then do become angry. It can also lead to segregation, even when this is self-imposed. For example, those people with red hair may feel more comfortable mixing with other red-haired people as they share similar experiences.

Box 8.2 Example of bias and changing prejudice
Thirteen years old Susan always saw her schoolmates as better than pupils at the local grammar school. However, when she was offered the chance to take the Eleven Plus exam again and passed this time, she adopted the attitudes of pupils in her new school and judged those from her old school as inferior.

Tajfel's (1978) classical studies have demonstrated the human tendencies described above and that being a member of a group can mean adopting group prejudices even if these are not held personally. It was noted that those who change groups also change prejudices accordingly. These studies also identified a bias, in that the group 'we' belong to is usually perceived more favourably than other groups.

A particularly concerning aspect of this process is that people from minority groups who are relatively powerless and already unpopular are most likely to be used as scapegoats, that is, blamed for events for which they have no control.

This inherited cognitive ability to differentiate between similarities and differences between people's appearance and behaviour is evident early in life. By school age children have been found to categorise themselves in terms of their similarities or dissimilarities to others and identify with groups based on shared features. It appears that by three and four years of age children display 'intergroup' attitudes towards other social groups. This becomes more evident until they reach seven years of age, after which there is a slight decrease in this behaviour during late childhood and early adolescence. The extent to which children display prejudice to those considered to be from an 'outgroup' appears to depend on how strongly a child identifies with their own 'ingroup' and if they feel the status of their own 'ingroup' to be threatened in some way (Gonultas & Mulvey, 2019). Piumatti and Mosso (2017) carried out research into adolescents' views of immigration. They found that those adolescents displaying greater impulsivity and lack emotional control focussed strongly on negative aspects of immigrants, ignored their positive attributes, and were most likely to engage in ethnic harassment.

Whether attitudes are conveyed explicitly or implicitly appears to influence the extent to which they will be adopted. For example, Pirchio et al. (2018) demonstrated that children's prejudice may result more from the implicit messages passed on by a caregiver's behaviour than what they are told by them. Gonultas and Mulvey (2019) explained that it is often to please their parents and other authority figures that children often mimic their prejudicial attitudes and behaviours. They point out that the extent to which prejudice is passed on is influenced by the quality of the relationship between caregiver and child. Caregivers, therefore, wittingly, and unwittingly, become 'agents of social control' in ensuring that children conform to the behaviour expected within their specific social environment. However, during late adolescence the influence of caregiver's prejudicial attitudes has been found to decline.

Gonultas and Mulvey (2019) also point out the influence that sibling and peer relationships have in shaping attitudes. They found that prejudice declined over time in adolescents involved in low-prejudice peer networks, whilst prejudice expressed by adolescents who formed part of a high-prejudice network increased over time. Gonultas and Mulvey (2019) express particular concern about the impact of the media on enhancing prejudice and discrimination in children and adolescents. They cite an experimental study conducted in Australia which suggested that when exposed to symbolic and economic threats included in advertisements, adolescents' negative attitudes toward immigrants increased. However, it is difficult to tease out cause and effect when seeking the influence of the media on prejudice and aggressive behaviour. Long-term studies suggest that those children and adolescents already holding prejudicial views and displaying aggression will be influenced by media portrayal of prejudicial, aggressive behaviour (Schaffer, 2003).

8.2 Deviance As a Social Construct

Having explored how deviance results from inherited human capacities for categorisation and group membership, it is necessary to consider further the complex role it plays in Western society. Bronfenbrenner's (1979) bi-ecological theory suggests that children and adolescents are members of numerous subgroups within this complex society. Early influences derive from direct contact with family, school, and other groups and later, less directly from their community and eventually decisions made at governmental level. Indeed, Western society, itself, is one group coexisting with other powerful groups at a global level. This means that decisions about what constitutes deviancy can create tensions within and between each group at every level. It is beyond the scope of this book to do justice to the macro-sociological theories which try to explain the workings of the wider forces. However, taking an interactionist perspective does help to understand some of the ways group processes may even create as well as reduce deviancy, which can impact on the wellbeing of children and adolescents.

Given the diversity of human nature, it is not always possible for any group to meet the exact needs of every individual member. Therefore, rules need to be followed which ensure the survival of the group even if some members do not agree. Power, in some form or another, to enforce these rules lies at the heart of socialisation. Interactionist theory was influenced by Max Weber's (1864–1924) explanations of different ways that power is exercised. Power can be obtained through controlling the basic survival needs of others, and/or threatening to punish them if they do not comply. When considering complex groups, such as Western society, Weber found three other forms of control in addition to this raw form of coercive power. One form, charismatic authority, is based on some individual's personal characteristics which allow them to become leaders. However, power gained this way is not always stable and the benefits it offers not guaranteed to last once the leader dies. A second form, traditional power, can be gained through making people feel secure by promoting familiar, traditional customs. This helps those who already have power to maintain their control. A third type of authority enables some people to have legal power over others because of their position within a legally or rationally established hierarchy which already exists.

It is easy to identify these different forms of power just by considering how they are used in families to socialise children and ensure their acceptance into the culture into which they are born. For example, parents exercise direct power to ensure acceptable behaviour by withholding or promising something desired by the child. The charismatic, fun, caring personality of some parents may be used to gain acceptable behaviour from their child. Also, they have a recognised legal authority to control their child's behaviour. However, parents only have limited power overall, as they are part of a social hierarchy which includes others in even more powerful positions. This means that others have the power to legally remove a child from their parents who fail to fulfil their socialisation duties effectively.

Understanding how these forms of power can be identified within groups at all levels is important as it enables some members to decide and control what form of behaviour is approved of and what is deemed as deviant. It can be used indirectly through promoting the ideas and beliefs of those in positions of power so often that they become accepted as 'common sense'. This way of controlling the assumptions of group members (hegemony) is a particularly effective way of ensuring that, what those in powerful positions define as deviant behaviour is clearly recognised within the socialisation process of children and adolescents.

The interactionist approach is extremely useful in identifying some of the complex social processes involved in judging human behaviour and focusing on the social context which creates 'deviancy'. For example, within Western society, the removal of a child's clothes by an unfamiliar adult is considered as abusive and deviant behaviour, whilst it is legally approved of when taking place in a medical context. However, judgements regarding deviance can change over time through pressure from certain interested groups. For example, within the UK, homosexuality is now no longer illegal, and pressure from many women's groups has meant changes in the law regarding domestic violence.

Interactionist theory became particularly popular within sociology in the 1960s and 1970s. It sought a deeper understanding of human interactions within the social processes resulting from the rules and sanctions created by powerful groups. Cicourel (1976) found that power based on class meant that the backgrounds of certain youths determined the extent to which their behaviour was classed as deviant. For example, the same kinds of actions were deemed as youthful antics if the youths came from a middle- or upper-class background, but delinquent if they came from a working-class background. A striking example of this is cited by Punch et al. (2013). They describe how the serious damage to valuable items caused by a young male member of the very rich Sainsbury family, when he was part of an elite student group at Oxford University, was passed off as just due to high spirits. Giddens

(2000) also offers examples of the imbalance of power between various groups at many levels within Western society. He suggests that these can include power of the young over those who are old, rich people over poor people, men over women, and ethnic majorities over ethnic minorities. The power of the healthy over the ill, and able-bodied over those who are disabled, could also be added to this list.

8.2.1 Primary and Secondary Deviance

Interactionist theory describes the complex process in which those in specific social groups label others as deviant to serve their own interests, or because they think it might be good for society. Becker (1973) who was influenced by the ideas of Lemert (1951) describes two different stages of deviance. The first, primary stage, includes the actual act or appearance considered deviant. The second stage develops when this act or appearance is recognised by others and labelled as deviant. This suggests that many acts considered as deviant may go unnoticed, but once they are witnessed, then sanctions are administered and a whole labelling process evolves.

For example, two adolescents may become involved in shoplifting. The first youth may intend to stop shoplifting after stealing the next item but be caught and formally charged. A rather exaggerated but relevant outcome could be that having been labelled a thief, appeared in court, and given a police record, he is shunned by those close to him, identifies more with others who have also broken the law, and is drawn further towards a life of crime. In contrast, the second youth may never be caught out in his stealing and later pursue a respectable career and enjoy a comfortable, respectable life. In both cases the primary deviant act has been committed but only in the first case is it recognised and then, secondary deviance occurs with severe consequences for the youth's future life.

Goffman (1968) identified the severe consequences on a person's self-esteem if given a negative label. He explained how this leads to the person being stigmatised and seen of less value than others which impacts on their sense of 'self-worth'. Such labels are then used to stereotype the person and others who have similar characteristics, leading to prejudice, discrimination, and disadvantage. The level of stigmatisation a person may suffer will depend on how serious the 'devious' behaviour or appearance is perceived to be by others. If seen as very serious, the label can become the person's 'master status' which begins to dominate over any other attributes they may have. This means that in the example offered above, the adolescent who was caught stealing may now be labelled as 'a thief' for the rest of his life. Goffman (1961) suggests that when a label becomes a master status, it can be internalised and dominate a person's self-identity and future behaviour. Labelling can, therefore, create a self-fulfilling prophecy process as illustrated in Fig. 8.1.

Through studies carried out by observing the behaviour of people living in total institutions, such as prisons, mental hospitals, and monasteries, Goffman (1961) clearly identified this process in an extreme form. He termed it the 'mortification of the self' as the procedures and rituals experienced through having to adapt to life within such institutions mean the person losing their original identity and taking on

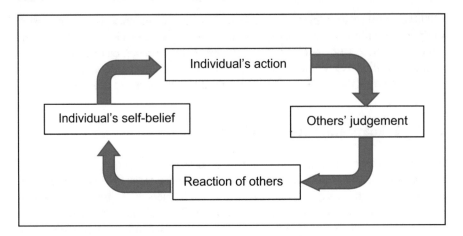

Fig. 8.1 The self-fulfilling prophecy process

a new one. This could also lead to difficulties in adapting to life outside the institu-tion. In cases such as prisons deviance can, therefore, be reinforced rather than reduced as prisoners accept their new identity.

Link and Phelan (2001) describe how the process of labelling leads to discrimi-nation as it involves a person or group being distinguished by some form of differ-ence based on what is already seen as important within a society, such as class, sex, and skin colour. Those with this attribute then become stereotyped, so that a division between 'them' and 'us' is created. This can then lead to those considered as 'them' to have less status and suffer discrimination. However, the ability to discriminate in this way will be determined by which group is already in a powerful position. For example, teachers hold positions of considerable power over students. Therefore (although they shouldn't!), teachers could stereotype students and treat them unfairly such that it affects a student's future career. In contrast the less powerful position of students means that although they may stereotype teachers and make their working life more difficult, this will not affect a teacher's future in quite the same way.

8.2.2 Amplification of Deviance and Moral Panics

The examples above illustrate how the labelling process is a powerful method of control both within and between groups. However, it has also become obvious that stigmatising people and groups can, unintentionally, increase deviance. This can be the case for adolescent males labelled as failures within the education system who reject the values of a society which they feel to have rejected them and form groups with similar others. Status within such groups may be achieved through acting in specific ways deemed deviant by mainstream society, but the greater the deviant act, the higher status achieved within the sub-group.

Young (1971) identified how the negative reactions of different powerful groups within society also amplify some forms of deviant behaviour. He studied marijuana use in Notting Hill and found that this 'peripheral activity' increased once users were labelled as 'drug takers' by the media and criminalised through increased legislation. Stigma from using marijuana meant the loss of jobs and social networks for users who became more reliant on the drug, as a pastime and source of income. Young (1971) pointed out that the creation of a specific drug squad (due to increased public concern) meant that it was possible to identify more users, resulting in more secondary deviance. Drug taking also increased amongst certain groups of young people, such as hippies. Hippies formed part of a movement emerging in the 1960s which challenged conventional values and sought a more 'back to nature' way of living. As some hippies' search for spiritual enlightenment involved taking hallucinogenic drugs all hippies came to be labelled as drug takers. This strengthened the shared identity within this group and created the expectation that anyone wanting to be a hippie would need to take drugs.

Although not the first to coin the term 'deviance amplification', Cohen (1972) used it after being influenced by Young's (1971) findings, to explain how deviancy amplification and moral panics allow those with more power in society to maintain their influence. Cohen (1972) found that in the 1950s and 1960s public anxiety was heightened by the way certain deviant events were reported so dramatically in the media. One example was the way newspapers reported a minor skirmish which took place between two adolescent groups, Mods and Rockers. Both groups attempted to flout traditional conventions but in very different ways. Mods adopted a highly detailed 'ultra-smart' appearance, rode scooters, and wore 'parka' jackets. In contrast, rockers rode motor bikes and dressed in black leather clothing. The main concern of those in both groups was being identified as member and having fun. However, some conflict, resulting in minor violence, developed between two groups of mods and rockers on a beach in the south of England, during a bank holiday.

Apparently, there was so little news to be reported at that time that newspapers gave considerable coverage to this event. This suggested it to be much more serious than it was and proof that British teenagers were becoming out of control. Such an interpretation touched a 'raw nerve' in public opinion. Many adults were still recovering from the effects of the Second World War and felt bewildered at the way adolescents were trying to establish a new identity for their generation. The result was great public fear of further violence, more young males identifying themselves as Mods or Rockers, and more fighting occurring between the two groups during subsequent bank holidays. As the media is owned and run by wealthy and powerful groups they benefitted financially from this kind of reporting. Also, some youths later claimed that they were paid by reporters to engage in the fighting.

> **Box 8.3 Personal account of the moral panic created by reports of fighting between mods and rockers**
> The amount of genuine public fear created by reports of these events can be testified by the first author. She clearly remembers, as a very young child, having a bank holiday trip to Scarborough (in the north of England) cancelled. Her parents had read frightening newspaper reports and were concerned about the rioting youths who had been predicted to be going to 'take over the town'. The result was that no mods or rockers appeared in Scarborough that weekend and there would have been quite a drop in tourist trade!

Public anxieties increased to such an extent that the reactions of those in authority, such as religious leaders, local councillors, magistrates, and politicians became more severe. There was greater police presence at seaside towns during bank holidays and any friction observed between Mods and Rockers was dealt with harshly. Cohen pointed out how such a minor skirmish had been transformed into a moral panic.

It appears that the more the media draw attention to certain deviant behaviour in dramatic, exaggerated ways, the more public anxiety is generated. It can also make such behaviour seem exciting to certain sub-groups such as young adolescent boys, who then copy the reported behaviour. Nijjar (2015) explains that moral panics occur every so often within the UK due to the stereotypical, stylistic media coverage of topics that threaten social values. This includes reporting the outraged reaction of those in authority such as editors, bishops, and politicians as well as the opinion of 'experts', who suggest reasons for the moral panic and potential solutions. The response to increased public concern and fear of challenges to current social rules often result in changes within legislation. Cohen, therefore, believed that control of what is covered by the media is a powerful way in which those already in positions of power can influence public opinion and justify measures that maintain their positions of authority.

Despite the appeal of Cohen's moral panic theory, Horsley (2017) considers it to be very much a product of its time and not relevant to the post-industrial capitalism currently dominating Western society. He sees it as patronising public concerns and underestimating public capacity for cynicism and points out how current, diverse forms of media means that traditional forms such as newspapers can be challenged and less influential. Horsley (2017, p. 11) also sees that those in power have to manage a tension between control and encouraging the 'ambition, competition and the pursuit of individualised desires' which he believes dominate post-industrial capitalism. He fears that accepting Cohen's theory creates a danger that really important issues may be dismissed as merely moral panics. However, Cohen also maintained that one of the challenging consequences of moral panics could be in recognising which issues needed to be taken seriously. It is also noticeable that points made by Horsley (2017) predated the COVID-19 pandemic, currently dominating the world at the time of writing this text. The way that the UK government have used the media to simultaneously scare, force, and cajole the public into complying with new social rules and legislation appears to reflect many of Cohen's concerns.

8.2.3 Current Relevance of Labelling Theory

Although the theory of moral panics may not be able to provide a sufficient explanation of the current, complex, competing power structures within Western society, it still provides a very useful way of understanding how perceptions of the changing status and roles of children and adolescents are generated within society and influence their wellbeing. For example, Nijjar (2015) studied how different newspapers covered the 2011 London riots in response to a fatal shooting by police of a British-born African-Caribbean male resident. The disorder was blamed by many sections of the press as the work of criminal youths with no sense of morality due to poor parenting. Young people's behaviour was referred to in lurid terms such as 'war and mass murder'. Just as Cohen would have predicted, politicians were cited who ignored the wider structural reasons for the youth's behaviour, focussing instead on a perceived lack of morals and discipline due to a decline in traditional family life. Nijjar (2015) found that some left-leaning newspapers did offer more complex explanations based on academic research, but all initially saw the riots as some individual traits of 'out of control' youths. Indeed, the Justice Secretary at the time, Kenneth Clarke, described the rioters as a 'feral underclass' suggesting they existed outside mainstream society. Much of the way the whole incident was reported still reflected the findings of Young (1971) and Cohen (1972).

Further examples of the implications of moral panics are offered by Clapton et al. (2013) in relation to media reports of 'satanic' child sexual abuse in the UK in the 1980s and 1990s. Although numerous children experiencing abuse had been removed from their families, it was the satanic practices said to be carried out by some families that became the focus of the media where it was described in terms of covens and devils. Later analysis found no evidence of satanic-based abuse but, at the time, such reporting had increased pressure on social services to root out such practices. Clapton et al. (2013) also cite further current child protection anxieties enhanced by media coverage, such as use of the internet, child trafficking, child 'grooming', and obesity.

Interestingly, there is a consistency about which issues are most likely to create moral panics. For example, Miller (2006) points out that reporting youth violence may create a panic whilst reporting class inequality does not, and referring to the dangers of 'rap' causes public anxiety whilst discussing the background of urban youth does not. It seems that concerns about children and adolescents can easily be turned into moral panics if they tap into existing adult anxieties about the state of an unknown future generation. Miller (2006) sees that the increased anxiety within societies based on moral panics stems from concern that young people will be unable to make mature future decisions. He offers examples of modern concerns about future control of nuclear energy, genocidal weaponry, biotechnology, and industrial pollution, alongside the remorseless news coverage of youth violence. Adult ambivalence towards children and adolescents, in terms of the desire to protect and yet control them, becomes particularly evident through moral panics. In the past their use of books, TV, and cinemas has been considered as potentially detrimental to their social development and monitored. However, monitoring the use and effect of new technology is less simple. Miller (2006) points out how their knowledge of new technology offers children and adolescents great power whilst leaving them vulnerable to its content. Increased proficiency in the use of technology by the young may threaten the power of adults to decide which social rules should be obeyed but, it also reduces their ability to offer protection.

8.3   Deviance and Agencies of Social Control

Socialisation involves exposure to group rules established by existing powerful agencies. Compliance is ensured by judging and monitoring the behaviour of children, adolescents, and their carers. Early socialisation begins through experiences within families, health and social care provision, and education. These systems are monitored by wider political and policing structures which legally enforce what is to be considered acceptable and what is deviant. It is useful to take an interactionist approach to appreciate how the wellbeing of children and adolescents is influenced by some of these different 'agencies of social control'.

8.3.1   Deviance, Crime, and Care

The interactionist explanations for criminal deviance help to explain how adverse experiences in childhood can lead to negative labelling and a later criminal career. As discussed previously, early experiences within the family have a powerful influence on children's development of self-identity and self-esteem. The quality of family relationships rather than family structure is particularly important as a low sense of self-worth has been identified as a causal factor in child and adolescent deviancy. Cross-cultural studies carried out by Vazsonyi et al. (2018) found that young people experiencing shared, close family activities were much less likely to be engaged in delinquency. Also, Shin et al. (2016) explain how links exist between different forms of familial childhood abuse and types of later criminal behaviour. Whilst physical abuse was related to all types of crime, impulsive property crime was found to result from child neglect. Property crimes, including vandalism and fraud, were also found to be impulsively carried out by those who had suffered early emotional abuse as an attempt to reduce stressful emotions, such as anger and hostility.

However, many family relationships are adversely influenced by the environment in which they exist, which is often through necessity rather than choice. For example, Bateman et al. (2018) point out how the youth justice population is dominated by vulnerable offenders from working-class backgrounds who have faced family poverty and neighbourhood deprivation. Young offenders are also more likely to have been excluded from school, victims of violence and practiced some form of self-harm. McAra and McVie (2016) describe the bidirectional causal relationship between victimisation and offending and how acquiring a conviction in childhood reduces future career prospects and increases the likelihood of later offences.

Children suffering abuse are often placed in some form of alternative care by social services which makes it even more likely that they will transition from the care system to criminal courts. For example, Bateman et al. (2018) explain how instability of placements, mixing with other vulnerable peers, and a readiness for police involvement all contribute to this process. They point to the influence of stigma attached to being in care and cite how social agencies within England and Wales admit that on occasions looked after child are 'needlessly criminalised'.

Bateman et al. (2018) also point out the over representation of black and minority ethnic (BAME) children and adolescents in the care and criminal systems. Such over representation also exists within wider Western society as, for example, Farrington et al. (2012) found a disproportionate number of both offenders and victims within male African Americans. Punch et al. (2013) explain that such inequality needs to be seen historically as it is more than just a result of inner-city poverty, rebellion, and lack of achievement leading to identification with a separate sub-culture.

On a more positive note, Bateman et al. (2018) point out the recent reduction in numbers of girls within the youth justice system. They explain how this follows a traditional trend as females have been less likely to follow a deviant career than males, through stricter socialisation and potentially more lenient treatment if arrested. In contrast, females are more likely to be victims of violence in their homes whilst males face such victimisation in public. In both cases there is greater probability that the aggressor will be male, as they are more physically powerful and aggressive than females (Punch et al., 2013). Violence committed by girls is often a way of asserting a 'sense of self' due to an inability to escape from an impoverished background and destructive relationships (McAra & McVie, 2016).

Overall, McAra and McVie (2016) believe that violence is a way that both disempowered young males and females attempt to gain status and a sense of self-worth and that perpetrators should be considered vulnerable rather than criminalised and punished. They advocate a more holistic approach, including greater understanding of violent adolescents' needs, rather than labelling and stigmatising them. However, they also admit that this requires a commitment to tackling social and economic inequalities and great 'courage and vision' by those responsible for policy making but, insist that it is necessary to create a more inclusive society.

8.3.2 Labelling in Education

The education system offers a prime example of an 'over-indulgence' of the human capacity to categorise experiences and make emotional and social judgements about others. As a result, it can have devastating consequences for some individuals given that it attempts to classify students on their ability to meet identified standards created by specific societies within specific historical periods. Some, concrete, agreed educational standards are assumed which, if not achieved, suggest deficiency within students with damaging consequences in terms of their self-esteem and future careers. Achievement within education offers more than an ability to read, write, and carry out maths. Educational success offers people a greater understanding of their place in society and, if successful, a greater ability to negotiate their position to gain more control over their lives. Ensuring their child receives 'a good education', particularly if this involves attending a private rather than state school, is one way that parents can help improve their child's future wellbeing. Such a situation makes it even more devastating for those children born into a position where such opportunities are limited. For example, failure within education is prevalent amongst those children and adolescents from poorer areas and linked to criminal deviancy. Middle-class values which dominate state schools are often unachievable for working-class students, creating status frustration and alternative values of toughness.

However, a critical appreciation is required of current classifications of what is included in a 'good education'. There is a need to consider who are qualified to make such judgments, what grounds they are based on, and the scientific rigour of supporting evidence. For example, a salutary lesson needs to be learned about the validity of the 'Eleven Plus' examination introduced to determine which children aged eleven were destined for an academic, technical, or practical future career. The origin of this exam was heavily influenced by the educational psychologist Sir Cyril Burt's work on the heritability of intelligence. Soon after Burt's death some of this work was discredited as based on falsified research data. Some, such as Rushton (2002), question these criticisms, suggesting that this data may have been gathered by other educational psychologists on Burt's behalf. Nevertheless, that the credibility of such an exam has been questioned suggests that it provides shaky ground on which to grade children which has considerable impact on their future self-esteem, education, and careers. Also, it is important to consider the different rates of development in children and how they have varied learning styles under various conditions. What is considered as a good education is influenced by tradition and maintained by those in power, such as politicians. Within the UK, academic achievement gained by means of a national curriculum is explained as necessary to produce a more able competitive work force and ensure the country excels within world competition. Teachers are forced into constant grading through governmental pressure for regular testing and publishing results as league tables. All this influences funding, resources, and staff morale which can have negative effects on experiences of children and adolescents.

There is limited space within this text to do full justice to the issues outlined above, but it is important to consider how an educational system based on constant classification of specific children's abilities offers a clear example of the impact of labelling on the lives of children and adolescents. This becomes particularly evident when considering those unable to meet rigorous educational standards and, therefore, labelled as having 'special educational needs'.

In contemporary Western society, professionals from medicine and psychology have the power to decide which children should be labelled as SEN (having special educational needs) and Arishi et al. (2017) explain that this is not always as objective or value-free as claimed. Diagnosing a specific debilitating condition involves an amount of socially determined bias. For example, Algraigray and Boyle (2017) point out that of children and adolescents labelled SEN, 60% have an ambiguous diagnosis. Also, the amount and type of resources available can influence decisions as to whether a child is seen as having such needs and able to be included or excluded from mainstream educational provision.

The effects of labelling a child or adolescent as having special educational needs are ambiguous as it can have both negative and positive effects. For example, knowing that a student has attended a 'special school' can influence future employment, but the label 'SEN' can also prove an 'admission ticket' to services not otherwise available (Arishi et al., 2017). It can also be used to improve communication between professionals, children, adolescents, and their families, as well as increasing public awareness of the need to support those who may require additional resources within education.

Despite some positive effects, labelling still needs to be considered in terms of just which labels are used and who can control their use. For example, Arishi et al. (2017) point out the different effects of using the labels 'dyslexia' and 'reading difficulties'. Being 'diagnosed' as dyslexic suggests some unavoidable medical condition and it is likely to illicit sympathy. Such a diagnosis can be obtained by means of expensive tests, which may be accessed by educationally aware parents, who are keen to avoid their child being stigmatised. In contrast, using a term such as 'reading difficulties' implies a deficiency in something that should be 'normal' and can create stigma, restrictions, and lowered expectations of teachers and parents. Arishi et al. (2017) also stress how labelling can exaggerate the differences between those with special educational needs and those who do not have these needs, such that there is failure to 'look beyond the label'. They suggest that this creates an imaginary subculture requiring conformity from those given the label SEN.

Such labelling risks creating outsiders which, according to Becker (1963), suggests a deviation from the mean, resulting from an inability to conform to certain socially required standards. Algraigray and Boyle (2017) believe that the label 'SEN students' raises broader concerns of social justice, equity, and human rights and helps to make artificially created differences within an unequal society seem normal. They explain how the very UK Disability Discrimination Act (1995) is based on concepts from medical science and expressed through powerful language. This allows professionals to identify and classify people as having special educational needs due to some form of dysfunction, creating exclusion from mainstream society, and impacting on students' wellbeing.

8.3.3   Labelling and Health

Although further reference to labelling will be made within later chapters on medicalisation and long-term, complex conditions, it is worth considering here just what a powerful effect this has on the health and healthcare experienced by children and adolescents. From an interactionist perspective ill health becomes a form of deviance given that people are expected to feel well. Doctors and other health professionals can be considered as 'agents of social control'; in that they have the power to decide if an illness or disability is legitimate and, therefore, requires special consideration from others in society. The symptoms of the illness or disability constitute 'primary' deviance and the diagnosis (a label) ascribed to these initiates 'secondary' deviance as it determines the reaction of others. For example, a child labelled as 'disabled' may be assumed to be unable to take part in many activities, denied opportunities to test out their abilities, and become passively compliant. Also, self-fulfilling prophecies may occur, such as if a child diagnosed with attention deficit hyperactivity disorder (ADHD), or teenager diagnosed with schizophrenia, loses their temper in frustrating circumstances, their actions are more likely to be viewed as cause for alarm. Therefore, a medical diagnosis is more than a convenient classification, but rather part of an interaction which, if becomes their 'master status', impacts on the patient's identity and influences their future interactions with others.

Cultural responses to medical labels define them as positive, neutral, or negative. For example, diagnoses, such as influenza and the common cold, experienced by most people are neutral labels whilst others less common such as epilepsy and schizophrenia attract negative responses including stigma. Indeed, overemphasis on certain labels can create health-based moral panics. For example, Moffat (2010) explains how increased references to childhood obesity in medical literature during the late 1990s made it a public-political issue resulting in media accounts of an 'obesity epidemic' such that it has become a legitimate medical and societal problem, attracting research funding. They stress how as the term 'obesity' is often linked to a lack of control leading to gluttony it is used to stigmatise and discriminate against overweight others. The impact of such stigma during childhood and adolescence is particularly detrimental as it can impact upon self-esteem and lead to either greater comfort eating or unhealthy dieting. A further complexity within the issue of childhood obesity is that it is more prevalent in children from low socioeconomic and ethnic minority groups; therefore, further media coverage risks exacerbating established stereotypes and greater marginalisation.

Chronically ill or disabled children and adolescents' experiences of perceived stigmatisation can be usefully explained through Goffman's concepts of 'discreditable' (potential) and 'discrediting' (existing) stigma. Discreditable stigma is faced by those who can hide signs of their condition/disability, which means they will often go to great lengths to do so, but always be in fear of exposure. In contrast, other ill/disabled children and adolescents who cannot conceal their condition/disability experience discrediting stigma by having to face daily negative reactions of others to their appearance and/or behaviour. Juvenile arthritis is a good example of when children and adolescents may, at different times, face both types of stigma. The variable nature of this condition can mean that on some occasions they face discreditable stigma, as although in pain, they may look physically well and work hard to fit in with their peers. However, at other times, those with this condition may face discreditable stigma, as they need to use crutches or wheelchairs and face other children's or adolescents' reactions. Fear of stigmatisation by peers is particularly acute during childhood and adolescents and Goffman pointed out that occasionally the fear of being stigmatised (felt stigma) can be greater than that which is experienced (enacted stigma).

The powerful effects of labelling in relation to child and adolescent health cannot be underestimated. Those working with very young children know to be wary of using expressions such as 'your bad leg' even in relation to a simple accidental fracture. Young children may take this literally as a judgement that their leg has done something wrong or 'gone bad'. This also highlights the way that once a diagnosis has been made it somehow becomes 'owned' by the patient, as for example when referring to 'Susan's asthma' or 'John's tumour'. Labelling may offer a way of recognising and responding to well-recognised physical conditions but can prove detrimental for those diagnosed with less understood conditions such as epilepsy and schizophrenia. Indeed, such diagnoses often take over the identity of a person to the extent that they are referred to as 'epileptics' or 'schizophrenics' (Link & Phelan, 2001).

Whilst some labels, such as being a 'child asthmatic', can be discarded as a child develops and symptoms cease, the case is not so simple in terms of mental health conditions. Rosenhan (1973) explains how diagnoses such as 'schizophrenic' or 'manic-depressive' are expected to last a lifetime and can lead to segregation, mortification, and self-labelling. O'Connor et al. (2020) point out how psychiatric diagnoses are not always reliable and can distract from the way distress is often caused by personal and social circumstances. They admit that diagnoses within mental health have been considered as a form of social control but explain that in practice, most clinicians will attempt to avoid or soften specific diagnoses, as acutely aware of how these may influence the future of children and adolescents.

Children and adolescents with mental health problems may face further discrimination if they need treatment within general healthcare settings. For example, Sukhera (2017) found that due to heavy workload and limited resources, staff working in paediatric emergency departments often labelled them as time-consuming, unpredictable, and/or unfixable, resulting in unintended discrimination. However, it is particularly important to be aware of the impact of labelling and stigma within mental health given that O'Connor et al. (2020) point to the current increased numbers of childhood emotional, behavioural, and neurodevelopmental disorders. Also, Bor et al. (2014) report a disturbing increase in child and adolescent mental health problems, particularly in relation to depression amongst adolescent girls.

8.3.4 Labelling, Parenting, and Family Life

As explained within previous chapters, within current Western society, 'ideal' parenting involves two devoted parents, dutifully placing their child's needs above their own and taking full responsibility for his or her future development and behaviour. Indeed, over-zealous reactions to the current pressure on parents to live up to such an ideal in a world increasingly perceived as risky have meant that moral panics of over-protective, paranoid parenting have been noted (see Furedi, 2008). However, many parents fear falling too short of such an 'ideal', given that social agencies, such as the media, are quick to stigmatise them by ascribing 'eye-catching' labels which may initiate further moral panics. Clapton et al. (2013) explain how this consistently increases the different types of child protection issues faced by under-resourced social services whose support for parents is often rejected by them in fear of being labelled a 'bad' mother or father. They offer the example of difficulties in identifying and reducing current concerns with the complex concept of 'emotional neglect'. They describe how the media (including popular soaps and fiction), charities, politicians, and fund raisers may contribute to increasing public anxiety and result in the greater prosecution of parents failing to emotionally nurture their children.

Parents are also often stigmatised for raising 'out of control' deviant adolescents to such an extent that this, too, creates a moral panic. Nijjar (2015) points out how long-standing social anxieties about the difficulties of controlling the behaviour of adolescents are used to explain many social troubles. She describes how those responsible for the 2011 London riots were reported to have been raised in 'troubled families' caused by increased 'single-parent families' (headed by mothers) which were to blame for the current 'moral collapse'. Other forms of family structure may also be stigmatised, for example, Prendergast and MacPhee (2018) explain that, despite current policy changes, same sex parents often experience stigmatisation and discrimination which impact on the whole family.

Box 8.4 Example of courtesy (associative) stigma

An example of courtesy stigma was offered by a past student. She described how, on her first day when starting school, each child was asked by their teacher to call out their names. After the student had called out her name, the teacher replied, in front of the whole class:

'Well so long as you do not cause as much trouble as your Uncle Andrew did, you will be alright!'

That other family members are also affected by parental stigma demonstrates how labelling can prove 'contagious. Goffman termed this 'courtesy' stigma, and it is also known as 'associative stigma'. Wenham (2020) explains how this can simply result from attending the same school as a sibling or other relative who had been considered by teachers to be 'difficult' or 'talented'. Being similarly labelled through such association can impact on a child's self-esteem.

Parents may suffer courtesy stigma through their children being perceived as 'different', due to some form of disability. Fearing that this may be considered as a failing within them, some parents may attempt to disguise the extent of the child's disability or, if this is not possible, limit their own social life. Mitter et al. (2019) describe how, despite rewarding aspects of caring for a learning disabled child, this can mean feeling of less value than other parents, resulting in lowered self-esteem and damaging family relationships. Other family members may also fear associative stigma so distance themselves from their relative with the learning disability. Similar experiences may be faced by families in which a member has been diagnosed with a mental health problem. When studying families of adolescents who self-harm, Ferrey et al. (2016) found that parents would often withdraw from social contact in fear of being stigmatised, and siblings were often worried that they would face stigma from peers.

Despite many, very positive, current attempts to improve public understanding of mental health problems and learning disabilities, it appears that such diagnoses still create distress from the reactions of others. One of a variety of explanations for such continued stigmatisation could be that they are a result of the innate capacities for categorisation within humans which not only helps to understand and predict the behaviour of others, but also helps to judge what responses are appropriate. The potentially unpredictable nature of interactions with those with a learning disability or mental health problem can make it difficult for others to know how to react appropriately, making them feel uncomfortable and out of control. This discomfort is relieved by blaming the learning disabled or mentally ill person as 'deviant' and stigmatising them. Stigmatising can, therefore, result from the respondent's need to feel 'back in control' and 'normal', rather than refer to something intrinsic within those with a learning disability or mental health problem. A further (unjustified and unacceptable) explanation from a functionalist perspective is that, as the behaviour of those labelled as having a learning disability or mental health problem is unpredictable, they are potentially less able to contribute to the continued functioning of society and, therefore, of less value. It is also interesting to note that there is ambiguity in the status of those who work with stigmatised groups such as those who are classed as mentally ill, learning disabled, and/or users of social services. Whilst often admired for undertaking jobs that can be challenging at times, staff also face possible stigmatisation through association resulting in low pay and/or lack of resources (Arishi et al., 2017).

However, despite the inevitability of attitude formation based on an innate human capacity to categorise experiences of others, some comfort can be gained from awareness that over time, constant exposure to contradiction to stereotypes, increased education, and concerted public awareness, changes can take place in the different balances of power within groups. Punch et al. (2013) offer a particularly heartening example of such changes. They report that due to experiencing stigma and discrimination, children from Afro-American families were found to have low self-esteem; however, after the huge social upheaval within the 1960s created changes within the socio-political climate, this has reversed, and they now see themselves much more positively. As well as seeking to reduce unjustified prejudice at a societal level it is important that those responsible for children and adolescents are mindful of their own inherited potential for making assumptions and constantly reflect upon their own beliefs to guard against causing distress for those in their care.

Summary

- Deviance is socially constructed as behaving or looking 'different' to most people is seen as breaking rules necessary for a groups' survival. Rules are enforced in different ways (often by the most powerful members). Group members whose behaviour or appearance is not compatible with group rules are identified as 'deviant' and depending upon the severity of their 'deviance', face negative attitudes from others, sanctions, and punishment.

- Interactionist theory explains that it is only when rule breaking is publicly recognised that it incurs sanctions. Being labelled as a 'deviant' can mean being stigmatised which impacts on an individual's future life. Public attitudes involve prejudging (often on little evidence) and stereotyping those thought most likely to break social rules and act towards them in discriminatory ways. Such negative public response can mean that those seen as deviant internalise this label and it becomes their 'master' status, dominating their self-identity. Public concern for certain kinds of deviancy (often enflamed by the media) can mean it becomes amplified through the resulting moral panics creating and self-fulfilling prophecies.
- Within Western society interactions between networks of complex subgroups combine to ensure individual compliance to social rules. Deviant behaviour judged as criminal through government legislation is identified and punished by means of a judicial system. Compliance to social rules is also ensured by other agencies such as social services and education as well as socialisation within family life. Stigma can be experienced by merely being associated with those labelled as deviant, even if this is through work. The potential prejudice resulting from such processes needs to be acknowledged, and assumptions made at societal and individual levels to avoid causing unfair discrimination and distress to others.

Case Study Questions

Read the family case study on page 265 and consider the following:

- What explanations can be given for Ben's shop lifting and how might this affect his future?
- How helpful would it be for Liam to be statemented as having special educational needs?
- How might Chrissy's family background impact on how well she later settles into school?

Reflective Questions:

- To what extent can deviancy be said to be socially constructed?
- How well do the theories of labelling and 'moral panics' explain deviancy?
- In what ways can being negatively labelled when young impact on a person at different stages of their lifespan?

References

Algraigray, H., & Boyle, C. (2017). The SEN Label and its Effect on Special Education. *Educational and Child Psychologist, 34*(4), 1–19. http://hdl.handle.net/10871/29376
Arishi, L., Boyle, C., & Lauchlan, F. (2017). Inclusive Education and the Politics of Difference: Considering the Effectiveness of Labelling in Special Education. *The Educational and Child Psychologist, 34*(4), 1–24. http://hdl.handle.net/10871/29377

Bateman, T., Day, A.-M., & Pitts, J. (2018). *Looked after Children and Custody: A Brief Review of the Relationship between Care Status and Child Incarceration and the Implications for Service Provision*. University of Bedford and Nuffield Foundation Report, 1–37. Retrieved April 15, 2021, from Nuffield-Literature-review-final.pdf (openrepository.com)

Becker, H. S. (1963). *Outsiders: Studies in the Sociology of Deviance*. Free Press.

Becker, H. S. (1973). *Deviance and Social Control*. Routledge.

Blakemore, S.-J., & Mills, K. L. (2014). Is Adolescence a Sensitive Period for Sociocultural Processing? *Annual review of Psychology, 65*, 1870–1207. https://doi.org/10.1146/annurev-psych-010213-115202

Bor, W., Dean, A. J., Najman, J., & Hayatbakhsh, R. (2014). Are Child and Adolescent Mental Health Problems Increasing in the 21st Century? A Systematic Review. *Australian & New Zealand Journal of Psychiatry, 48*(7), 606–616. https://doi.org/10.1177/0004867414533834

Bronfenbrenner, U. (1979). *The Ecology of Human Development: Experiments by the Nature of Design*. Harvard University Press.

Cicourel, A. V. (1976). *The Social Organization of Juvenile Justice*. Heinemann.

Clapton, G., Cree, V. E., & Smith, M. (2013). Moral Panics, Claims-Making and Child Protection in the UK. *British Journal of Social Work, 43*(4), 803–812. https://doi.org/10.1093/bjsw/bct061

Cohen, S. (1972). *Folk Devils and Moral Panics: The Creation of the Mods and Rockers*. Martin Roberts.

Cooley, C. H. (1902). *Human Nature and Social Order*. Charles Scibner.

Farrington, D. P., Loeber, R., & Berg, M. T. (2012). Young Men Who Kill: A Prospective Longitudinal Examination from Childhood. *Homicide Studies, 16*(2), 99–128. https://doi.org/10.1177/1088767912439398

Ferrey, A. E., Hughes, N. D., Simkin, S., Locock, L., Stewart, A., Kapur, N., Gunnell, D., & Hawton, K. (2016). The Impact of Self-Harm by Young People on Parents and Families: A Qualitative Study. *BMJ Open, 6*, 1–27. e009631. https://doi.org/10.1136/bmjopen-2015-009631.

Furedi, F. (2008). *Paranoid Parenting: Why Ignoring the Experts may be Best for your Child* (3rd ed.). Continuum.

Giddens, A. (2000). *Sociology*. Polity Press.

Goffman, E. (1961). *Asylums*. Penguin.

Goffman, E. (1968). *Stigma*. Penguin.

Gonultas, S., & Mulvey, K. L. (2019). Social-Developmental Perspective on Intergroup Attitudes towards Immigrants and Refugees in Childhood and Adolescence: A Roadmap from Theory to Practice for an Inclusive Society. *Human Development, 63*, 90–111. https://doi.org/10.1159/000503173

Horsley, M. (2017). Forget 'Moral Panics'. *Journal of Theoretical and Philosophical Criminology, 9*(2), 84–98. http://hdl.handle.net/10034/620884

Kagan, J. (1981). *The Second Year: The Emergence of Self-Awareness*. Harvard University Press.

Kagan, J. (2018). Three Unresolved Issues in Human Morality. *Perspectives on Psychological Science, 13*(3), 346–358. https://doi.org/10.1177/1745691617727862

Kagan, J., & Snidman, N. (1991). Temperamental Factors in Human Development. *American Psychologist, 46*, 856–862.

Komorosky, D., & O'Neal, K. K. (2015). The Development of Empathy and Prosocial Behavior through Humane Education, Restorative Justice, and Animal-Assisted Programs. *Contemporary Justice Review, 18*(4), 395–406. https://doi.org/10.1080/10282580.2015.1093684

Kotler, J. S., & McMahon, R. J. (2005). Child Psychopathy: Theories, Measurement, and Relations with the Development and Persistence of Conduct Problems. *Clinical Child and Family Psychology Review, 8*(4), 291–235. https://doi.org/10.1007/s10567-005-8810-5

Lemert, E. M. (1951). *Social Pathology; A Systematic Approach to the theory of Sociopathic Behavior*. McGrawhill.

Link, B. G., & Phelan, J. C. (2001). Conceptualizing Stigma. Annual Review. *Sociology., 27*, 363–385. http://www.jstor.org/stable/2678626

Lorenz, K. (1966). *On Aggression*. Methuen.

Marshall, L. E., & Marshall, W. L. (2011). Empathy and Antisocial Behaviour. *Journal of Forensic Psychiatry & Psychology, 22*(5), 742–759. https://doi.org/10.1080/14789949.2011.617544

McAra, L., & McVie, S. (2016). Understanding Youth Violence: The Mediating effects of Gender, Poverty and Vulnerability. *Journal of Criminal Justice, 45*, 71–77. https://doi.org/10.1016/j.jcrimjus.2016.02.011

Miller, T. (2006). A Risk Society of Moral Panic. The USA in the Twenty first Century. *Cultural Politics, 2*(3), 299–318.

Mitter, N., Alia, A., & Scior, K. (2019). Stigma Experienced by Families of Individuals with Intellectual Disabilities and autism: A Systematic Review. *Research in Developmental Disabilities, 89*, 10–12. https://doi.org/10.1016/j.ridd.2019.03.001

Moffat, T. (2010). The "Childhood Obesity Epidemic": Health Crisis or Social Construction? *Medical Anthropology Quarterly, New Series, 24*(1), 1–21. https://www.jstor.org/stable/40606173

Nijjar, J. (2015). 'Menacing Youth' and 'Broken Families': A Critical Discourse Analysis of the Reporting of the 2011 English Riots in the Daily Express Using Moral Panic Theory. *Sociological Research Online, 20*(4), 10. http://www.socresonline.org.uk/20/4/10.html. https://doi.org/10.5153/sro.3793

O'Connor, C., Downs, J., McNicholas, F., Cross, L., & Shetty, H. (2020). A Content Analysis of Diagnostic Statements in a Psychiatric Case Register. *Children and Youth Services Review, 113*(1049482), 1–10. https://doi.org/10.1016/j.childyouth.2020.104948

Pirchio, S., Passiatore, Y., Panno, A., Maricchiolo, F., & Carrus, G. (2018). A Chip Off the Old Block: Parents' Subtle Ethnic Prejudice Predicts Children's Implicit Prejudice. *Frontiers in Psychology, 9*(110), 1–9. https://doi.org/10.3389/fpsyg.2018.00110

Piumatti, G., & Mosso, C. (2017). Relationships Between Individual Endorsement of Aggressive Behaviors and Thoughts with Prejudice Relevant Correlates Among Adolescents. *Europe's Journal of Psychology, 2017, 13*(1), 47–59. https://doi.org/10.5964/ejop.v13i1.1223

Plomin, R. (2019). *Blueprint: How DNA Makes Us Who We Are*. MIT Press.

Prendergast, S., & MacPhee, D. (2018). Family Resilience Amid Stigma and Discrimination: A Conceptual Model for Families Headed by Same-Sex Parents. *Family Relations. Interdisciplinary Journal of Applied Family Science, 67*(1), 26–40. https://doi.org/10.1111/fare.12296

Punch, S., Marsh, I., Keating, M., & Harden, J. (2013). *Sociology. Making Sense of Society* (5th ed.). Pearson Educational Ltd..

Rosenhan, D. L. (1973). On Being Sane in Insane Places. *Santa Clara Lawyer, 13*(3), 379–399. http://digitalcommons.law.scu.edu/lawreview/vol13/iss3/3

Rushton, J. P. (2002). New Evidence on Sir Cyril Burt: His 1964 Speech to the Association of Educational Psychologists. *Intelligence, 30*(6), 555–567. https://doi.org/10.1016/S0160-2896(02)00094-6

Schaffer, H. R. (2003). *Social Development*. Blackwell.

Shin, S. H., Cook, A. K., Morris, N. A., McDougle, R., & Peasley Groves, L. (2016). The Different Faces of Impulsivity as Links Between Childhood Maltreatment and Young Adult Crime. *Preventive Medicine, 88*, 210–217. https://doi.org/10.1016/j.ypmed.2016.03.022

Sukhera, J., Miller, K., Milne, A., Scerbo, C., Lim, R., Cooper, A., & Watling, C. (2017). Labelling of Mental Illness in a Paediatric Emergency Department and its Implications for Stigma Reduction Education. *Perspectives in Medical Education, 6*, 165–172. https://doi.org/10.1007/s40037-017-0333-5

Tajfel, H. (1978). Social Categorization, Social Identity and Social Comparison. In H. Tajfel (Ed.), *Differentiation Between Social Groups*. Academic Press.

Tajfel, H., & Turner, J. C. (1986). The Social Identity Theory of Intergroup Behavior. In S. Worchel & W. G. Austin (Eds.), *Psychology of Intergroup Relations* (pp. 7–24). Nelson-Hall.

Van Teijlingan, E. R., & Humphris, G. (Eds.). (2019). *Psychology and Sociology Applied to Medicine* (4th ed.). Elsevier.

Vazsonyi, A. T., Javakhishvili, M., & Ksinan, A. J. (2018). Routine Activities and Adolescent Deviance Across 28 Cultures. *Journal of Criminal Justice, 57*, 56–66. https://doi.org/10.1016/j.jcrimjus.2018.03.005

Wenham, L. (2020). 'It was more a Fear of the School thinking that I'd be a Troublemaker'— Inappropriate use of Internal Exclusion through Labelling by Association with Siblings. *Journal for Critical Education Policy Studies, 18*(3), 154–187. http://www.jceps.com/archives/10176

Young, J. (1971). *The Drug Takers: The Social Meaning of Drug Use*. MacGibbon and Kee.

'Medicalisation' and Surveillance of Children and Adolescents' Lives

9

9.1 Changing Attitudes Towards 'Difference' in Appearance and Behaviour

'Medicalisation' refers to the way that, within Western society, many aspects of a person's appearance, behaviour, life stages, and daily living are increasingly seen as health issues. For example, children's lives are monitored from birth by adults, who measure their development and seek medical attention and possible interventions when this does not appear to be consistent with what is considered typical. Ensuring this 'normalisation' of children is explained by professionals as necessary to protect them from future distress, disability, and harm. However, although some medical interventions, such as operating to prevent a severe physical disability, can be easily justified, others such as surgery to ensure a child's ears do not 'stick out' are more questionable.

The positive impact that advances within medical knowledge and treatments has had in reducing child and adolescent mortality rates and improving physical health generally cannot be overstated. However, despite the undeniable, often lifesaving benefits of many procedures within medicine and health promotion, the increasingly intense monitoring and search for a potential 'ideal' health status can have a negative impact on mental wellbeing. For example, Morrall (2009) expresses concern about the way that the medical profession and pharmaceutical companies are increasingly encouraging a 'medical hegemony' (accepted way of thinking) through promoting an 'ideal' appearance and lifestyle. He points out how such ideas are then exploited by the manufacturers of health and beauty products as well as the sport, fashion, advertising, and entertainment industries. That new discoveries and increased technology within medicine have raised the possibility of manipulating genes, which could be used to ensure that future children physically conform to what is considered 'normal' in their specific culture is a cause for alarm. Timimi et al. (2011) warn against such practices as they reflect elements of the past eugenic movement, which aimed to eradicate many forms of human 'differences' through forced sterilisation. All this suggests that it is important to consider who decides when some form of 'difference' becomes a medical issue and under what circumstances.

9.1.1   Bad, Mad, or Sad? Pathologising Children's and Adolescents' Behaviour

Within Western society, prior to the eighteenth century, religious beliefs (including demonic possession) informed explanations of why some children and adolescents seemed 'different', and physical force was used to correct their unacceptable behaviour. The gradual decline of religious influence and increased confidence in science have meant that a medical approach is now taken to explain and treat such behaviour, which is seen as due to a mental illness rather than being possessed or naturally evil. Although interpreting unusual behaviour as due to a mental illness is perceived as kinder and more humane it can still have adverse consequences, such as forced medication and stigma. Morrall (2001) concludes, that it is better to be considered as 'mad' and drugged rather than burnt as a witch. Nevertheless, questions still need to be asked about just how more humane it is to 'label' children and adolescents as mentally 'ill' rather than 'bad' and the positive and/or negative impact of such labels.

Both approaches reveal the continued tension between nurturing or disciplining children and adolescents to ensure that they conform to what adults perceive to be the ideal way for them to look and behave. Their appearance and behaviour, therefore, are judged on a ranked scale, suggesting that some form of 'perfection' is possible. Those children and adolescents whose behaviour falls short of such perfection are deemed 'difficult' and, according to Wright (2009), considered as 'bad, mad or sad'. Each label has different consequences. However, although those considered as bad usually follow a pathway through the juvenile criminal system, all will at some point receive attention from medical professionals attempting to change the way they behave.

According to Wright (2009) bad children are perceived as out of control, socially irresponsible, or having an anti-social or sociopathic pathology. Concern about delinquent youths has, therefore, meant the increased involvement of many professionals including psychologists, physicians, and lawyers. The introduction of juvenile courts within the UK in 1908, which were more sensitive to stages of child development and potential rehabilitation, offered some benefits over the adult criminal system but also meant relinquishing some rights. For example, juveniles cannot opt to be tried by a jury and are subject to compulsory probation service interventions.

Children and adolescents who display atypical emotional responses and behaviours are often perceived as 'mad' due to some 'chemical imbalance, diet, or gene disturbance' (Wright, 2009). A diagnosis is sought for their behaviour through testing, and assessments leading to some form of intervention to modify their actions.

Children and adolescents displaying 'difficult' behaviour may now be classified as suffering from a specific disorder. For example, in 1965 disorders such as oppositional defiance disorder and conduct disorders (based purely on their observed behaviour) were added to the section on mental disorders within the International Classification of Diseases (ICD). Oppositional defiance disorder includes negative, hostile, or defiant behaviour. Conduct disorders include behaving aggressively to people and animals, deliberately destroying property, deceit, theft, and seriously violating the basic rights of others or age-appropriate societal norms and rules (Costello & Angold, 2004). Attempts to treat such disorders are often varied and can include behaviour training, medication such as Ritalin, or both.

Children and adolescents who Wright (2009) describes as 'sad' have often experienced abuse, trauma, neglect, or bereavement. Their behaviour is usually diagnosed as due to 'anxiety' and/or 'depression' and therefore, a mental health issue. Wright (2009) reports the successful use of variety of therapeutic techniques in relation to treating such conditions. However, here, as with diagnoses of other mental health conditions, there is always the risk of stigma leading to further prejudice and discrimination amongst peers. Heary et al. (2017) report that negative attitudes to mental illness have been found in children as young as five years of age then fluctuate as children develop. Adolescents with mental health issues were found to be particularly vulnerable to stigma. For example, Heary et al. (2017) found that some peers judged adolescents suffering depression as 'weak' rather than sick. Also, adolescents diagnosed with attention deficit disorder (ADHD) were perceived by peers as dangerous and more likely to get into trouble than those diagnosed with a physical condition such as asthma. Sadly, adolescents expected that they too would suffer prejudice from other peers if they befriended an adolescent diagnosed with ADHD.

In some ways, medical interventions can be perceived as forms of internal control replacing the incarceration and exclusion experienced by those previously labelled 'bad' or 'mad'. Also, the very basis of mental health can become questionable. Unlike physical health, it is very difficult to define what it is to be in good mental health. Van Teijlingen and Humphris (2019) suggest that some mental health diagnoses may be based on flawed data within mental health research. They also point out how different conditions can change over time. For example, they point out how the current diagnosis of 'gender dysphoria' now replaces that previously described as 'gender identity disorder' (1994), which in turn replaced the term 'transsexualism' (1980). That 'gender dysphoria' is now considered a medical condition rather than choice of behaviour can have a serious impact on public expectations. It may suggest that for some, 'suffering' this disorder is not a choice, but it is important to consider how both views may influence vulnerable adolescents struggling to develop an emerging sexual identity. Decisions to medically change biological sex may appear straightforward but include hormone treatments with the potential to cause future fertility problems and serious side effects which can compromise the heart.

9.1.2   Atypical Child Development and the 'Sick Role'

Classifying children and adolescents as suffering from some form of 'condition', requiring treatment because they do not fit expectations of typical development, appears to be due to concern that they should be fit to carry out their future social responsibilities. Such a view underpins the sick role theory suggested by Talcott Parsons (1951). Parsons noted that different types of deviance were increasingly being classified as 'illnesses' within Western society with medical treatments and psychotherapy used instead of exclusion or punishment.

Parsons saw illness as a form of deviance in that it reduces the human organism's ability to adapt to their environment and requires remedial action (Chris, 2019). He recognised that allowing special concessions to sick individuals until they became well again helps maintain control of sickness and offers social benefits through ensuring that, after recovery, members continue contributing to society. Parsons described how once a doctor diagnosed a person's illness, they were able to take on the sick role and allowed to take time out from their duties to recuperate. Parsons recognised that the 'sick role' process involves both rights and obligations. For example, a person deemed ill is not held responsible for their feelings and behaviour and allowed temporary relief from their social-role obligations, including time away from school, work, and family duties. However, once legitimately termed 'sick' a person is obliged to see the illness as undesirable, want to get better, and seek medical help. Failing to observe these obligations can, under some circumstances, mean the intervention of legal action (such as sectioning) to force them to accept medical care. The sick role can be considered as a form of social control as legitimate diagnoses become crucial and only medical experts can provide them. For example, absence from school or work requires a doctor's note.

Medical professionals, therefore, have a very powerful role in ensuring that people can continue to carry out their social obligations. Parsons saw how their role also includes rights and obligations. For example, medical professional autonomy and dominance allow practitioners access to patients' personal information and the right to carry out intimate physical investigations. However, they must always act in ways to meet patients' health needs and adhere to rules of conduct established by their professional organisation. This includes using their high degree of knowledge and expertise to make emotionally detached and objective decisions.

However, in the case of children and adolescents the implications of the sick role become more complex as medical professionals are involved with parents as well as patients. They have the power to gain intimate information from child and adolescent patients and their parents, including specific parenting skills. Both children and parents eventually come under the medical 'gaze' and are ultimately judged in terms of the sick role principles, as parents may be considered as potentially responsible for causing their child's 'deviant' behaviour. For example, such concerns were used by Bilksy et al. (2018) to justify their investigation into the extent to which parental responses reinforced adolescents' panic attacks.

When applying Parsons' theory to parents it becomes evident that they are forced to take on the sick role by proxy. They are desperate to find a diagnosis for their child's behaviour, but once this is achieved, they find that, to some extent, their lifestyle has become medicalised. For example, once a child is diagnosed with a condition such as juvenile arthritis, ADHD, or within the autistic spectrum, parents feel relief as they may have felt that others suspected them to be responsible for their child's 'illness'-related behaviour. In line with the principles of Parsons' sick role theory parents are allowed and even obliged to take time away from their normal duties to care for their 'ill' child. However, they must aid the improvement of their child's health through seeking medical help, agreeing to advice given, and participating in administering treatment as instructed by medical professionals. A failure to comply with medical dictates can not only be considered as irresponsible parenting, but also leads to legal action and, in extreme cases, the removal of the sick child. Table 9.1 illustrates the roles of children/adolescents, parents, and doctors in terms of Parsons' (1951) sick role theory.

However, Parsons' sick role theory has been criticised as it seems to apply well to acute forms of illness, but it is not always possible for individuals to recover from a chronic illness and/or disability. It also tends to assume that patients always passively follow doctors' instructions when, in fact, many patients do not do so and even seek alternative 'cures'. It also has been accused of ignoring the impact of social inequalities on illness as some parents' financial status allows them to take on the sick role whilst others cannot afford to take time off work. A feminist approach would also add that it perpetuates the power of the male-dominated medical profession and drug companies and fails to account for the way different people make sense of illness. Nevertheless, Shilling (2002) claims that Parsons' theory is not meant to literally reflect reality but rather to be used as a tool for investigating

Table 9.1 The sick role applied to children and adolescents and parents

Rights of sick children and adolescents	Rights of parents	Rights of doctors
Not held responsible for their 'illness' and related behaviour. Exemption from normal duties such as school, college, and family obligations	Not held responsible for causing their child's 'illness' and related behaviour. Relief from normal duties and possibly work to care for their 'ill' child	Control assignment of the 'sick role'. Allowed access to intimate physical and personal information from child and adolescent as well as personal information from parents about their child and parenting skills. Professional autonomy and dominance.
Obligations of sick children and adolescents	Obligations of parents	Obligations of doctors
Must attempt to get well (improve behaviour) Must accept treatments and comply with instructions from doctors and parents	Must desire for their child to get well Must seek medical help, agree to advice and be complicit in administering treatment as instructed by medical professionals.	Act in ways to meet the health needs of the patient and respect parents' views. Adhere to professional conduct rules Utilise high degree of knowledge and expertise Make emotionally detached and objective decisions

reactions to sickness within Western society and the dominant role of the medical profession in this process. He points out how Parsons' theory illustrates how the main concern within medicine is to restore an individual's functional efficiency to ensure their social usefulness.

Parsons later recognised that patients may seek alternative health information to that given by health professionals and added this to his theory as a residual capacity (Shilling, 2002). Even so, despite parents' desperate searching for other forms of help, such as using the internet and alternative health providers, only doctors can ultimately legitimise the diagnosis. The sick role theory, therefore, does demonstrate the power of the medical profession to influence, directly and indirectly, the lives of all members of society. This is particularly important when considering children and adolescents as they have less power and social status than adults. When interpreted as a health issue, deviant behaviour can, therefore, create life-changing consequences for a child or adolescent and their family.

Parsons' 'sick role' theory was applied by Cresswell (2020) to help explain some of the dynamics within healthcare which impact on the lives of children and adolescents who self-harm. Adolescents are particularly vulnerable to self-harming, with girls most at risk. This is particularly concerning given that the large number of those who have self-harmed in adolescence and later committed suicide has remained distressingly consistent over the last fourteen years (Cresswell, 2020). Suicide was considered as legally deviant behaviour until the Suicide Act of 1961, and along with self-harm still elicits negative attitudes within healthcare, particularly within emergency departments. Cresswell (2020) found that when this was a first attempt, patients were seen sympathetically but after carrying out further attempts they were considered bad patients. This was even more likely if such attempts were linked to substance abuse and/or personality disorder, with patients often implicitly 'punished' through rougher handling during treatments. Cresswell (2020) explains that, when considered in terms of the sick role theory, these suicide attempts were perceived as a choice and, therefore, less legitimate than other mental health conditions. However, although not addressed by Cresswell, an additional explanation for healthcare staffs' attitudes could be that it results from their heavy and emotionally draining workload. Although this does not justify such reactions, it must be extremely difficult for staff, who, for example, may have been fighting hard to save a child's life but had to inform distraught parents of his/her death, to then attend to self-inflicted injuries for which no reasons seem obviously apparent to them.

Cresswell (2020) raises some other interesting questions about the fine line between 'mental health' problems and 'criminal behaviour'. For example, Section 136 (s136) of the Mental Health Act (1983) can be used by the police to justify removing someone who appears to have a mental disorder to a place of safety. This can often end up as a short stay in a prison cell given that the priority of policing is public safety. The blurring of boundaries between the police and mental health professionals suggests how closely they work together along with social workers to ensure social control.

9.2   Healthism and Medicalising Children's and Adolescents' Lives

It is difficult to underestimate the power of the medical profession given that it appears to offer people the opportunity for a prolonged, healthy life and reduces their anxiety about the inevitability of death. This is particularly important for parents, who work hard to ensure their child's survival. However, Nettleton (2000) suggests that the increasing need for health experts undervalues lay beliefs and means that professionals can monitor, interfere, define, and use force if necessary, over many social interactions. The more that social experiences are regarded as health issues the more the medical profession can be blamed for medicalising everyday aspects of life and promoting ideas of an ideal healthy body, mind, and appearance.

9.2.1   Increased Medicalisation of Daily Living

Adopting a medical approach to improving an undesirable appearance and/or problematic behaviour is increasingly seen as normal. However, Illich (1977) was particularly critical of the way modern, scientific medicine is practised within industrialised countries. He believed that patients may suffer from medical errors and treatments which create more problems than cures, and that many aspects of life and human behaviour are increasingly seen as 'medical' problems. All this leads to society becoming constantly dependent upon 'medical' experts. The adverse effect of such over-medicalisation was identified by Illich as 'iatrogenesis' which Peer and Shabir (2018) explain as originating from the Greek words, 'iatros' (physicians) and 'genesis' (origin). Table 9.2 describes three forms of iatrogenesis identified by Illich (1977).

The first form of iatrogenesis identified by Illich (1977) includes potential mistakes resulting from wrong diagnoses made by doctors, the use of drugs which have problematic side effects and hospital procedures and other medical processes which can cause pain, distress, and even fatalities. Peer and Shabir (2018) report how suspicion of medical procedures was evident within the Western world from the eighteenth century. This became particularly evident in the 1960s due to insufficient

Table 9.2 Types of iatrogenesis identified by Illich (1977)

Clinical iatrogenesis	Harm resulting from medical interventions, including unnecessary invasive tests and surgery; mistakes during invasive tests and surgery; drug addiction and side effects; mistakes; and accidents due to hospital procedures.
Social iatrogenesis	Harm resulting from medicalising aspects of everyday life, especially social problems, including children and adolescents who are difficult to control and feel anxious or depressed; fertility; pregnancy and abortion.
Cultural iatrogenesis	Harm resulting from society's over-dependence on medicine which allows medical 'expects' to control most aspects of social and political life and reduces the independence and rights of children, parents, and sub-groups.

testing of new drugs which became highly apparent when thalidomide was prescribed to pregnant women and caused damaging effects on foetus development. Peer and Shabir (2018) explain that this kind of iatrogenesis is the fifth leading cause of death in the world. They also cite World Health Organisation findings of 8% to 12% hospital errors within European Union member states. This becomes even more concerning given that only a small number of drug-related errors are thought to be reported.

Although it cannot be denied that many modern drugs have the potential to save lives, they can also compromise personal autonomy and be used instead of alternative, less risky ways of overcoming illness. Peer and Shabir (2018) point out how drug companies have a powerful hold over the medical profession by their transnational standing, funding of research, and links with financial companies. Also, within healthcare the benefits of using new technology to save lives must be weighed up against the damaging effects some surgical procedures and invasive diagnostics may have on the quality of life saved.

The increased risk of potential iatrogenesis within paediatric medicine is discussed by Teti et al. (2017) who point out that doctors are responding to not only the health needs of their patients but also the decisions parents make on behalf of their child or adolescent. This can create a dilemma, particularly if there is conflict between patients and parents' wishes, as well as their own views based on medical knowledge and experience. Teti et al. (2017) also explain how such iatrogenesis can create distress for staff who they see as potential secondary victims and stress the need for the interests of children and adolescents to take priority over adult concerns.

In addition to medical iatrogenesis Illich also identified the existence of social iatrogenesis, which involves the medicalisation of universal life stages, challenging events, and social problems. This can be due to concerns about a child because they have not yet reached the typical development milestones for their age and/or are exhibiting difficult behaviour. It also includes medical concerns and interventions in relation to adolescents facing difficulties in their transition to adulthood such as moody behaviour, sexual activity, and gender preferences as well as menstruation irregularity and pregnancy in females. Once such behaviour of children and adolescents becomes scrutinised by medical professionals, they may be diagnosed with specific conditions requiring remedial treatment. Examples of the links between specific behaviour and potential conditions are offered in Table 9.3.

Table 9.3 Examples of potentially medicalised child's and adolescent's behaviour

Behaviour displayed	Potential medicalised condition
Clumsy movements	Dyspraxia
Difficulty reading	Dyslexia
Refusing to obey commands	Oppositional defiance disorder (ODD)
Impulsive and erratic behaviour, difficult to control	Attention deficit hyperactive disorder (ADHD)
Lack of empathy	Autistic, Asperger's Syndrome, or borderline personality disorder
Violence and violating the rights of others	A Conduct disorder

Despite general acceptance that some behavioural problems may have a biological base, concerns have been expressed about the increase in diagnosis of such conditions. For example, Timimi (2010) believes that this can be due to a lack of recognition that differences in developmental progress and challenging behaviour may be caused by family and wider social issues which can change over time as children and adolescents develop.

A third form of iatrogenesis identified by Illich is cultural iatrogenesis. This refers to the way that so many aspects of everyday behaviour are defined and treated as health issues that people have become increasingly dependent on experts to control their own wellbeing and that of their family. For example, to be a good parent within the UK means adhering to the dictates of prescribed parenting programmes and individuals such as 'Super Nanny' whose advice is based on the child rearing beliefs of this specific cultural epoch.

Illich believed that the over medicalisation of life denies individual autonomy and freedom and can create negative cultural values and judgements. These can be particularly traumatic for families, when, for example, children may be taken into care if parents fail to agree with medical decisions. It can also mean the creation of potential moral panics such as those currently related to childhood obesity and include increased screening which may create anxiety and self-fulfilling prophecies. Medicalisation also increases financial pressures on health service budgets, which may mean that medical decisions are determined by financial restrictions and government sanctions. It also masks the social rather than medical causes of some illnesses such as poverty and appears to be a form of social control.

However, whilst Illich (1977) criticises medicalisation as resulting from large, impersonal societies and suggests a need for smaller community-based societies, he does not offer any real alternatives or suggestions as to how these may be created. Also, Illich tends to view patients as passively accepting medicalised lives, when often parents and patients do not follow expert advice. Also, the internet offers information to a better educated population, which can challenge medical opinion and, currently within the UK, self-management is encouraged to reduce escalating costs within the health service.

The claims of Illich (1977) that many 'health' problems are socially created and doctors should only be responsible for conditions with an obvious organic cause must also be seen within their historical and cultural context. His views, along with those of Szasz (1974) and Zola (1975), formed part of an antipsychiatry movement in the 1970s due to concerns about the increased surgery and medication within the mental health services. Although, rather extreme, such views have drawn attention to the powerful position of the medical profession within Western society and particularly in legitimising when children and adolescents are to be considered 'typical' (healthy) and 'atypical' (suffering physical or mental ill health).

The extent of this power, as well as limits, has become starkly obvious in recent times with the onset of the worldwide pandemic due to COVID-19. It appears as if the previously half-veiled position of raw conflict between economics, politics, and the medical profession has suddenly become glaringly obvious. Given the undoubtedly physical nature of the COVID-19 virus, with its potentially fatal consequences on both individual health and health services, data based on medical science has been used to influence most aspects of every individual's life. This has produced many examples of iatrogenesis due to faulty treatment, lack of protective clothing, and other resources as well as speeding up of vaccine testing processes. Government decisions, including self-isolation, highly restricted hospital and care home visiting, and periods of 'shut-downs', claimed to be based on scientific evidence have created other forms of iatrogenesis ranging from increased anxiety and depression to domestic violence and murder. However, during this pandemic the power of the medical profession can also be seen to have been muted by politically motivated government dictates which have censured publication of health data, manipulated the media coverage, and sought to influence public health advice. Many decisions have been based on maintaining economic prosperity despite the cost of many human lives. When competing with politics and economics, even the preciously guarded medical profession struggles to maintain its powerful hold and provide a health service dedicated to saving human life at all cost.

9.2.2 Healthism, Perfectionism, and Appearance

Healthism refers to current taken for granted attitudes about what constitutes a healthy lifestyle within Western society. In the past, being healthy meant preventing illness but now it involves judgements made about parents' and adolescents' lifestyle choices. Nettleton (2000) maintains that ideas about what it means to be healthy are shaped by government sponsored health promotion which both reflects and contributes to increasing consumerism within society. Such ideas determine what is considered as healthy eating, exercise, and appearance. She suggests that past, internal spiritual concerns have been replaced by an individualistic concentration on outward physical appearance. According to Nettleton (2000), having a healthy body is now seen to offer higher public status, improved self-image, a sense of moral superiority, and increased cultural capital. Parents are made to feel even more responsible for ensuring their family meals conform to what is deemed healthy. Also, they and their older children are encouraged to join fitness clubs and gyms (marketed as health producers) and pressured through advertising to buy expensive branded sports clothing and equipment.

That healthism promotes a sense that there is an ideal 'healthy' lifestyle suggests it is based on philosophical principles of perfectionism. Kumar (2020) points out the moral and political implications of perfectionism which require humans to constantly strive towards achieving the best possible state of mental, spiritual, physical, and material wellbeing. Such striving is seen as a moral duty, requiring that individual desires are denied, to ensure that members make the most useful contribution to improving society. M'hamdi (2021) explains how this sense of perfectionism encouraged within public health promotion can create a tension, as the interests of the community may conflict with those of individual members. For example, the current trend to ensure that school dinners conform to what is deemed healthy may not suit the taste of some children. Also, it may not always be possible for some children to take part in physical education which is compulsory within schools. Despite the often, obviously beneficial nature of such state interventions into public life, perfectionism assumes a society in which everyone has an equal starting point. The unequal power base within Western society means that promoting the idea that all children have the potential to achieve perfection can lead to unfair elitism and paternalism.

Nevertheless, Western ideals of being physically fit and having an attractive appearance are often used as a measure of social worth. However, there is a need to take account of inequalities in terms of inherited physical qualities, social position, access to necessary resources, and standard of living. Not striving towards healthism is increasingly seen as a form of deviance and risks stigma, which has huge implications for children and adolescents with a chronic illness and/or disability. Morrall (2001) points out how any deformity resulting from an accident, illness, or difficult birth may be considered in need of modification through drugs or surgery. Timimi et al. (2011) agree and express concern that if taken to extremes, such future thinking could mean that those with a learning or physical disability may be perceived as having a form of genetic weakness which must not be allowed to be passed on.

Concerns have also been expressed about the practice of overzealously following healthiest advice regarding diet. Great pressure is placed on parents to monitor their children's weight given the current moral panics about child and adolescent obesity. However, caution is required as, in the case with any moral panic, unintended consequences may emerge. For example, an overzealous response can mean parents inadvertently encouraging family members to become unhealthily obsessed with healthy eating. To illustrate this, Hangau-Bresch (2019) points to a potentially new condition based on a pathological obsession with healthy food, identified in 1997 as 'Orthorexia'.

Also, contradictions can be found within the concept of healthism in relation to appearance and some types of physical exercise. Beltrán-Carrillo et al. (2018) point out how adolescent girls striving to achieve the ideal slim body promoted through healthism are increasingly resisting participating in school sports for fear of developing a masculinised body. Indeed, Hangau-Bresch (2019) concludes that following the pernicious ideal of purity with regard to food and exercise can mean that healthism is increasingly pushing the boundary of what is considered as culturally healthy.

Health is, therefore, used to judge appearance and behaviour. Children and adolescents have little control over the extent to which healthism may increasingly dictate their lives. Morrall (2001) explains that although healthism appears to offer greater individual control and autonomy, in fact, it increases oppression and feeds consumerism. He refers to how health service propaganda medicalises what is normal. There appears to be an increasing reticence to accept the 'cards' that nature has dealt each individual and a drive to use any means available to conform to a socially approved ideal.

Van Teijlingen and Humphris (2019) identify commercial forces which increase health consumerism and the search for a perfect appearance. They point out how information gained from the internet, mobile technology, and other forms of media increasingly encourages self-diagnosis and suggests treatments. Van Teijlingen and Humphris (2019) also offer examples of private services providing blood testing, screening procedures, and plastic surgery. This is particularly concerning as what kind of appearance is considered as ideal changes over time. It is in the financial interest of those promoting and catering for a consumerist society to constantly create new fashions to encourage further sales of commodities and services aiding the 'newest' look.

The role of social media in exacerbating the importance of appearance on self-esteem was specifically considered by Trekels et al. (2018). They found adolescents to be particularly concerned about their appearance when using Facebook and saw it as affecting levels of popularity, self-esteem, and romantic success. Whilst this was the case for both sexes, the effects appeared to have an even greater impact on girls. That children and adolescents are continually at risk of submitting to pressure to modify their appearance has become increasingly recognised, with legislation establishing age restrictions on such procedures as tattooing, teeth whitening, and sunbed use. Recently concern about the number of vulnerable young people undertaking cosmetic surgery has led to legislation restricting the use of botulinum toxin and cosmetic fillers. It is, therefore, now an offence in England to administer botulinum toxin, or a subcutaneous, submucous, or intradermal injection of a filler for a cosmetic purpose to anyone under the age of eighteen years of age if not approved by a doctor.

> **Box. 9.1 The Botulinum Toxin and Cosmetic Fillers (Children) Act 2021**
> Evidence cited by Lord Bethell, the government health minister responsible for this Act, explained how the numbers of young adolescents seeking cosmetic treatments were increasing at an alarming rate. For example, in 2017 approximately over 29,300 dermal filler procedures were carried out on adolescents under eighteen years of age. Also, in 2020, an estimated 41,000 botulinum toxin procedures were conducted on those from this same age group.

As children and adolescents are particularly vulnerable to feeling different from their peers in any way, it is important to try and protect them from the constant bombardment of unrealistically ideal human images displayed through the media and the increasing normalisation of cosmetic interventions.

Concerns for current and future children are raised by Morrall (2001) who points out how it is becoming possible for potential parents to choose and purchase eggs and sperm from the most 'healthy' and attractive donors. He also speculates that, given the development of increasingly sophisticated medical technology there may be a future possibility to select and pay for the specific genetic coding of children. This raises the frightening spectre of 'designer babies' with the risk that, whatever have been previously created will eventually be judged as 'out of date' and less 'fashionable' than the latest 'batch'!

9.3 Over-medicalisation of Children's and Adolescents' Lives

9.3.1 Surveillance and Diagnoses

Whilst the legislation protecting children and adolescents from health risks such as unnecessary cosmetic surgery is very welcome, it must be admitted that in other areas of children's and adolescents' lives, there is a fine line between protection and control. In addition to being influenced by family members, peers, and media, children are monitored by professionals from birth to ensure that they meet expected developmental milestones. This process means that they and their caregivers are placed under surveillance by health care staff, teachers, and social workers whose assessments reflect the historical and cultural context in which they exist.

Beltrán-Carrillo et al. (2018) describe the development and concerning use of new forms of digital surveillance, such as health monitoring technology which can consistently track the body size and health of children and adolescents. According to Oravec (2020) such devices purportedly offer enhanced wellbeing through a sense of personal control over physical fitness yet, result in the 'datafication' and 'professionalisation' of self-care and may, in fact, reduce self-control. Continual digital monitoring may even create some harm to health (iatrogenesis) through increasing anxiety and potential addiction to the gamification used within these systems. Oravec (2020) offers the example of how data on physical ability tracked and displayed through products such as Fitbit can be shared with others on their website to encourage joint challenges, but potentially may lead to social shaming. She cautions against the use of rewards for achieving personal goals set without medical advice, which if not met may impact on the user's self-esteem. There is always the possibility of inaccuracies in data collected from such devices and Oravec (2020) is particularly concerned about infringement of human rights through possible purchasing of data and potential future use by organisations, including schools and colleges.

The prospect of potential digital monitoring of mental as well as physical health in schools becomes particularly concerning when considering suggestions made by Williams (2013) that these are the best places to carry out mental health surveillance through routine testing. Williams (2013) argues that this is necessary, given that mental health costs more than double those of cancer diagnosis and treatment, with the origins of three quarters of adult disorders evident in childhood. He suggests that screening in schools and offering early intervention could be effective strategies to reduce mental health issues in children and later adulthood. Williams (2013) points out how fluoxetine has proved to be a cost-effective treatment for depression in childhood and adolescence and suggests that early diagnosis and using this have the potential to reduce the stigma of having a mental health condition. However, the role and responsibility of parents are recognised by Williams (2013) who recommends that they be given the opportunity to refuse to let their child undergo mental health assessments.

An example of a mental health assessment tool designed to be used with children and adolescents is 'Teen Screen'. This was developed by the pharmaceutical industry during President Bush's administration in the USA as a potential means of screening all school children. The developers of this assessment tool argued that it would be useful in detecting symptoms of poor mental health which are evident two to four years before the disorder is recognised, which is important, given that mental health issues evident during adolescence are likely to persist into adulthood. They added that poor mental health is linked to obesity, risk taking, over-use of computers, poor sociability, poor school attendance and schoolwork, violence, and suicide. They also claimed that a quarter of adolescents attending appointments within primary care discuss emotional problems linked to chronic physical conditions, mental health problems, and suicide.

Nevertheless, concerns arise from the mass use of such screening tools, particularly as, although meant to be undertaken voluntarily, they may at times be used without parental consent. Also, Morrall (2001) points out how screening is never 100% accurate. Other considerations which need addressing in relation to screening for mental health include problems in defining what it actually means to be emotionally healthy, how adults or children can ever know that they possess good mental health, and the impossibility of accurately measuring mental health. This is particularly pertinent during adolescence given the intense biological and social-role changes experienced during this period. Defining mental health becomes further problematic when considering the varied cultural interpretations of behaviour during childhood and adolescence.

Concern about the over-surveillance of children's lives is expressed by Timimi et al. (2011) who caution against mental health diagnoses being based on statistical norms and devised to speedily identify those failing to meet cultural standards so that this can be rectified by experts. They point to the proliferation of new conditions based on children's difficult behaviour and seeking of possible 'quick fixes'. Timimi et al. (2011) speculate on the outcome of such a trend as eventually meaning that those who do not like doing maths are diagnosed with a developmental-arithmetic disorder, those who argue with their parents have an oppositional-defiant disorder, and if children and adolescents criticise the definition and treatment of these kinds of disorders they may be suffering from a 'noncompliance with treatment disorder'!

9.3.2 Rights of Children and Adolescents and Ethical Dilemmas in Practice

Parents and the state share responsibility to meet children's and adolescents' needs. However, it can prove difficult to decide on just what constitutes these needs as they can change over time and between cultures. For example, Woodhead (1997) explains how the Universal Convention of Rights of the Child (UCRC) (1989), accepted by most countries, emphasises children's need for protection, whilst the OAU African

Charter on Rights and Welfare of Children (1990) prioritises their need to develop a sense of responsibility, duty, and obedience towards work and family.

Current legislation within the UK, including the Children Act 1989 and Children Act 2004, follows the UCRC (1989) interpretation of children's needs as well as their rights. Although, within this legislation, parents are deemed responsible for children's care and families are perceived as the best place for care provision, local authorities are given the power to remove children from the family home if suspected of suffering harm. Local authorities are also given the responsibility of ensuring co-operation between relevant agencies, such as the police, health service, and voluntary sectors as well as ensuring that children's and adolescents' views are respected. Other government initiatives, such as Every Child Matters (2004), aim to develop more 'joined up' services and listen to the views of children. Although these acts and initiatives stress the rights of children, their impact is limited by funding, austerity measures, and the constantly changing needs of children and adolescents (Dickinson, 2019).

The limited power of children and adolescents to exercise their rights is particularly evident within healthcare and can create ethical dilemmas. For example, it is difficult for children and adolescents to refuse treatment. Also, doctors who treat children suffering a terminal illness may face pressures from parents desperate that their child be kept alive at all costs. This can result in the need for invasive treatment, causing a child pain and distress whilst reducing the opportunity for a dignified death. Although the need to take account of children's wishes is recognised, doctors must balance this against the wishes of parents and public interest (Worthington, 2006). Such decisions can be particularly difficult when the economic value of treatments is considered in terms of the National institute of Clinical Excellence (NICE) guidelines for cost effectiveness.

The UK National Health Service (NHS) is guided by principles within the UNCR (1989) and Children Act (2004), as well as National Service Frameworks (NSFs) which offer general guidance rather than directives about autonomy and consent within healthcare. It is left to practitioners to decide if an older child or adolescent is deemed competent for their wishes to be taken seriously. This can prove particularly difficult if the wishes of the older child or adolescent conflict with parents' views about treatment and confidentiality. Consent becomes even more problematic if both parents do not agree. In such cases courts will follow advice within the Children Act (1989) and Children Act (2004), to decide on what is in the best interests of the child.

Issues of children's rights have also to be acknowledged when considering the current provision of family-centred healthcare which assumes that parent's wishes are always in the child's best interest. Family-centred care recognises that ill children need the security of their family, who in turn are affected by their child's illness. Caring for the whole family is, therefore, seen as in the best interests of the child. However, Davies et al. (2019) point out that priority is often given to parent's views about treatment during consultations, as many healthcare professionals assume that children and adolescents are unable to make rational decisions. Interestingly, an anomaly arises here, as noted by Worthington (2006), when treating adults within healthcare, their refusal to accept treatment must be accepted even if they offer no rationale for their decision.

Although the UCRC (1989) defines all those under the age of eighteen years to be a child, the specific age and developmental stage of children and adolescents need to be considered to ensure that their wishes are acknowledged within health-care provision. Griffith (2016) suggests that it should be recognised that those con-sidered 'of tender years' require consistent parental consent, those under sixteen years of age should be considered 'Gillick competent', and those aged sixteen and seventeen years should have the same rights as adults to consent to treatment.

Of the stages referred to by Griffith (2016), it is the 'Gillick competent' view that raises the most complex dilemmas for healthcare professionals. The concept of a child under sixteen years of age being considered as 'Gillick competent' in consent-ing to medical examinations and treatment originates from a ruling within the House of Lords. This was in response to the case Gillick v West Norfolk and Wisbech AHA (1986), in which a mother objected to the ability of a doctor to give contraceptive advice (in line with Department of Health guidelines) to her daughter who was under sixteen years of age. As a result, it was ruled that providing they were consid-ered to have sufficient maturity and intelligence, a child under sixteen years has the legal competence to consent to medical examination and treatment. Professionals were required to consider the complexity of the health issues and the child's devel-opment. To assess levels of maturity meant taking account of the child's experiences and decision-making ability, including resisting peer and family pressures. Levels of intelligence required measurement of the child's ability to understand the com-plex issues involved, including weighing up risks and benefits as well as long-term consequences.

Once a child has been deemed 'Gillick competent' parents cannot overrule their consent as it has been accepted in the same way as that of an adult. However, if a child refuses a medical examination or treatment it is within the law for those accepted as having parental responsibility to consent instead. This raises some inter-esting issues as Griffith (2016) states that to date no court has supported a child's refusal to accept life sustaining treatment. It appears that some children have the right to comply with medical treatment, even against their parents' wishes, whilst none has the right to refuse. The Children Act 2004 puts the onus on professionals to inform and persuade children into accepting procedures deemed by medical pro-fessionals to be in their best interests.

Immunisation creates further complexities regarding children's and adolescents' rights to consent within healthcare. Again, the dilemma arises of having to weigh up the child's best interest against the needs of the general public. Consent is necessary, as within the UK immunisation is not compulsory unless it is seen as necessary to avoid significant harm to a child. If that is seen to be the case the state can intervene under the Children Act (1989). Griffith (2016) offers an example of a recent case where, due to parental disagreements, courts intervened and insisted that the MMR vaccine be given to sisters aged eleven and fifteen years of age. The judge decided that it was in the best interests of the children to have the vaccine. In doing so he ignored the wishes of the children on the grounds that they were influenced by their mother. Nevertheless, despite court rulings it can prove very difficult to carry out their dictates when those who resist refuse to attend or submit their bodies to the necessary physical procedures. Griffith (2016) adds that as a result, the two girls had not received the vaccination.

Griffith (2016) does explain that in exceptional cases it is possible under the Family Proceedings Rules (1991) for a person refusing to adhere to an order to be jailed for contempt, or the child be removed by a representative of the court and forcibly immunised. However, he does explain that both would be considered detrimental to the child's welfare. He also points out that consent is needed for touching which places the nurses administering the injection in a difficult position. They are not legally compelled to carry out the immunisation and must decide if it is necessary to continue injecting a resistant child.

The complexity of rights and consent within healthcare discussed above have huge implications for the current UK government which has considered mass vaccination of children and adolescents against COVID-19. This is a particularly controversial decision as scientific data has shown that children and adolescents are able to spread the virus but be less likely than adults to suffer its severe adverse effects. Such decisions, therefore, appear to be based on the needs of the adult population rather than in the interests of children. This is particularly concerning now that children aged twelve years and above have been offered the vaccine with the need for any parental consent being overruled. It is extremely worrying that, despite the unknown long-term effects of such vaccinations, consideration is now being given to vaccinating much younger children. In accordance with current legislation and policies, such vaccinations should only take place after gaining both parents' consent. However, that during the pandemic the government have adopted emergency legislative powers raises the fear that the wishes of parents of even very young children may be ignored. Should this be the case highly disturbing questions arise about whose best interest all this is serving, that of the child or rather that of adults? The whole subject of children's and adolescents' rights appears to be questionable and increasingly complex for those responsible for making decisions about their health and wellbeing.

9.4 Biopsychosocial Basis of Health in Childhood and Adolescence

9.4.1 Biopsychosocial Explanations for Health in Childhood and Adolescence

Despite awareness of the medicalisation of life within Western society it is important to also note the huge contributions that medicine and public health measures have made to many areas of health. For example, impressive reductions have been made in rates of infant mortality and childhood morbidity. Indeed, Morrall (2001, p. 108) cautions against 'throwing the baby out with the bath water' and admits that new technology and drugs do have their place providing they are seen within their social context and agendas. He points out how distress and pain are a reality for those suffering acute and chronic illness. Greater understanding and relief from some distressing aspects of life stages such as menstruation and childbirth are very welcome. However, arguments become more complex when considering socially and culturally based 'health' matters, such as reactions to those suffering teenage, 'puppy fat', acne, or moodiness.

The socio-cultural basis of many diseases is discussed by Peer and Shabir (2018) who also refer to the impact of humans on the environment, including creating air and water pollution and toxic chemical waste. Also, there is growing awareness that socio-environmental factors create stress which is linked to an increasing number of 'health' conditions. For example, Van Teijlingen and Humphris (2019) found poverty and poor housing to be particularly responsible for respiratory problems in childhood and vulnerability to mental health problems in adolescence. This suggests a need to acknowledge and address the impact of intolerable social conditions on wellbeing. There is a need for greater awareness about how the social position of many families, particularly those experiencing poverty, poor housing, and unemployment, restricts their ability to make healthy decisions.

When considered at a macro level, the way Western society is structured means that there is an imbalance of power between people based on their access to status and wealth, which influences the level of control they have over their lives. Those who have more power can ensure that they benefit as much as possible from the current knowledge and resources available. The position of parents within this stratified society affects the lives of their children. For example, a doctor will be respected and well paid so able to raise children in a spacious home in a desirable neighbourhood. The education and training for doctors is of a high standard and means mixing with other professionals also held in high esteem. This allows them to pass on to their children knowledge gained from their own education and experience, guide them through career choices, and introduce them to other types of professionals who can offer additional advice and knowledge. All this creates a form of cultural capital that offers an advantage for those children to go on and achieve good health and high-status professions in later life.

Combined levels of status, income, and cultural capital, therefore, impact on the standard of living experienced by children and adolescents. Those children whose parents may be unemployed and living in poorly built homes in deprived areas are likely to experience a poor standard of living which proves stressful and impairs physical health. However, even the benefits of a good standard of living cannot completely shield children from distressing life events, such as bereavement, parental separation, illness, and disability. How children and adolescents react to such adverse events will also be determined by a variety of psychosocial factors. For example, individual differences exist in children's resilience, with some able to survive extremely distressing events.

Levels of resilience may have a genetic component but also be influenced by the degree of attachment, support, and cohesiveness within family life, the type of peer relationships, community facilities, and educational opportunities available as well as access to good social services. The mental and physical wellbeing of children and

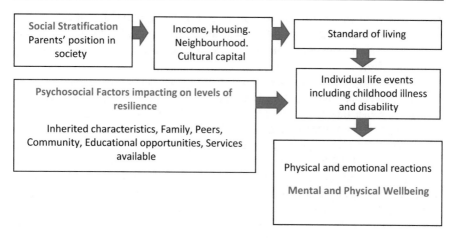

Fig. 9.1 Biopsychosocial impact on the wellbeing of children and adolescents

adolescents, therefore, is heavily influenced by their families' position within the social hierarchy and the levels of biological, psychological, and social preventative mechanisms available. Fig.9.1 attempts to capture this complex process.

9.4.2 Attitudes Towards Childhood, Adolescent Wellbeing, and Therapeutic Approaches

Adopting a biopsychosocial explanation of physical and mental health suggests societal as well as individual responsibility for the wellbeing of all children and adolescents. It also requires more than seeking to 'fix a faulty machine' when trying to help reduce problematic behaviour. Timimi (2010) points out how any form of difference is seen as the fault of the child or adolescent, with the acceptance of the myth of natural teenage rebellion liable to become a self-fulfilling prophecy. He believes that the aggressive capitalism underpinning Western values influences the way children's and adolescents' behaviour is seen within a proliferation of psychiatric diagnostic categories. Such monitoring of children's behaviour is considered by those in power as essential as control at this micro level ensures order is maintained at a macro level. Timimi et al. (2011) explain how new technology within this medicalised society encourages the constant scanning of each other for potential deviancy and ensures compliant children.

Algraigray and Boyle (2017) offer the example of how the classification of children and adolescents with problematic behaviour as disabled is made by professionals responsible for managing the disability industry, rather than those who have disabilities. They explain how such 'ableism' constantly compares and treats those with disabilities as different from those without a disability. Algraigray and Boyle (2017) stress how pathologising difference without acknowledging individual differences can lead to assuming similarities between those who are labelled disabled, rather than recognising shared similarities with non-disabled children and adolescents. Medicalising disability and problematic behaviour can lead to a readiness to prescribe medical treatments regardless of the context in which the behaviour occurs (Timimi, 2018).

Current therapeutic approaches tend to try help individuals adjust to the position they are placed in, within a highly stratified society, therefore, altering what is in their mind rather than problems created by their social and physical environment. For example, Timimi (2018) is highly critical of the Children and Young Peoples–Improving Access to Psychological Therapies (CYP–IAPT) project. This new UK government-funded initiative is based on a similar adult model and aims to improve existing Child and Adolescent Mental Health Services (CAMHS). This project reflects the National Institute of Health and Care Excellence (NICE) guidelines, by presuming that there is an identifiable cause for the problematic behaviour of children and adolescents, which once diagnosed can be matched to an appropriate therapeutic method. However, Timimi (2018) criticises such assumptions and points to the lack of evidence that such matching works. He expresses concern that such thinking suits the current trend to offer readymade, branded, quick fit solutions to specific types of behaviour without taking account of the child or adolescent's social experience within a particular economic and political culture.

Attention deficit hyperactivity disorder (ADHD) illustrates well how children's problematic behaviour has been labelled as an illness, often requiring drug treatment. In contrast, Timimi (2017) insists that it is better understood as a cultural construct, particularly as the same type of behaviour is judged differently in cross-cultural studies. Also, Whitely et al. (2018) suggest how the educational environment can be influential, given that those diagnosed with ADHD are often the youngest children in a classroom. Timimi (2017) is particularly concerned about the increased diagnoses of ADHD and use of stimulant drugs as treatment within the USA and even the UK. He describes how within the UK, stimulant prescriptions for ADHD rose from approximately 6000 a year in 1994 to over 1 million by 2013.

The use of such medication for ADHD is even more problematic given that it is impossible to ensure that such a diagnosis is accurate. Normally a 'condition' would be identified by symptoms, but those relating to ADHD may be slight, absent, or only evident within specific settings. Although a genetic basis has been suggested, Timimi (2017) points out that it is difficult to decide the point at which normal child behaviour becomes pathological. He also adds that the term ADHD only ever describes rather than explains symptoms so can never be a true diagnosis.

When considering how to 'treat' those with challenging behaviour it is necessary to take account of potential adverse environmental factors such as socio-economic disadvantage, marital discord, and maternal depression. Timimi (2017) points out that contextual factors and human relationships are more important than any specific therapeutic technique. He suggests that a variety of common factors within all therapies can be successful, provided a therapeutic alliance has been formed between the practitioner, child or adolescent, their family, and possibly any other agencies involved. He insists that to avoid existing power dynamics within families and between clinicians and patients, sessions need to be patient-directed and accepted by their family, despite pressures of the 'system' within which professionals work. Timimi (2017) stresses the need to avoid over-intervention, as this can make patients and their family lose confidence in their existing abilities and feel unable to cope.

Similarly, Kelly et al. (2012) recognise the importance of therapeutic interactions between children, parents, and professionals within family-centred care when treating physical health. They explain that professionals need to respect the different values and beliefs of patients and their families and actively listen to children and adolescents. They suggest that professionals provide age-appropriate information, encourage questioning and discussion, talk to both child/adolescent and parents as well as provide space and opportunity for them to process information and act on the patient's views as much as possible.

Timimi (2017) suggests that adopting the principles informing the 'Nurtured Heart Approach' (NHA) by Glasser and Easley (2007) can help to avoid medicalising children's and adolescent's challenging behaviour. Given that children crave attention, regardless of how it is gained, this approach gives priority to relationship building rather than over controlling adult behaviour. Timimi (2017) also insists that it is vital for practitioners to nurture a therapeutic alliance and ensure that the child or adolescent and their family are at centre of the process. Whilst great changes are needed at a structural level within society, such an alliance and constant awareness of the context in which the child and family are embedded currently offer the best means of promoting the wellbeing of children and adolescents.

Summary

- There is a need to consider whether it is kinder to now see deviance/differences as due to children and adolescents being 'mad' rather than 'bad' as they would have been in the past. Pathologising child and adolescent behaviour can be perceived as a means of control. Application of Parsons' (1951) theory of the sick role illustrates how such attitudes help to ensure children, adolescents, and their parents continue to contribute to the good of society.
- Illich's (1977) theory of iatrogenesis helps to explain how over-reliance on medicine can mean suffering the effects of treatment errors, experience aspects of daily life as health issues, and constantly need to consult experts. A culture of 'healthism' has emerged with medicine, and health promotion constantly attempting to control children and adolescents' diet, exercise, and appearance. Healthism assumes some mythical ideal of perfectionism requiring an equality which does not exist within Western society.
- Over-medicalisation means children's and adolescents' lives are under constant surveillance, with a readiness to offer a diagnosis of an increasing number of newly discovered mental health conditions. Acknowledging the rights

of children and adolescents creates ethical dilemmas in practice as conflicts between the views of parents, children, adolescents, and professionals can occur. Current legislation offers only a guide in relation to child and adolescent consent within healthcare. Professionals must decide when a child is mature and intelligent enough to give consent to procedures against their parents' wishes. However, if children and adolescents refuse to accept medical advice they must be 'persuaded' to comply.

- Biopsychosocial explanations are necessary to understand health and wellbeing in childhood and adolescence. Being born into a socially stratified society impacts on children and adolescents' standard of living. Despite therapeutic approaches attempting to change behaviour, injustices and inequalities in wider society need to be addressed.

Case Study Questions

Read the family case study on page 265 and consider the following:

- What might be influencing Gemma's concern about gaining too much weight?
- What issues need to be considered if Liam is diagnosed with ADHD?
- How might Gemma's doctor react to her request for some form of birth control?

Reflective Questions

- To what extent are the UK government able to demand mass vaccination against the COVID-19 across all ages?
- What are the implications of schools being used to test students' level of wellbeing?
- How might a diagnosis of a mental health condition during childhood or adolescence impact across the different stages of an individual's lifespan?

References

Algraigray, H., & Boyle, C. (2017). The SEN Label and Its Effect on Special Education. *Educational and Child Psychologist, 34*(4), 1–19. http://hdl.handle.net/10871/29376

Beltrán-Carrillo, V. J., Devís-Devís, J., & Peiró-Velert, C. (2018). The Influence of Body Discourses on Adolescents' (non)Participation in Physical Activity. *Sport, Education and Society, 23*(3), 257–269. https://doi.org/10.1080/13573322.2016.1178109

Bilksy, S. A., Cloutierb, R. M., Byniona, T.-M., Feldner, M. T., & Leen-Feldnera, E. W. (2018). An Experimental Test of the Impact of Adolescent Anxiety on Parental Sick Role Reinforcement Behavior. *Behavioural Research and Therapy, 109*, 37–48. https://doi.org/10.1016/j.brat.2018.07.009

Chris, J. J. (2019). Social Control: History of the Concept. In M. Deflem (Ed.), *Handbook of Social Control*. John Wiley & Sons. Ltd.

Costello, E. J., & Angold, A. (2004) In, J., Hill & B., Maughan (Eds.), Conduct Disorders in Childhood and Adolescence. : Cambridge University Press.

Cresswell, M. (2020). Self-Harm and Moral codes in Emergency Departments in England. *Social Theory & Health, 18*, 257–269. https://doi.org/10.1057/s41285-020-00137-x

Davies, C., Fraser, J., & Waters, D. (2019). Establishing a Framework for Listening to Children in Healthcare. *Journal of Child Health Care*, 1–10. https://doi.org/10.1177/1367493519872078

Dickinson, R. (2019). Reflecting on the Children Acts of 1989 and 2004. The MJ & Co. Retrieved July 18, 2021, from https://themj.co.uk/Reflecting-on-the-Children-Acts-of-1989-and-2004/216219

Glasser, H., & Easley, J. (2007). *Transforming the Difficult Child: The Nurtured Heart Approach*. Worth Publishing.

Griffith, R. (2016). What Is Gillick Competence? *Human Vaccines & Immunotherapeutics, 12*(1), 244–247. https://doi.org/10.1080/21645515.2015.1091548

Hangau-Bresch, C. (2019). Orthorexia: Eating Right in the Context of healthism. *Medical Humanities, 46*, 311–322. https://doi.org/10.1136/medhum-2019-011681

Heary, C., Hennessy, E., Swords, L., & Corrigan, P. (2017). Stigma towards Mental Health Problems during Childhood and Adolescence: Theory, Research, and Intervention Approaches. *Journal of Child and Family Studies, 26*, 2949–2959. https://doi.org/10.1007/s10826-017-0829-y

Illich, I. (1977). *Limits to Medicine—Medical Nemesis. The Expropriation of Health*. Penguin.

Kelly, M., Jones, S., Wilson, V., & Lewis, P. (2012). How Children's Rights are Constructed in Family-Centred Care: A Review of the Literature. *Journal of Child Health Care, 16*(2), 190–205. https://doi.org/10.1177/1367493511426421

Kumar, V. (2020). Perfectionism: An Ethical Theory of the Soul. *Research Review, International Journal of Multidisciplinary, 5*(6), 128–130. https://doi.org/10.31305/rrijm.2020.v05.i06.026

M'hamdi, H. I. (2021). Neutrality and Perfectionism in Public Health. *The American Journal of Bioethics. Published online ahead of printing*, 1–12. https://doi.org/10.1080/1526516 1.2021.1907479

Morrall, P. (2001). *Sociology and Nursing*. Routledge.

Morrall, P. (2009). *Sociology and Health*. Routledge.

Nettleton, S. (2000). *The Sociology of Health and illness*. Polity Press.

Oravec, J. A. (2020). Digital Iatrogenesis and Workplace Marginalization: some Ethical Issues involving Self-Tracking Medical Technologies. *Information, Communication & Society, 23*(14), 2030–2046. https://doi.org/10.1080/1369118X.2020.1718178

Parsons, T. (1951). *The Social System*. Routledge and Kegan Paul.

Peer, R. F., & Shabir, N. (2018). Iatrogenesis: A Review on Nature, Extent, and Distribution of Healthcare Hazards. *Journal of Family and Medical Primary Care, 7*(2), 309–314. https://doi.org/10.4103/jfmpc.jfmpc_329_17

Shilling, C. (2002). Culture, the 'Sick Role' and the Consumption of Health. *The British Journal of Sociology, 53*(4), 621–638. https://doi.org/10.1080/0007131022000021515

Szasz, T. (1974). *Ideology and Insanity*. Penguin.

Teti, S. L., Ennis-Durstine, K., & Silber, T. J. (2017). Etiology and Manifestations of Iatrogenesis in Pediatrics. *APA Journal of Ethics, 19*(8), 783–792. https://doi.org/10.1001/journalofethics.2017.19.8.stas2-1708

Timimi, S. (2010). The McDonaldization of Childhood: Children's. Mental Health in Neo-liberal Market Cultures. *Transcultural Psychiatry, 47*(5), 686–706. https://doi.org/10.1177/1363461510381158. http://tps.sagepub.com/content/47/5/686

Timimi, S. (2017). Non-diagnostic Based Approaches to Helping Children Who Could Be Labelled ADHD and Their Families. *International Journal of Qualitative Studies on Health and Well-being, 12*(Suppl. 1), 1–8, Thematic Cluster on ADHD. https://doi.org/10.1080/1748263 1.2017.1298270

Timimi, S. (2018). The Diagnosis is Correct, but National Institute of Health and Care Excellence Guidelines are part of the Problem not the Solution. *Journal of Health Psychology, 23*(9), 1148–1152. https://doi.org/10.1177/1359105318766139

Timimi, S., Gardener, N., & McCabe, B. (2011). *The Myth of Autism*. Palgrave.

Trekels, J., Ward, L. M., & Eggermont, S. (2018). I "Like" the Way You Look: How Appearance-Focused and Overall Facebook Use Contribute to Adolescents' Self-Sexualization. *Computers in Human Behavior, 18*, 198–208. https://doi.org/10.1016/j.chb.2017.12.020

Van Teijlingen, E., & Humphris, G. (Eds.). (2019). *Psychology and Sociology Applied to Medicine* (4th ed.). Elsevier.

Whitely, M., Raven, M., Timimi, S., Jureidini, J., Phillimore, J., Leo, J., Moncrieff, J., & Landman, P. (2018). Attention Deficit Hyperactivity Disorder Late Birthdate Effect Common in both High and Low Prescribing International Jurisdictions: Systematic Review. *Journal of Child Psychology and Psychiatry, 60*(4), 380–391. https://doi.org/10.1111/jcpp.12991

Williams, S. N. (2013). Bring in Universal mental Health Checks in Schools. *British Medical Journal, 347*, f5478. https://doi.org/10.1136/bmj.f5478

Woodhead, M. (1997). The Cultural Construction of Children's Needs. In A. Prout & A. James (Eds.), *Constructing and Reconstructing Childhood* (2nd ed.). Falmer Press.

Worthington, R. (2006). Standards of Healthcare and Respecting Children's Rights. *Journal of the Royal Society of Medicine, 99*(4), 208–210. https://doi.org/10.1177/014107680609900426

Wright, A.-M. (2009). Every Child Matters: Discourses of Challenging Behaviour. *Pastoral Care in Education, 27*(4), 279–290. https://doi.org/10.1080/02643940903349344

Zola, I. K. (1975). In the Name of Health and Illness: On Some Socio-Political Consequences of Medical Influence. *Social Science & Medicine, 9*(2), 83–87. https://doi.org/10.1016/0037-7856(75)90098-0

The Impact of Long-Term Conditions During Childhood and Adolescence

10

When compared to early last century, children's healthcare priorities have changed dramatically. As health and social care systems and therapeutic interventions have improved, the life expectancy of children with long-term conditions (LTC) has increased and the psychosocial wellbeing of children, adolescents, and families have become increasingly the focus of interventions. Often, LTC have a course that varies over time specific to the aetiology and physiology of the illness. However, there are shared challenges for children, adolescents, and families which include recognising symptoms and taking appropriate actions, using medications effectively, managing complex regimens, developing strategies to deal with the psychological consequences of the illness, and interacting with the health and social care systems over time. These demands are to be navigated against Western societies' attitudes and behaviours to those with LTC and disability.

This chapter will firstly explore issues of definition, identifying the nuances and categorisations of LTC. In acknowledging definitional debate in the literature, this chapter will refer to LTC when considering children and adolescents living with conditions beyond three months of duration of varying prognoses, complexities, and limitations. We will highlight how those with LTC and their families cope with related stressors and manage their developmental wellbeing. The impact of LTC and disability during childhood and adolescence will then be discussed alongside the concepts of stigma, ableism, and otherness.

It is to be noted that the more recent studies that have listened to children's and adolescents' accounts of their experiences have encouraged recognition that their lives are not homogeneous and need to be studied in all their diversity.

© The Author(s), under exclusive license to Springer Nature Switzerland AG 2022
J. M. Waite-Jones, A. M. Rodriguez, *Psychosocial Approaches to Child and Adolescent Health and Wellbeing*, https://doi.org/10.1007/978-3-030-99354-2_10

10.1   Issues of Definition and Prevalence

A childhood LTC is a health problem that lasts three months or more, impacts the child's or adolescents' day-to-day activities, and necessitates regular hospital treatment, home healthcare, and/or extensive medical care (Petersson et al., 2013). LTC can relate to all bodily systems, including the following.

The Endocrine System: For example, diabetes is an increasingly prevalent LTC in children and adolescents. In 2019, it was estimated that 36,000 children and adolescents are living in the UK with diabetes; this statistic has increased from 31,500 in 2015 (Diabetes UK, 2019). Type 1 diabetes melitus accounts for 90% of diabetes childhood cases. This condition affects the body's ability to produce insulin. The condition is not associated with deprivation. However, Type 2 diabetes, where the body does not produce enough insulin or is insulin resistant, although less common, is associated with deprivation. The condition is more often seen in obese or overweight children and adolescents and is more highly prevalent in children and adolescents from South Asian and Afro-Caribbean backgrounds. If diabetes is not managed, there can be several complications including eye and kidney disease, heart disease, and stroke (RCPCH, 2019).

The Respiratory System: For example, chronic lung disease, cystic fibrosis, and asthma. Asthma is the most prevalent LTC found in children and adolescents (Ferrante & La Grutta, 2018), with 1.1 million children currently in receipt of treatment (Asthma UK, 2021). Asthma is listed within the top ten reasons for UK childhood emergency hospital admissions for children and adolescents in the UK (Keeble & Kossarova, 2017). The UK is also one of the countries in Europe with the highest asthma-related mortality rates (Shah et al., 2019). Many emergency admissions are preventable if there is good condition management and early intervention. The National Review of Asthma Deaths highlighted that 46% of those children and adolescents who had died had not been in receipt of appropriate asthma care (Royal College of Physicians, 2014).

Musculoskeletal System: The musculoskeletal system includes the bones and the muscles. Musculoskeletal conditions can develop over the lifespan, be resultant of injury, or be congenital. Musculoskeletal conditions include more than 150 conditions and affect movement, the LTC are associated with persistent limitations and disability.

Musculoskeletal LTC include conditions affecting

- joints, for example, osteoarthritis, rheumatoid arthritis, psoriatic arthritis, ankylosing spondylitis
- bones, for example, osteopenia and associated fragility fractures, traumatic fractures
- muscles, for example, sarcopenia
- the spine, for example back and neck pain.
- multiple body areas or systems, for example pain disorders and inflammatory diseases such as connective tissue diseases and vasculitis that have musculoskeletal manifestations, for example systemic lupus erythematosus.

Analysis of the Global Burden of Disease (GBD) data identifies 1.71 billion people globally have musculoskeletal conditions (Cieza et al., 2020). While the prevalence of musculoskeletal conditions varies by age and diagnosis, Juvenile Idiopathic Arthritis (JIA) is the most reported musculoskeletal condition in the child and adolescent literature. In the UK, about 15,000 children and young people are affected by arthritis.

Blood Disorders: For example, leukaemia and other blood cancers, haemophilia, HIV, sickle cell anaemia, and thalassaemia. In 2018, approximately 160,000 children aged 0–9 years were newly infected with HIV globally; this brought the total figure to 1.1 million of 0–9-year-olds with this LTC, 90% of this population residing in sub-Saharan Africa (Unicef, 2018). Cancer, however, remains the leading cause of death in children and adolescents in the UK with an average 240 deaths per year due to childhood cancer (Cancer Research UK, 2021).

There are many diverse types of childhood cancers, the most common include:

- Leukaemia
- Brain and other central nervous system (CNS) and intracranial tumours
- Lymphomas

The UK incidence rates of these cancers have risen by 15% over the last 20 years. However, more children are now surviving for more years post-diagnosis, thanks to advances in technology and the increased number of clinical trials leading to further treatments and better cancer care for children and adolescents (Cancer Research UK, 2021).

Neurological Disorders: Aside from cancers, genetic, congenital, and developmental disorders, epilepsy is the most common significant long-term neurological condition of childhood with 112,000 children and young people in the UK currently living with this LTC (Joint Epilepsy Council of the UK and Ireland, 2011). Unfortunately, even with treatment many children and adolescents continue to have seizures (Chen et al., 2010). Epilepsy is also linked to an elevated risk of mental health difficulties with 37% of children with epilepsy also experiencing a co-existing mental health disorder; a higher prevalence of mental health co-morbidity than found in other LTC (Davies et al., 2003).

Cognitive Health: Amongst children and adolescents aged 5–19 years, 13% are considered to have at least one mental health disorder. In addition, 286,000 children have a learning disability in the UK. Each country in the UK has different policies and systems to identify and support children and young people with disabilities and learning difficulties, which are collectively labelled as 'Special Educational Needs and Disabilities' (SEND) in England and Northern Ireland, 'Additional Support Needs' (ASN) in Scotland, and 'Additional Learning Needs' (ALN) in Wales. However, there are different criteria applied to these labels.

- England: A child or adolescent has SEND if they are considered to have significantly greater difficulties in learning as compared to others of their age, or they have a disability which limits their ability to use facilities that others their age can do with ease.

- Northern Ireland: Criterion is like that used in England but includes a more rigorous framework to help schools to support children with SEND.
- Scotland: A child or adolescent has an Additional Support Need (ASN) if 'for whatever reason, the child or young person is, or is likely to be, unable without the provision of extra support to benefit from school education provided or to be provided for the child or young person'. This wider definition allows any factor which causes a barrier to learn, including being bullied, a young parent or carer, or with a parent in prison to be considered.
- Wales: In 2018, the Additional Learning Needs and Education Tribunal (Wales) Act broadened their criterion which was like that used in England to provide support for children and adolescents with Additional Learning Needs (ALN) (whether the learning difficulty or disability arises from a medical condition or otherwise) where there is a need for additional learning provision.

Children and adolescents with SEND/ASN/ALN are more at risk of experiencing poorer outcomes, such as:

- Increased risk of mental health difficulties (Emerson & Hatton, 2007)
- Lower educational attainment (Jones et al., 2013)
- Challenging behaviour (Gutman & Vorhaus, 2012)
- Difficulties forming healthy relationships with others (Gutman & Vorhaus, 2012)

There is an association between deprivation and higher SEND prevalence in the UK (DoE, 2017).

It is important to note that LTC may also be referred to as chronic conditions. Van Cleave et al. (2010, p. 624) state that child and adolescent chronic health conditions include:

Any physical, emotional, or mental condition that prevented him or her from attending school regularly, doing regular schoolwork, or doing usual childhood activities or that required frequent attention or treatment from a doctor or other health professional, regular use of any medication, or use of special equipment.

10.1.1 Life-Limiting Conditions

In general, chronic illnesses are of an extended duration, cannot be managed without treatment, and most often cannot be cured. Within this population, there will also be young people categorised as living with life-limiting, life-shortening, medically complex, or life-threatening conditions. The terminology is vast.

Life-limiting conditions (LLC) are categorised into four groups (TfSL, 2021):

- Group 1 = Curative treatment may be feasible but can fail (e.g. cancer and organ failure and as such these conditions may also be categorised as life threatening)

- Group 2 = Premature death is inevitable; there may be extended periods of intensive treatment to extend life (e.g. cystic fibrosis)
- Group 3 = Progressive, without curative treatment options and where treatment is exclusively palliative and may extend over many years (e.g. mucopolysaccharidoses)
- Group 4 = Irreversible, non-progressive causing severe disability (e.g. multiple disabilities following brain injury).

The *Make Every Child Count, estimating current and future prevalence of children and young people with life-limiting conditions in the United Kingdom* study identified the national prevalence of LLC in children (aged 0–19 years) in England. It had increased over 17 years from 26.7 per 10,000 in 2001/2 to 66.4 per 10,000 in 2017/18. The prevalence of LLCs was highest for congenital abnormalities with prevalence of LLCs significantly higher among boys (72.5 per 10,000 vs girls 60.0 per 10,000 (2017/18)) and amongst children of Pakistani origin (103.9 per 10,000). This is important in terms of flexibility of service models and provisions to meet the needs of all children. More children than expected with an LLC also live in areas of higher deprivation (Fraser et al., 2020).

Various terms also exist to define health needs complexity including 'medically complex children', 'special healthcare needs', and 'complex chronic conditions'. Complexity can be categorised by economic, clinical, or family impacts, with the current NHS definition concentrating on medical criteria. However, often children and adolescents themselves and many clinicians view complexity as an interplay of medical, psychological, emotional, social, and environmental factors. Thus, there is a need to develop a broader, universally accepted definition (Aitchison et al., 2021).

10.2   Impact on Child and Adolescent Wellbeing

Children and adolescents with LTC are often expected to go through the same developmental stages as their healthy peers (unless there are neurological/degenerative issues incumbent with their LLC or impacts of treatment). However, studies suggest that regardless of diagnosis, children and adolescents with LTC are more limited in their participation in everyday activities and often follow atypical developmental patterns (Lambert & Keogh, 2015). Table 10.1 highlights broadly the effects LTC can have on children's and adolescents' wellbeing.

10.2.1 The Impact of LTC on Developmental Stages

Children and adolescents learn to manage complex developmental tasks alongside the demands of their LTC. Many however struggle with self-esteem, body image, social roles, and peer-related issues. In addition, living with an LTC is correlated with educational disengagement and significantly lower educational outcomes (Hopkins et al., 2014). This array of difficulties can mean children and adolescents

Table 10.1 The effects of LTC on children's and adolescents' wellbeing

Wellbeing category	Effects
Physical	Features of LTC or treatments can impact growth pubertal delay. Undernutrition can be resultant of many LTC. Obesity can occur when LTC reduce physical activity. Visible signs of LTC or the impacts of treatment also 'mark' individuals as different which can be difficult to manage at a stage of development whereby children and adolescents want to be like their peers. Body image issues can be related to height, weight, pubertal stage, and scarring—issues can continue into adulthood.
Emotional and mental health	Children/adolescents cope well with the emotional effects of LTC. However, they may experience lower levels of emotional wellbeing than peers without LTC. They may feel different to and isolated from their peers, frustrated by the demands of their LTC and efforts needed to work with support. They experience many sources of stress. Although prevalence for mental health issues is lower than adult cases, monitoring for depression, anxiety, and adjustment disorders is needed.
Social, educational, and vocational aspects	LTC can impact cognition and learning, highlighted by deficient performance at school and LTC-related absences. Social isolation and loneliness because of school absenteeism and unable to participate in extracurricular and leisure activities are notable risks.

with LTC experience problems with coping and can then also suffer from psychological disorders (Petersson et al., 2013). Peer relationships and family support are important to help negotiate developmental wellbeing. Where LTC limit children's and adolescents' ability to make friends and to socialise, they can be left to feel inadequate and can struggle feeling they do not belong with a peer group. Despite constantly striving for 'typical' childhoods, children and adolescents often report feeling different from their peers and will exert much energy to try to 'fit in'. Unfortunately, this can be difficult and mean that they then engage with passive coping strategies such as withdrawal, avoidance of activities, and non-adherence to treatment regimens. Living with an LTC for children and adolescents is often 'a balancing act' where they try to perform to peer norms but also feel different as a consequence of their LTC (Spencer et al., 2013).

10.3   Coping and Adjustment to LTC by Children and Adolescents

LTC and their associated treatment regimens present children, adolescents, and their families with significant stress which can lead to emotional and behavioural difficulties, then affecting condition management. In addition, some LTC are also impacted by the stress children and adolescents have in other areas of their lives. It is important to consider how children and adolescents cope with these multiple stressors to then target supportive interventions to promote better adjustment.

Lazarus and Folkman (1984) suggest coping relates to the thoughts and behaviours individuals use to manage the internal and external demands of events/

situations they appraise as stressful. There has been debate as to whether this definition can extend to children and adolescents. However, coping in children and adolescents is stipulated to be a group or central mass of 'purposeful', 'volitional' efforts used to regulate aspects of the self and environment under stress. Compas et al. (2001, p. 89) offer the following definition: 'conscious and volitional efforts to regulate emotion, cognition, behaviour, physiology, and the environment in response to stressful events or circumstances'. This definition reflects the important links that exist between coping and the regulation of psychological and physiological processes, including emotion, behaviour, and cognition, as well as the efforts to regulate interactions with others and the environment.

The evidence on children's and adolescents' coping with stress highlights how coping can be resultant of both controlled and automatic processes. Included within the category of automatic stress responses are reactions associated with temperament and conditioning, including emotional and physiological arousal, automatic thoughts, and conditioned behaviours. Effective coping responses are alternatively considered to be controlled and volitional, where children will purposefully and increasingly take actions to manage and adjust to stressors in their lives. However, these effective coping responses develop over the lifespan and so children and adolescents can still often experience automatic and temperament fuelled stress reactions until they learn other ways to respond.

10.3.1 Coping Strategies Used by Children and Adolescents with LTC

There are three distinct groups of coping strategies used by children and adolescents, primary control engagement coping, secondary control engagement coping, and disengagement coping.

▶ Coping strategies used by children and adolescents with long-term conditions

▶ **Primary control engagement coping**—aims to change the stressor/emotional responses. One good example would be the use of active problem solving where an individual first defines the problem, considers an array of solutions, and then identifies and enacts the best solution to then solve the problem. Where primary control coping is enacted as a response to an emotional reaction, the coping strategy employed could be emotional expression and then related communication with others whereby it is hoped that the individual will receive emotional support, including empathy and understanding to relieve or lower the emotionality of the situation.

▶ **Secondary control engagement coping**—the aim is for adaptation. This is achieved by enacting strategies such as acceptance (e.g. thinking this is something that they will need to live with and so it is best to accommodate it) and positive reinterpretation (e.g. trying to find positivity in something that may immediately only appear as negative).

▶ **Disengagement coping**—aims to escape the stressor or the emotions that the stressor has created. This is accomplished using passive and maladaptive responses such as avoidance (e.g. ignoring the problem or 'burrowing one's head in the sand'), pretending that the stressor does not exist and for some adolescents there can be engagement in substance use to forget or 'block out' the stressor (Carver & Connor-Smith, 2010).

Studies highlight how engagement coping is associated with health benefits and improved measures of quality of life. Disengagement coping however can be problematic, especially amongst those experiencing long-term stress. Disengagement strategies can lead to prominent levels of distress, anxiety, and depression (Nielsen & Knardahl, 2014).

We all respond to stress differently. However, our cognitive appraisal of both the threat of the stressor(s) and our coping resources is situational. An important influencing factor is our perceived controllability of the stressor(s). Perceived control is defined as the extent we think that the stressor(s) can be attributed to internal (personal) sources, external (situational/environmental) sources, or to the cause or predictability of an event (Eisenbarth, 2012). In a seminal review of children's coping with medical stressors, Rudolph et al. (1995) offered a multifaceted model of control and coping that continues to aid our contemporary understanding of children and adolescents and their successful adaptation/adjustment to LTC. The model details primary control (active coping strategies to control events), secondary control (active coping strategies to adapt to events), and relinquished control (an absence of a coping strategy effort) as constituting appraisals of control and coping subtypes. The framework therefore includes both coping responses or types of strategies and coping goals. The authors consider a coping response as an intentional action, whereas a coping goal is instead the objective of a coping response or strategy which is usually the resolution or reduction of stress (see Table 10.2). Both the type of coping response and coping goal can be related to the perceived or actual controllability of the source of the stressor(s) (Table 10.3).

In accordance, Jaser and White (2010) found that adolescents experiencing diabetes-related stress were most likely to use secondary control coping strategies, followed by primary control coping and disengagement coping strategies to 'cope'. Where adolescents used more primary control coping strategies there was evidence of higher competence levels, higher quality of life, and better metabolic control. Similarly, where adolescents used more secondary control coping strategies, they had higher quality of life and better metabolic control. As their diabetes-related stress increased, however, they were less likely to use these adaptive strategies. Relinquished control or 'disengagement coping' strategies, such as avoidance and denial, were then associated with lower levels of resilience, teamed with lower levels of competence and poorer metabolic control.

Table 10.2   The effects of LTC on families and treatment adherence

Impact of LTC on families	Parenting difficulties are exaggerated by LTC. LTC can limit the child's autonomy, increasing and maintaining dependence on family care givers. Time to provide for needs can also impact finances and parent ability to work. Parents can struggle emotionally with guilt, frustration, anxiety, and depression. Siblings can experience adjustment difficulties.
Treatment adherence	Health and social care professionals are motivated to achieve the best outcomes for the child or adolescent which can mean focusing on current behaviours for the benefit of now and the future. Children and adolescents alternatively are only focused on the 'here and now' with more interest in achieving developmental goals (which includes maintaining peer relationships) than improving their health. This often leads to conflicting priorities between the child/adolescent, professionals, and parents/family carers. In focusing on external benefits, professionals can highlight treatment goals related to appearance, ability to socialise or join in leisure activities. In agreeing short-term goals, for example being well enough to attend a party, there can be increased adherence. Involvement in treatment/care planning can assist children/adolescents to feel they have some control over their LTC which can influence motivations for self-management. It is important that children/adolescents understand their LTC, why they need treatments and other interventions via developmentally appropriate information. Families can be instrumental to treatment adherence. Those who belong to supportive families who openly communicate experience lower levels of family stress and have better adherence to regimens and improved long-term health outcomes. Peers may also be an additional source of support.

Table 10.3   The constructs of control and coping applied to diabetes stress

Construct	Description	Example
Coping response	Intentional action	Adopting behaviours to reduce diabetes-related stress
Coping goal	Objective of coping response	Increased resilience, higher competence levels, higher quality of life, better metabolic control
Primary control	Active coping strategies to control events	Problem solving, emotional expression
Secondary control	Active coping strategies to adapt to events	Acceptance, distraction
Relinquished control	Absence of a coping effort	Avoidance, denial

Further studies have reported on the effectiveness of the distinct types of coping strategies in relation to the appraised controllability of stressor(s). In general, primary coping is more effective when the stressor(s) are perceived to be highly controllable, whereas secondary coping is more effective in stressful situations that are perceived as long lasting, where the person has little control and the situation is likely to not change dramatically, for example in living with a LTC that is life limiting in its condition trajectory, for instance in children and adolescents with neuromuscular conditions such as muscular dystrophy. With muscular dystrophy conditions there can be a gradual loss of muscular strength and mobility, slowly and increasingly limiting the individual's mobility and then due to issues of rigidity there are impacts on other bodily symptoms. In these situations, there can be much uncertainty regarding the longevity of the condition and the rate of degeneration. With increasing loss of movement and impacts on activity and speech the affected child or adolescent can indeed experience many stressors impacting on wellbeing. Positive appraisal of these stressors accompanied by active coping strategies can influence the person to adapt or discover new ways of being. If this can be achieved, then the levels of stress experienced can be reduced. Where children and adolescents can be flexible in their appraisals of stressful events and situations and the controllability of outcomes their wellbeing and adaptation can be increased.

There is mounting evidence that children and adolescents with LTC cope and adjust better to the demands of their conditions if they draw on active coping strategies, for example problem solving, cognitive reappraisal, positive thinking, and acceptance. However, where children and adolescents instead relinquish control to try and cope and they then use denial, social withdrawal, and wishful thinking they have poorer outcomes including feeling anxious, sad, and experience somatic symptoms. In addition, parents can feel less stressed/cope better if they witness their children with LTC seek and accept support from friends and family, stay optimistic, and where appropriate use problem-focused behaviours (Rodriguez et al., 2012).

10.3.2 Stress and Coping Adopted by Family Caregivers

A major source of stress perceived by family caregivers of children and adolescents with LTC is their responsibility for treatment management (Rodriguez & King, 2009). This stress is felt irrespective of type of LTC and severity. Whereas for children and adolescents with LTC, it is their perceived lack of control over their condition, its progression, being restricted because of the condition, feeling dissimilar to peers, treatment side effects, and pain that can influence emotional and behavioural difficulties that cause them the most stress.

Amongst the most common LTC in children are cancer, diabetes, and asthma and as a result these are the most researched LTC when exploring psychological wellbeing. Although the nuances of relationships and interrelationships between family caregivers/parents and children remain a needed area of study in this context, it has been found that all parties find the process of receiving a cancer diagnosis, its treatment (including pain and hair loss and school absenteeism), and the condition uncertainties highly stressful. When treatment fails or cancers return, there is also a substantial risk of depression for both parent and child (Bikmazer et al., 2020).

These condition-focused studies have also identified protective and risk factors that can mitigate/moderate psychological outcomes. Primary and secondary control coping or 'productive coping' is related to resilience and satisfaction, whereas disengagement coping or 'non-productive' coping is associated with the development of psychopathology. Where families receive instrumental support and children are provided with developmentally appropriate information about their LTC and care/treatment plan there is better adjustment and more optimal measures of wellbeing (Alperin et al., 2019). For example, where children are supported to take their asthma inhaler treatments and are given developmentally appropriate information on the use of their steroid and reliever medications, they can feel empowered to take responsibility. A routine can be established to take inhalers in the morning and evening, for instance, incumbent with their routine of washing and dressing. Good management may negate the need for emergency use of reliever medication. However, if the child has had the informational support they be empowered and will know how to respond to breathlessness without heightened panic. Where medication is routinised, children can feel confident and in control and so appraisal and coping can be both active and productive. Where there is little guidance and information provided to children, they can be dependent on parental direction, feel a lack of control and uncertainty about when to take their medication and about what to do and how to act if they experience breathlessness/wheeze. This unknowingness and lack of regime can heighten the stress the child experiences and can lead to poor condition management.

Most common LTC can begin with an acute phase that leads to diagnosis followed by extensive periods of stress linked with treatment, periods of recovery and the striving for wellness and living with hope. As such, we can identify how stress can be experienced across the full disease trajectory of LTC. To design and deliver targeted and supportive interventions it is important that we both understand what issues cause stress in children and adolescents with LTC but also what stressors children and adolescents focus their coping efforts upon. In addition, health and social care professionals need to be mindful of what sources of support are available to children and families and what factors could impede their effective coping.

10.3.3   Sources of Support for Children and Adolescents with LTC

Parents are a source of support for their children with LTC and role models for effective or ineffective coping and as such children can mirror to what extent parents are emotionally managing the child's illness situation (see Wiebe et al. 2005 for a discussion around parental coping and children with diabetes, Rodriguez & King, 2009, 2014 with respect to parents of children with life-limiting conditions and Sieberg et al., 2011 for a similar discussion relating to chronic pain). Thompson et al. (1989) developed a transactional model of stress and coping, within an ecological system's theory perspective, to explore LTC as a major source of stress for both child and family. The model highlights how the relationship between illness and psychological adjustment depends on biomedical, developmental, and psychosocial processes. Using this perspective, the coping strategies, of both parent and child, are moderators of the illness–adjustment relationship, with greater influence on outcomes than illness characteristics and demographics (Thompson & Gustafson, 1996).

For example, if we again consider the COVID-19 pandemic, it has presented families around the world with extraordinary challenges related to physical and mental health, economic security, social support, and education. Brooks et al. (2020) highlight how the pandemic is associated with notable increases in self-reported levels of problematic mental health indicators among parents and young people. Skinner et al. (2021) undertook a longitudinal, multi-centre study of parenting, adolescent development, and young adult competence to explore any associations between personal disruption during the pandemic and reported changes in mental health of young adults and their mothers since the pandemic began. The study also considered family functioning three years prior through adolescence. Families ($n = 484$) from five countries (Italy, the Philippines, Sweden, Thailand, and the United States) participated. More than half of the young adults reported an increase in anxiety or sadness during the pandemic, and one third reported increases in externalising behaviours. It was reported in Italy, the Philippines, Sweden, and the United States that life disruptions during the pandemic were related to increases in internalising and externalising behaviours for both young adults and their mothers. There were associations with prior pandemic behaviours, that is, 'Higher levels of youth disclosure', 'more supportive parenting', and 'lower levels of destructive adolescent-parent conflict'. This study therefore suggests that qualities of the parent child relationship during adolescence around the world may serve to protect children from increases in maladaptive behaviour during major negative life events, not just during childhood and adolescence but also into young adulthood. Mothers also benefit from these protective effects, suggesting that strong parent adolescent relationships characterised by open communication, support, and positive conflict resolution are enduring resources that can promote family resilience during times of unprecedented stress.

10.4   COVID-19 and Children and Adolescents with Long-Term Conditions

The COVID-19-pandemic is a source of significant stress for children and adolescents with LTC and their families. The Royal College of Paediatrics and Chid Health (2020) have developed parent information sheets, highlighting those at greatest risk should isolate to minimise their risk of infection. In addition, as suggested by Dalton et al. (2020), adults have been advised to be honest with their children when asked about the disease but to try not to overwhelm them with their own fears. In the absence of information, children and adolescents will try make sense of the situation on their own. Great Ormond Street Children's Hospital (GOSH) have also developed several information sheets about COVID-19 for children with LTC. These child-friendly information leaflets can be downloaded from the GOSH website (https://tinyurl.com/gosh-covid). They include leaflets on COVID and asthma, COVID and cystic fibrosis, COVID and haematology oncology, COVID and immunology, COVID and kidney transplant, COVID and non-invasive or tracheostomy ventilation. The charity Together for Short Lives has also produced guidance for families (https://tinyurl.com/together-covid). Additionally, Southampton children's hospital developed a useful child-friendly poster explaining COVID-19 to children, which is available on the Royal College of Paediatrics and Child Health website (https://tinyurl.com/Southampton-covid).

10.4.1   Risks to Wellbeing

There is evidence that children and adolescents with attention-deficit/hyperactivity disorder (ADHD) and autism spectrum disorder (ASD), who have better day-to-day wellbeing when they have structure and routine, have been more affected by the changes caused by the pandemic than any other group. Carers have reported an increase in behavioural difficulties (Zhang et al., 2020). Mental health services for children and adolescents with LTC are limited, especially those targeted towards health anxiety. Services have been further reduced due to the pandemic. A study based in Singapore reported how psychological services for children and adolescents' youth eating disorders are now only being offered to the most urgent cases. This has meant community and charitable services have needed to try and bridge the gap for those who have experienced reduced access to psychological therapies (Davis et al., 2020). In addition, a recent UK survey including more than two thousand young people with a history of mental health problems discovered 51% of the participants had experienced a deterioration in their mental health due to the pandemic, reporting psychological distress and loneliness (Young Minds, 2020). Children and adolescents with cancer have also reported heightened worries about social isolation and how their propensity for catastrophising has increased (Brooks et al., 2020; Ng et al., 2020). Studies of children from China have also noted related clinginess, distraction, irritability, and fear of asking questions about the pandemic (Jiao et al., 2020). There has also been a reduction in primary care services and access to GP appointments. There is increasing evidence to suggest that children with certain LTC have been negatively impacted by these changes, including those with inflammatory bowel disease (Martinelli et al., 2020), cancer (Parasole et al., 2020; Vasquez et al., 2020), and type 1 diabetes (Dayal et al., 2020).

10.4.2   Benefits to Wellbeing

Despite children and young people with LTC experiencing health-related concerns and stressors, not least due to the need to shield and access to services being altered, they have also experienced some benefits to their wellbeing. Children and adolescents with LTC have often had lifetime experiences of hospitalisations and changes to education and peer networks. This experience has served them well in the pandemic because they have had the prior experience of being away from day-to-day school life and have learnt ways to cope. In addition, for some children with LTC returning to school and needing to wear masks, for example those with cystic fibrosis, this normalisation of practice for all has meant they are not singled out as different (Ladores, 2020). In addition, the many weeks at home with parents has meant children and adolescents with LTC have had parents and siblings at home so they have been even more involved in their support, A study based in Austria suggests that there has been an increase in social connectedness within families, reducing family stress and fatigue (Nitschke et al., 2021).

10.5   Chronic Pain and Persistent Stress in LTC

Chronic pain (pain lasting more than three months in duration) is a significant source of stress and a debilitating factor for many children and adolescents with an LTC. Various physiological systems underpin chronic pain, including central sensitisation (heightened neural activity within the central nervous system that encourages increased nociceptive signalling). The stress model of chronic pain suggests that chronic pain can result from increased levels of cortisol (a stress hormone) in the brain (a sustained endocrine response) and lowered hippocampal volume following repeated stressors (Vachon-Presseau et al., 2013).

10.5.1 Impact of Chronic and Reoccurring Stress

Constant or recurrent stress in a person's life can subject them to increased levels of cortisol which means their bodies can be in a constant state of arousal or 'sensitisation'. With repeated exposure to adverse childhood experiences (ACEs, as discussed in Chap. 4 on attachment, are known to contribute to long-term harmful effects on physical and mental health across the lifespan; research suggests that having an LTC can be conceptualised as a traumatic experience, and therefore an ACE), there can be significant wear and tear on the body's sympathetic and parasympathetic response systems (often referred to as 'allostatic load' in the literature) (Rogosch et al., 2011).

Allostatic load and over-activation of the hypothalamic–pituitary–adrenal (HPA) axis, a factor implicit with allostatic load of the HPA axis, describes a complex feedback system of neurohormones that are sent between the hypothalamus, pituitary gland, and adrenal glands. This negative and positive feedback system regulates the physiological mechanisms of stress reactions and is related to the development and/or maintenance of chronic pain in children and adolescents. This can be irrespective of their history of ACEs and we know that multiple ACEs can result in poorer outcomes (Lupien et al., 2006).

The research that has explored allostatic load relative to LTC stress has been undertaken with adult populations. Where individuals in addition experience social stressors (e.g. bullying) the same neural processes involved in the processing of physical pain can be found to be activated (Eisenberger, 2012). Looking at these combined processes of physical and socio-emotional stress experiences, theories exploring the neurobiology of ACEs (chronic stress) identify similar physiological processes involved with pain processing in chronic pain. To illustrate, dysregulation influenced by allostatic load can affect different bodily systems incumbent with chronic pain (endocrine and immune systems predominantly). Therefore, where people are experiencing both chronic pain and other chronic stressors, they could also experience greater neurological and neuroendocrine function problems. There remains a dearth of studies however in this field associated with neuroendocrine processes and chronic pain in children and adolescents with LTC and a history of ACEs.

There are numerous studies that have looked at the wellbeing of children and adolescents cross-sectionally and longitudinally and have identified that when there is an history of multiple ACEs then there is more likelihood of mental health difficulties. There are also many studies that show how emotional difficulties are linked to the experience of heightened pain and disability in children and adolescents with chronic pain problems. Therefore, children and adolescents with an LTC and both chronic pain and a history of other stressors could be more vulnerable to emotional and behavioural difficulties which then can impact their coping. Studies have been undertaken that have looked at the trajectories of children and adolescents reporting mental health difficulties and chronic pain. There appears to be a strong association between psychological symptoms and chronic pain conditions and so it is possible there could be a bidirectional relationship (Kerker et al., 2015). Kascakova et al. (2020) explored the association between childhood trauma, anxiety, and long-term pain conditions in general and clinical populations (including, e.g., those with hypertension, asthma, and arthritis and other LTC). Anxiety and pain were associated with individuals having experienced emotional abuse and emotional and physical neglect regardless of their clinical status. However, where individuals reported emotional and physical abuse and emotional neglect, they had an increased chance of also suffering from an anxiety or adjustment disorder with concurrent long-term pain compared to the general population.

Further studies are needed to investigate if exposure to ACEs via psychological comorbidities puts children and adolescents with LTC at a higher risk of chronic pain or pain-related disability. Where children and adolescents have a history of ACEs, they often appraise innocuous or ambiguous experiences as more threatening than reality, this can influence their perceived ability to cope. This negative appraisal can result in cognitive distortions influencing threat appraisal, coping efficacy, and subsequent impairment. Such has important implications for behavioural intervention (Cohen et al., 2006).

10.5.2 Coping with Stress Resulting from Adverse Childhood Experiences

When faced with a stressful situation we draw on both internal and external coping resources. External resources for children and adolescents are firstly their family caregivers. However, often when children experience chronic pain this is also an issue for their parents. These family units may have histories of ACEs and heightened risk of current ACEs including job loss, and marital conflict. These families are often found to have ineffective pain coping strategies and disharmonious relationships. Stressful home lives can impact social functioning (interpersonal attachment, family relational styles), meaning children and adolescents may struggle to access positive support systems (modelling parental coping styles) that would help relieve their stress.

Zeng and Hui (2018) investigated the prevalence rate and associations of ACEs amongst young children with disabilities. They also investigated the child and family risk factors that mediated the number of ACEs. They used data from a US national database from June 2016 to February 2017, sampling 364,150 households identifying households where there was at least one child aged 0–17 with a health concern. Eligible households (*N* = 68,961) received an age-specific survey to complete (ages 0–5, 6–11, or 12–17). In total 72.8% completed the survey. The survey requested parents or guardians to detail the child's current health condition. A child was identified as having a disability if they had one of the following conditions: developmental delay, traumatic brain injury, cerebral palsy, Down syndrome, epilepsy, Tourette syndrome, speech, or language disorder, learning disability, autism, attention deficit disorder (ADD) or attention-deficit/hyperactivity disorder (ADHD), intellectual disability, anxiety, depression, orthopaedic impairment, deafness, and blindness. The most prevalent ACEs for these children were lack of basic food and housing (40.9%), parental divorce (24.3%), alcohol/drug problems (11.1%), parent or guardian incarceration (10.6%), and adult abuse (6.8%).

Service models and policies within Western societies often necessitate that many cares are delivered in the community with parents being relied upon to provide complex care and treatments. Cross-system collaboration between early intervention service and the social welfare system is warranted for young children with LTC and their families as these children may encounter various ACEs that then mediate the outcomes of early childhood and indeed impact their wellbeing across their lifespan. Again, more research is needed to explore the impact the family environment may have on children and adolescents with LTC experiencing chronic pain and a history of ACEs (Hoftun et al., 2013). Unfortunately there is also a need for studies to evaluate the effectiveness of psychological interventions for symptoms of mental illness, including anxiety and depression in children and adolescents with LTC (Bennett et al., 2015). Studies that have been undertaken using trial methodologies are considered in general to be of low quality and underpowered, using outcome measures that may not be sufficiently dependable in younger populations (Moore et al., 2020).

10.6   Developmental Differences in Coping with LTC

Few studies have investigated age and developmental patterns in children and adolescents coping with LTC. Quantitative studies of coping in children with cancer have found no significant age-related effects. However, there is suggestion that adolescents may draw on more cognitive and secondary control coping strategies than younger children, perhaps because they have greater cognitive resources they can draw upon to enact this type of coping (Aldridge & Roesch, 2007). Several LTCs involve impaired cognitive function in children and adolescents, resulting from the disease process or treatments. Studies report significant cognitive impairment in childhood cancer survivors, those with type 1 diabetes, congenital heart disease, and sickle cell disease. As such, this could be why children with certain LTC struggle to enact complex cognitive coping strategies that are needed to cope with stressful situations effectively. Where children can use complex coping strategies (cognitive reappraisal and acceptance) they are likely to have maintained healthy development of regions of the prefrontal cortex, whereas these areas of the brain can be vulnerable in some LTC (Compas, 2006). Campbell et al. (2009) found higher levels of primary and secondary control coping were associated with better executive functioning (e.g. working memory, cognitive flexibility, and self-monitoring), whereas disengagement coping was correlated with poorer executive functioning. In addition, coping style mediated the relationship between executive function and emotional or behavioural difficulties. In addition, children and adolescents with early onset of type 1 diabetes are likely to have poor neuropsychological performance, with particular deficits in attention and executive function (Gaudieri et al., 2008). Heightened levels of glucose can impact the formation of myelin and neurotransmitter regulation during critical periods of brain development (Lin et al., 2010).

10.7   Self-management of LTC in Children and Adolescents

Self-management is a dynamic, interactive, and daily process enacted to manage LTC (Lorig & Holman, 2003). Self-management refers to 'the ability of the individual, in conjunction with family, community, and healthcare professionals, to manage symptoms, treatments, lifestyle changes, and psychosocial, cultural, and spiritual consequences of health conditions' (Richard & Shea, 2011, p. 261). Good self-management involves the individual monitoring of their illness and developing and operationalising effective strategies to maintain quality of life. Self-management is considered different to self-care, which is linked to healthy lifestyle behaviours for general wellbeing development and health maintenance (Richard & Shea, 2011).

10.7.1 Self-management Frameworks

Several self-management frameworks have increased our understanding of what constitutes self-management in LTC, however the specific processes or mechanisms of self-management are still to be depicted and there remains few studies that explore self-management from the perspectives of children and adolescents with LTC. Corbin and Strauss (1988) first identified the processes of self-management noting the efforts involved with living with an LTC. They suggested three tasks of self-management: medical management, (treatment adherence—taking medications and attending medical appointments), behavioural management (lifestyle, role adaptation), and emotional management (processing emotions influenced by LTC). In relation to this framework, Lorig and Holman (2003) suggested the processes of self-management included problem solving, decision making, making use of resources, partnering with healthcare providers, taking action, and improving self-efficacy. These tasks and processes of self-management are considered applicable to all LTCs. However, Ryan and Sawin (2009) discuss that self-management includes the processes of enhancing knowledge and beliefs (self-efficacy, outcome expectancy, goal congruence), regulating skills and abilities (goal-setting, self-monitoring, reflective thinking, decision making, planning and action, self-evaluation, emotional control), and social facilitation (influence, support, collaboration). Although these processes are more specified, they do not consider how there can be many emotional or existential challenges in living with an LTC. For example, if we take children with oncology conditions, they may have experienced the loss of peers, the fear of treatment and its impacts and may worry about their own futures and how their futures may be different or shortened. Communication with children and adolescents around these interlinked emotional and existential challenges may be limited due to parental distress and both parental and professional protectiveness (Rodriguez et al., 2018; Watts et al., 2020). Qualitative studies exploring lived experiences, however, highlight how emotional and existential processes, such as reconciling emotions and deriving meaning from the illness experience, impact upon self-management (De Ridder et al., 2008). Further studies are necessary to explore this array of concepts with children and adolescents.

10.7.2 Digital Solutions in LTC Management for Children and Adolescents

Studies over the last ten years have become increasingly focused on developing and evaluating digital solutions and mHealth applications or 'apps' aimed at supporting LTC management and behavioural change for children and adolescents. Behaviour changes interventions include a battery of techniques designed to change health behaviours. For children and adolescents with LTC, these interventions often target adherence to treatment and education about their condition. For example, to promote the management of diabetes, a behaviour change intervention would encourage behaviours needed for blood glucose monitoring, the selection of healthy food choices, engagement with physical activity, and attendance at routine clinical appointments. Behaviour change interventions are important because habits can be formed that can impact lifespan behaviours and condition management over many years. In a recent review, Hamine et al. (2015) investigated the self-management of diabetes, cardiovascular disease, and chronic lung disease. One key finding was mHealth can facilitate adherence to processes involved in good LTC management. Although, many authors suggest applications to be used for adolescents and young adults, Fedele et al. (2017) identified that mHealth interventions can be acceptable as behavioural change interventions in younger populations. There are, however, efforts needed to engage children and adolescents with LTC to use associated applications and so the content and aesthetics of applications are in major area of contemporary LTC research. In addition, Huang et al. (2014) suggest that digital interventions can be more cost effective than other approaches. They evaluated a web-based and short message service (SMS) text message-delivered LTC management app as a supportive transition solution. Griffiths et al. (2017) add that the adoption of communication technologies (mobile phone calls, SMS, email, and Voice over Internet systems) can promote child and adolescent engagement with self-management, improve relationships, and the trust they hold for healthcare professionals.

10.7.3 Impact of Digital Applications on Lived Experience of LTC

It is important that we consider how condition trajectories can alter lived experience and symptomology and how there may be issues with digital applications being able to keep apace of changes. There is also the question around family acceptability and health professional education and ease in facilitating and supporting their use. There is much research yet to be done on digital application impact on LTC management and child and adolescent wellbeing across condition trajectories and services. Where they might be more efficacious is in areas of practice where there appears to be a dearth of support or long waits to receive support, for example where children and young people are struggling with mental health difficulties. In addition, digital mental health technologies are a solution to improve reach and access to psychological therapies, at a low cost. The National Institute for Health and Care Excellence (2019), for example, supports the use of digital cognitive behavioural therapy (CBT) for depression. However, although most children and adolescents have internet access there remains a minority of hard-to-reach families living in digital poverty without the funds to pay for devices or internet access. In addition, due to the novelty of many applications there is still research to be executed that explores the acceptability of digital interventions outside of the research context. It is important that applications, however, are not adaptations of adult-centric interventions; children and adolescents have developmental and age-related needs, interests, and preferences. The presentation of difficulties may also be very different to adult populations. It is also worth mentioning that where there is use of virtual interventions, accessed in the community, there may be issues of confidentiality and compatibility with different systems. There may also be difference in disease demands and so digital support needs to consider such nuances. For example, an application to encourage children and adolescents with diabetes to engage in regular self-testing seems unproblematic but if a similar approach were taken for children and adolescents with juvenile arthritis to monitor their symptoms, this could then create anxiety and over concern with their condition, potentially reinforcing their 'sick role' status.

10.8   Stigma and the Development of Children and Adolescents with LTC

Stigma is broadly defined as *perceived or enacted disapproval, discrimination, or rejection associated with an attribute or characteristic that is different or undesirable* (Link & Phelan, 2006). Adult and child studies together highlight that illness-related stigma influences negative psychosocial outcomes (Cianchetti et al., 2015). Stevelink et al. (2012) developed a model of illness-related stigma in adults. In this model poorer psychosocial outcomes result from individuals experiencing, perceiving, and anticipating negative social reactions. Such stigma experiences cause the internalisation of stigma, creating negative thoughts, impacting perceived identities, and then promoting maladaptive behaviours, such as not participating in social events. Negative psychosocial outcomes ensue, for example, emotional and behavioural difficulties related to depression and anxiety.

10.8.1 Mediating Factors Impacting on Illness-related Stigma

In considering the model developed by Stevelink et al. (2012), there are modifiable mediating factors that impact the relation between illness-related stigma and psychosocial outcomes in children and adolescents. In particular, 'maladaptive behaviours' may be further influenced by the perception of illness intrusiveness. Illness intrusiveness in this context is defined as the extent to which an LTC is thought to cause disruptions in lifestyle, activities, values, and interests (Devins, 2010). Illness intrusiveness is a well-established construct and reliable predictor of psychosocial outcomes in child and adolescent populations. The construct is independently associated with psychosocial outcomes, more so than objective measures of disease severity (Ramsey et al., 2014). Both social and cognitive variables impact increased perceptions of intrusiveness. Illness intrusiveness stems from an individual's perception of their illness and their environment and can be exacerbated by negative cognitions such as illness-related stigma and associated negative perceptions of the self (Dancey et al., 2002). For example, an adolescent with epilepsy may want to be the same as their peers, learn to drive, go out socialising, enjoy a drink of alcohol but their condition may disallow them from learning to drive and their treatment regimen may limit where they socialise and limit or prevent their intake of alcohol. Peer awareness may limit the stigma or felt stigma and associated negative perceptions of the self, but this level of illness intrusiveness can sometimes make it difficult for adolescents to feel apace of and part of their youth culture, interests, and milestones.

There is, however, a dearth of studies that have investigated illness-related stigma, and potential mediators, in children and adolescents with LTC. This is surprising given that we know from seminal developmental psychology theory and practice that children and adolescents especially can be vulnerable to the views of others and therefore may be vulnerable to illness-related stigma. In a study undertaken by Waite-Jones and Madill (2008) a sibling explained how his brother (with juvenile arthritis) had, had to 'grow up backwards', in that most children learn to get on with peers first and then adults as they mature. However, those with long-term conditions spend much of their early childhood interacting with adults which means they have then to learn how to relate to peers—which can make stigma worse. Through adolescence, individuals strive to belong to a peer group and need to manage their social networking alongside the demands of their LTC (Arnett, 2001). They must navigate the changing nature of their health and the potential negative peer evaluation of such.

10.8.2 Independence and Vulnerability of LTC

Among older adolescents with LTC, those attending college or university, especially if they live away from home, may be particularly vulnerable. Studies undertaken with students with epilepsy and inflammatory bowel disease highlight correlations between stigma and lowered measures of self-esteem and self-efficacy, and a desire to not disclose or discuss their LTC with others and social withdrawal (Cianchetti et al., 2015; Taft et al., 2013). Where children and adolescents perceive they have low social support, outcomes include poor treatment regimen adherence, depression and anxiety, and lower measures of health-related quality of life (Warner et al., 2016). However, it is also the case that adolescents with LTC may choose to not move away from home to attend college or university because of their condition-related anxieties and treatment needs. This can mean they also do not get the opportunities of their peers to experience developmental milestones related to gaining increasing independence from their parents. As a result, comparisons of developmental wellbeing amongst adolescents with LTC living at home and away and against peers without LTC need critical evaluation.

10.9 Difference and Ableism

The notions of perceived, actual, and self-stigma are promoted by 'difference'. Difference is at the centre of many debates within disability studies and is relevant to the lived experience of children and adolescents with LTC. Some argue that difference does not exist whereas others acknowledge there are differences but it is the views of others that construct bodies as different and disabled (Price & Shildrick, 2002). An alternative view is that disabled people are 'essentially' different from non-disabled people, so the 'difference' is part of the 'essence' of a disabled person. For Morris (1991) having an impairment does render an individual as fundamentally different from someone who does not have one. However, this difference exists beyond the socially constructed effects of disablism, making the presence of an impairment the key difference between disabled and non-disabled people or between people with and without LTC.

Goodley (2012) defines disablism as: 'a set of assumptions and practices, often internalised, that trigger inequality and the othering of disabled people. This, in turn, undermines disabled people's physical, psychological, and emotional well being.' Disablism then manifests in society as lower expectations, stereotypical labelling, and assumptions about the competencies of children and adolescents with LTC/disabilities (Hehir, 2002).

Similar to disablism, the concept of ableism refers to a set of beliefs that produces disability or difference as a counter-image to able-bodiedness and therefore considered deviant or an unwelcome difference (Campbell, 2009). According to feminist disability studies and anti-oppressive studies, ableism is currently the most dominant disability narrative in Western societies (Ahlvik-Harju, 2015).

The body is at the crux of ableism; the body highlights otherness by comparison categorisation, where normative ableist logic sifts out the wanted from the unwanted bodies then constructs such in terms of the unwanted and different. This ableist narrative is also referred to as 'the normalcy narrative' or 'a comforting narrative' despite such narratives being far from comforting (Ahlvik-Harju, 2015). According to Fiona Kumari Campbell (2009, p. 5), ableism is a:

> Network of beliefs, processes and practices that produces a particular kind of self and body (the corporeal standard) that is projected as the perfect, species typical and therefore essential and fully human.

Ableism in narrative circulation can be understood in terms of epistemic injustice, which, in general, concerns prejudices that influence individual and social identities (Fricker, 2007). This injustice crosses paradigms with children and adolescents with LTC remaining invisible across many areas of research, policy, and discourse (Watson, 2012).

Barriers of involvement lead to children with LTC and disabilities being overlooked as legitimate research participants. This impacts on our understanding of child and adolescent development and indeed has created the homogenisation of childhood, and assumptions about children and adolescents' capacity to contribute to research. Our assumptions in the context of research are reinforced by ableist and adultist attitudes.

Back in the 1990s and 2000s some researchers highlighted how there was a lack of diversity in the theorising of childhood (Davis & Watson, 2001). The Western concept of 'the child' who meets developmental milestones stipulated by linear theoretical models has led to children with LTC and disabilities to be viewed as vulnerable 'others'. Priestley's (1998) and Watson et al.'s (1999) studies that explored the lives of children living with LTC and disability were among the first to challenge this Western and homogenised thinking of childhood, not least by highlighting the many facets of childhood and how the childhood experience of childhood and disability intersects with factors such as gender, race, and sexuality. Since there have been many discussions around the heterogeneity of childhood from a range of disciplines. Holt and Holloway (2006, p. 136) highlight we should recognise *multiple differentiations of childhoods* as the lives of children and adolescents are *dissected and connected by a variety of axes of difference*.

The requirement to think in more complex terms about childhood and LTC in research and practice has continued (Mallett & Runswick-Cole, 2014). However, there persists shared assumptions about body movement, speech, and social interaction and therefore children with diverse bodies, minds, and emotions remain overlooked for research studies. Children and adolescents have been considered incapable to participate because of how they speak, walk, or look (James, 1993). This prejudice is further demonstrated by practices of research by-proxy, where professionals, parents, and other family carers are invited to speak on behalf of children with LTC and disabilities and account for their lived experiences. In addition, there is also a gender issue notable here, as parent by-proxy usually means 'mother'.

Ableist thinking has reinforced the notion of the 'typical' self and body that denotes us as human (Campbell, 2009). How and in what ways prejudice of the body influences our perceptions of an individual's capability and value of contribution has been investigated by several authors (e.g. Scully, 2008; Toombs, 1997). Speech is also a basis for ableist assumptions around if children and adolescents should have a 'say'. Children with LTC may have complex communication needs and as result can be overlooked or excluded or researched by proxy because they are categorised as non-verbal. These assumptions are a result of ignorance, all children can communicate, but in different ways. Lewin and Luckin (2010) illustrated this effectively when they highlighted how children and adolescents can communicate via body language, pictures, signs, assistive technology, and/or ICT and indeed draw on several methods. It is the fault of researchers who set about their studies to capture just speech or the written word (Cocks, 2008).

10.10   Impact of Adultism on Children and Adolescents with LTC

Adultism is a further form of prejudice enforced by adults over children, additionally contributing to the lack of child and adolescent involvement in policy and research. Adultism refers to the perception that children are not able to provide their own reliable opinion or perspectives on matters and their lived experiences (Sinclair, 2004). This is because children are not as physically mature as adults (James et al., 1998) and therefore are thought to be vulnerable (Davis & Watson, 2001). Interestingly and as stated earlier in this book, 'childhood' is a relatively new construction emerging between 1850s and 1914 (James, 1993). But it is from our acceptance of the concept of childhood that we allow adultism. Adultism however when coupled with ableism results in the greater prejudice towards children and adolescents with LTC and disabilities. Therefore, it is important that we begin to change how we perceive children and adolescents and the contributions they can make to society, and research. When we identify that those children and adolescents with LTC and disabilities can be legitimate participants, our research approach and methods will progress and become orientated towards the child/adolescent, empowering their genuine involvement in research and in doing so will strengthen our research findings and the value of interventions that are developed for practice.

Summary

- An LTC impacts the life of the child or adolescent and their families. The diagnosis, treatment, and ongoing management of LTC are stressful for children and families. The range of health and social care needs needed across months, years, and lifespans can impact on daily family routines and social activities leading to adaptations to ensure good condition management.
- Lifestyle changes and differences can be the source of much chronic stress with long-term emotional and behavioural consequences. The stressors are multifaceted and can include stress related to daily role functioning (e.g. missing school), stress related to treatment (e.g. painful procedures), and stress related to uncertainty (e.g. wondering what caused the illness or

condition). Coping involves purposeful efforts to regulate cognitions, emotions, behaviours, physiology, and interactions with others. Considerable evidence across LTC suggest secondary control coping, or accommodative coping leads to better adjustment in children and adolescents. The use of disengagement coping, including cognitive and behavioural avoidance, is related to poorer adjustment. The use of avoidance, denial, and wishful thinking does not facilitate effective regulation of emotional distress and further may disrupt or derail of engagement coping strategies aimed at adjusting to uncontrollable stress. As children mature and develop, they learn to draw on more cognitive-based coping strategies and can become more autonomous in their disease management. As interventions become increasingly focused on self-management and user-led digital technology, we are hopeful that children and adolescents will become increasingly resilient and gain control over how they effectively live their lives with their LTC.

- A significant number of children and adolescents with chronic pain have a history of adverse experiences (ACEs). To date, much of the research examining the relationship between ACEs and chronic pain has been conducted on adults and so evidence remains lacking on specific neurobiological processes (e.g. allostatic load, cortisol secretion, sympathetic/parasympathetic nervous system activation) related to the presence and severity of chronic or persistent pain in those with a history of ACEs. More research on this topic would also allow healthcare providers to better predict and treat those children and adolescents with LTC who may be at greater risk for psychological and/or pain-related impairment.

- A core concern for children and adolescents with LTC is the desire to be like their peers and to 'fit in'. Peer acceptance and social connectivity are critical issues for all children and adolescents and are amplified for those with LTC. Fear of rejection and the stigma associated with LTC and disability often prevent them from disclosing their illness to peers and may prevent them from fully integrating in their peer group.

- Disablist, ableist, and adultist discourse continues to make children with LTC and disability to feel different enhancing stigmas, leading them to be viewed as vulnerable and without capability to participate fully in society. Related discourses transfer to practice and research where we see the voice of children and adolescents with LTC is limited. Awareness of how difference does not equate to vulnerability or weakness is needed. Researchers should aim to achieve diversity in their populations under study, aiming to include the child and adolescent voice, considering a variety of data collection methods so that all who want to be heard can be heard. It is only through research involvement that children and adolescents with LTC can help us to combat the homogenisation of childhood and enable us to develop complex and supportive interventions to assist individuals and families to live with and effectively manage LTC.

Read the family case study on page 265 and consider the following:

- How might the stigma faced by Lily and her family differ if Liam is diagnosed as having ADHD in contrast to the diagnosis of asthma given to Gemma and juvenile arthritis given to Ben?
- In what ways may Ben's recent shoplifting activities be a result of having juvenile arthritis?
- How effective could the use of self-help apps on mobile phones be in helping Gemma to control her asthma?

Reflective Questions:

- How can stress be linked to the pain associated with long-term conditions?
- Why is it important to listen to the views of children and adolescents as well as parents and professionals when researching the impact of long-term conditions on wellbeing?
- What issues are raised by the past desire to better 'normalise' the lives of children and adolescents with long-term conditions?

References

Ahlvik-Harju, C. (2015). Disturbing Bodies—Reimagining Comforting Narratives of Embodiment through Feminist Disability Studies. *Scandinavian Journal of Disability Research, 18*(3), 222–233.

Aitchison, K., McGeown, H., Holden, B., Watson, M., Klaber, R. E., & Hargreaves, D. (2021). Population Child Health: Understanding and Addressing Complex Health Needs. *Archives of Disease in Childhood, 106*(4), 387–391.

Aldridge, A. A., & Roesch, S. C. (2007). Coping and Adjustment in Children with Cancer: A Meta-analytic Study. *Journal of Behavioral Medicine, 30*(2), 115–129.

Alperin, B. R., Smith, C. J., Gustafsson, H. C., Figuracion, M. T., & Karalunas, S. L. (2019). The Relationship Between Alpha Asymmetry and ADHD Depends on Negative Affect Level and Parenting Practices. *Journal of Psychiatric Research, 116*, 138–146.

Arnett, J. J. (2001). Conceptions of the Transition to Adulthood: Perspectives from Adolescence Through Midlife. *Journal of Adult Development, 8*(2), 133–143.

Asthma UK. (2021). Retrieved September 05, 2021, from https://www.asthma.org.uk/

Bennett, S., Shafran, R., Coughtrey, A., Walker, S., & Heyman, I. (2015). Psychological Interventions for Mental Health Disorders in Children with Chronic Physical Illness: A Systematic Review. *Archives of Disease in Childhood, 100*, 308–316.

Bikmazer, A., Orengul, A. C., Buyukdeniz, A., Okur, F. V., Gokdemir, Y., & Perdahli Fis, N. (2020). Coping and Psychopathology in Children with Malignancy and Bronchiectasis. *Pediatric Pulmonology, 55*(1), 214–220.

Brooks, S. K., Webster, R. K., Smith, L. E., Woodland, L., Wessely, S., Greenberg, N., & Rubin, G. J. (2020, March). The Psychological Impact of Quarantine and How to Reduce It: Rapid Review of the Evidence. *Lancet, 395*(10227), 912–920.

Campbell, F. K. (2009). *Contours of Ableism: The Production of Disability and Abledness.* Palgrave Macmillan.

Campbell, L. K., Scaduto, M., Van Slyke, D., Niarhos, F., Whitlock, J. A., & Compas, B. E. (2009). Executive Function, Coping and Behavior in Survivors of Childhood Acute Lymphocytic Leukemia. *Journal of Pediatric Psychology, 34*, 317–327.

Cancer Research UK. (2021). Retrieved September 05, 2021, from https://www.cancerresearchuk.org/

Carver, C. S., & Connor-Smith, J. (2010). Personality and Coping. *Annual Review of Psychology, 61*, 679–704.

Chen, H., Chen, Y., Yang, C., & Chi, C. (2010). Lived Experience of Epilepsy from the Perspective of Children in Taiwan. *Journal of Clinical Nursing, 19*(2010), 1415–1423.

Cianchetti, C., Messina, P., Pupillo, E., Crichiutti, G., Baglietto, M. G., Veggiotti, P., Zamponi, N., Casellato, S., Margari, L., Erba, G., Beghi, E., & TASCA study group. (2015). The Perceived Burden of Epilepsy: Impact on the Quality of Life of Children and Adolescents and Their Families. *Seizure, 24*, 93–101.

Cieza, A., Causey, K., Kamenov, K., Hanson, S. W., Chatterji, S., & Vos, T. (2020). Glob Estimates of the Need for Rehabilitation Based on the Global Burden of Disease Study 2019: A Systematic Analysis for the Global Burden of Disease Study 2019. *The Lancet, 396*(10267), 2006–2017.

Cocks, A. (2008). Researching the Lives of Disabled Children: The Process of Participant Observation in Seeking Inclusivity. *Qualitative Social Work, 7*(2), 163–180.

Cohen, R. A., Hitsman, B. L., Paul, R. H., McCaffery, J., Stroud, L., Sweet, L., Gunstad, J., Niaura, R., MacFarlane, A., Bryant, R. A., & Gordon, E. (2006). Early Life Stress and Adult Emotional Experience: An International Perspective. *The International Journal of Psychiatry in Medicine, 36*(1), 35–52.

Compas, B. E. (2006). Psychobiological Processes of Stress and Coping: Implications for Resilience in Childhood and Adolescence. *Annals of the New York Academy of Sciences, 1094*, 226–234.

Compas, B. E., Connor-Smith, J. K., Saltzman, H., Thomsen, A. H., & Wadsworth, M. E. (2001). Coping with Stress During Childhood and Adolescence: Problems, Progress, and Potential in Theory and Research. *Psychological Bulletin, 127*(1), 87.

Corbin, J. M., & Strauss, A. (1988). *Unending Work, and Care: Managing Chronic Illness at Home.* Jossey-Bass.

Dalton, L., Rapa, E., & Stein, A. (2020). Protecting the Psychological Health of Children through Effective Communication about COVID-19. *The Lancet Child & Adolescent Health, 4*(5), 346–347.

Dancey, C. P., Hutton-Young, S. A., Moye, S., & Devins, G. M. (2002). Perceived Stigma, Illness Intrusiveness and Quality of Life in Men and Women with Irritable Bowel Syndrome. *Psychology, Health & Medicine, 7*(4), 381–395.

Davies, S., Heyman, I., & Goodman, R. (2003). A Population Survey of Mental Health Problems in Children with Epilepsy. *Developmental Medicine and Child Neurology, 45*(5), 292–295.

Davis, C., Ng, K. C., Oh, J. Y., Baeg, A., Rajasegaran, K., & Chew, C. S. E. (2020, July). Caring for Children and Adolescents with Eating Disorders in the Current Coronavirus 19 Pandemic: A Singapore Perspective. *Journal of Adolescent Health, 67*(1), 131–134.

Davis, J. M., & Watson, N. (2001). Countering Stereotypes of Disability: Disabled Children and Resistance. In M. Corker & T. Shakespeare (Eds.), *Disability and Postmodernity: Embodying Disability Theory* (pp. 159–174). Continuum.

Dayal, D., Gupta, S., & Raithatha, D., & Jayashree, M.. (2020, May 13). Missing During COVID-19 Lockdown: Children with New-onset type 1 Diabetes. *Res Square.*

De Ridder, D., Geenen, R., Kuijer, R., & van Middendorp, H. (2008). Psychological Adjustment to Chronic Disease. *The Lancet, 372*(9634), 246–255.

Devins, G. M. (2010). Using the Illness Intrusiveness Ratings Scale to Understand Health-related Quality of Life in Chronic Disease. *Journal of psychosomatic research, 68*(6), 591–602.

Diabetes UK. (2019). Us, Diabetes and a Lot of Facts and Stats. Diabetes UK: 2019–2002. Retrieved August 04, 2021 from https://www.diabetes.org.uk/resources-s3/2019-02/1362B_Facts%20and%20stats%20Update%20Jan%202019_LOW%20RES_EXTERNAL.pdf

DoE. (2017). Retrieved September 15, 2021, from https://www.gov.uk/government/publications/send-code-of-practice-0-to-25

Eisenbarth, C. (2012). Does Self-esteem Moderate the Relations Among Perceived Stress, Coping, and Depression? *College Student Journal, 46*(1), 149–157.

Eisenberger, N. I. (2012). The Neural Bases of Social Pain: Evidence for Shared Representations with Physical Pain. *Psychosomatic Medicine, 74*(2), 126.

Emerson, E., & Hatton, C. (2007). Mental Health of Children and Adolescents with Intellectual Disabilities in Britain. *The British Journal of Psychiatry, 191*(6), 493–499.

Fedele, D. A., Cushing, C. C., Fritz, A., Amaro, C. M., & Ortega, A. (2017). Mobile Health Interventions for Improving Health Outcomes in Youth: A Meta-Analysis. *JAMA Pediatrics, 171*(5), 461–469.

Ferrante, G., & La Grutta, S. (2018). The Burden of Pediatric Asthma. *Frontiers in Pediatrics, 6,* 186.

Fraser, L., Gibson-Smith, D., Jarvis, S., Norman, P., & Parslow, R. (2020). *Make every Child Count. Estimating Current and Future Prevalence of Children and Young People with Life-Limiting Conditions in the United Kingdom*. Martin House Research Centre.

Fricker, M. (2007). *Epistemic Injustice. Power & the Ethics of Knowing*. Oxford University Press.

Gaudieri, P. A., Chen, R., Greer, T. F., & Holmes, C. S. (2008). Cognitive Function in Children with type 1 Diabetes: A Meta-Analysis. *Diabetes Care, 31*(9), 1892–1897.

Goodley, D. (2012). Jacques Lacan + Paul Hunt = Psychoanalytic Disability Studies. In D. Goodley, B. Hughes, & L. Davis (Eds.), *Disability and Social Theory* (pp. 179–194). Palgrave Macmillan.

Griffiths, F., Bryce, C., Cave, J., Dritsaki, M., Fraser, J., Hamilton, K., Huxley, C., Ignatowicz, A., Kim, S. W., Kimani, P. K., Madan, J., Slowther, A.-M., Sujan, M., & Sturt, J. (2017). Timely Digital Patient-Clinician Communication in Specialist Clinical Services for Young People: A Mixed-methods Study (the LYNC study). *Journal of Medical Internet Research, 19*(4), e7154.

Gutman, L. M., & Vorhaus, J. (2012). *The Impact of Pupil Behaviour and Wellbeing on Educational Outcomes*. Dept for Education.

Hamine, S., Gerth-Guyette, E., Faulx, D., Green, B. B., & Ginsburg, A. S. (2015). Impact of mHealth Chronic Disease Management on Treatment Adherence and Patient Outcomes: A Systematic Review. *Journal of Medical Internet Research, 17*(2), e3951.

Hehir, T. (2002). Eliminating Ableism in Education. *Harvard Educational Review, 72*(1), 1–32.

Hoftun, G. B., Romundstad, P. R., & Rygg, M. (2013). Association of Parental Chronic Pain with Chronic Pain in the Adolescent and Young Adult: Family Linkage Data from the HUNT Study. *JAMA Pediatrics, 167*(1), 61–69.

Holt, L., & Holloway, S. (2006). Editorial: Theorising Other Childhoods in a Globalised World. *Children's Geographies, 4*(2), 135–142.

Hopkins, L., Green, J., Henry, J., Edwards, B., & Wong, S. (2014). Staying Engaged: The Role of Teachers and Schools in Keeping Young People with Health Conditions Engaged in Education. *The Australian Educational Researcher, 41*(1), 25–41.

Huang, C. Y., Costeines, J., Kaufman, J. S., & Ayala, C. (2014). Parenting Stress, Social Support, and Depression for Ethnic Minority Adolescent Mothers: Impact on Child Development. *Journal of Child and Family Studies, 23*(2), 255–262.

James, A. (1993). *Childhood Identities: Self and Social Relationships in the Experience of the Child*. Edinburgh University Press.

James, A., Jenks, C., & Prout, A. (1998). *Theorising Childhood*. Polity Press.

Jaser, S. S., & White, L. E. (2010, May). Coping and Resilience in Adolescents with Type 1 Diabetes. *Child: Care, Health and Development, 37*(3), 335–342.

Jiao, W. Y., Wang, L. N., Liu, J., Fang, S. F., Jiao, F. Y., Pettoello-Mantovani, M., & Somekh, E. (2020, June). Behavioral and Emotional Disorders in Children during the COVID-19 Epidemic. *Journal of Pediatrics, 221*, 264–266.

Joint Epilepsy Council of the UK and Ireland. (2011). Retrieved September 15, 2021, from https://d3imrogdy81qei.cloudfront.net/instructor_docs/373/29_05_2016_Joint_Epilepsy_Council_Prevalence_and_Incidence_September_11.pdf

Jones, E., Gutman, L., & Platt, L. (2013). *Family Stressors and Children's Outcomes*. Dept for Education.

Kascakova, N., Furstova, J., Hasto, J., Madarasova Geckova, A., & Tavel, P. (2020). The Unholy Trinity: Childhood Trauma, Adulthood Anxiety, and Long-term Pain. *International Journal of Environmental Research and Public Health, 17*(2), 414.

Keeble, E., & Kossarova, L. (2017). Focus on: Emergency Hospital Care for Children and Young People. Focus On Research Report. *QualityWatch*, 2018-10.

Kerker, B. D., Zhang, J., Nadeem, E., Stein, R. E., Hurlburt, M. S., Heneghan, A., Landsverk, J., & Horwitz, S. M. (2015). Adverse Childhood Experiences and Mental Health, Chronic Medical Conditions, and Development in Young Children. *Academic pediatrics, 15*(5), 510–517.

Ladores, S. (2020, May 19). The Unique Challenges and Lessons Imparted by the Cystic Fibrosis Community in the Time of COVID-19 Pandemic. *Journal Patient Experience, 7*(4), 442–443.

Lambert, V., & Keogh, D. (2015). Striving to Live a Normal Life: A Review of children and Young People's Experience of Feeling Different When Living With a Long-term Condition. *Journal of Pediatric Nursing, 30*(1), 63–77.

Lazarus, R. S., & Folkman, S. (1984). *Stress, Appraisal, and Coping*. Springer.

Lewin, C., & Luckin, R. (2010). Technology to Support Parental Engagement in Elementary Education: Lessons Learned from the UK. *Computers & Education, 54*(3), 749–758.

Lin, E. H., Rutter, C. M., Katon, W., Heckbert, S. R., Ciechanowski, P., Oliver, M. M., Ludman, E. J., Young, B. A., Williams, L. H., McCulloch, D. K., & Von Korff, M. (2010). Depression and Advanced Complications of Diabetes: A Prospective Cohort Study. *Diabetes Care, 33*(2), 264–269.

Link, B. G., & Phelan, J. C. (2006). Stigma and Its Public Health Implications. *The Lancet, 367*(9509), 528–529.

Lorig, K., & Holman, H. (2003). Self-management Education: History, Definition, Outcome, and Mechanisms. *Annals of Behavioral Medicine., 26*(1), 1–7.

Lupien, S. J., Ouellet-Morin, I., Hupbach, A., Tu, M. T., Buss, C., Walker, D., Jens, P., & Mcewen, B. S. (2006). Beyond the Stress Concept: Allostatic Load—A Developmental Biological and Cognitive Perspective. In D. Cicchetti & D. J. Cohen (Eds.), *Developmental Psychopathology: Developmental Neuroscience* (pp. 578–628). John Wiley & Sons Inc.

Mallett, R., & Runswick-Cole, K. (2014). *Approaching Disability: Critical Issues and Perspectives*. Routledge.

Martinelli, M., Strisciuglio, C., Fedele, F., Miele, E., & Staiano, A. (2020, August 20). Clinical and PSYCHOLOGICAL Issues in Children with Inflammatory Bowel Disease During COVID-19 pandemic. *Inflammatory Bowel Disease, 26*(9), e95–e96.

Moore, S. A., Faulkner, G., Rhodes, R. E., Brussoni, M., Chulak-Bozzer, T., Ferguson, L. J., Mitra, R., O'Reilly, N., Spence, J. C., Vanderloo, L. M., & Tremblay, M. S. (2020). Impact of the COVID-19 Virus Outbreak on Movement and Play Behaviours of Canadian Children and Youth: A National Survey. *International Journal of Behavioral Nutrition and Physical Activity, 17*(1), 1–11.

Morris, D. B. (1991). *The Culture of Pain*. University of California Press.

National Institute for Health and Care Excellence. (2019). Retrieved October 03, 2021, from https://www.nice.org.uk/Media/Default/About/what-we-do/our-programmes/evidence-standards-framework/digital-evidence-standards-framework.pdf

Ng, D. W. L., Chan, F. H. F., Barry, T. J., Lam, C., Chong, C. Y., Kok, H. C. S., Liao, Q., &, Fielding, R. (2020, June 04). Psychological Distress during the 2019 Coronavirus Disease (COVID-19) Pandemic among Cancer Survivors and Healthy Controls. *Psychooncology*. https://doi.org/10.1002/pon.5437

Nielsen, M. B., & Knardahl, S. (2014). Personality and Social Psychology Coping Strategies: A Prospective Study of Patterns, Stability, and Relationships with Psychological Distress. *Scandinavian Journal of Psychology, 55*, 142–150. https://doi.org/10.1111/sjop.12103

Nitschke, J. P., Forbes, P. A., Ali, N., Cutler, J., Apps, M. A., Lockwood, P. L., & Lamm, C. (2021). Resilience During Uncertainty? Greater Social Connectedness during COVID-19 Lockdown is Associated with Reduced Distress and Fatigue. *British Journal of Health Psychology, 26*(2), 553–569.

Parasole, R., Stellato, P., Conter, V., De Matteo, A., D'Amato, L., Colombini, A., Pecoraro, C., Bencivenga, C., Raimondo, M., Silvestri, S., Tipo, V., Petruzzelli, L. A., Giagnuolo, G., Curatolo, A., Biondi, A., & Menna, G. (2020, August). Collateral Effects of COVID-19 Pandemic in Paediatric Hematooncology: Fatalities Caused by Diagnostic Delay. *Paediatric Blood Cancer, 67*(8), e28482.

Petersson, C., Simeonsson, R. J., Enskar, K., & Huus, K. (2013). Comparing Children's Self-report Instruments for Health-related Quality of Life Using the International Classification of Functioning, Disability and Health for Children and Youth (ICF-CY). *Health and Quality of Life Outcomes, 11*(1), 1–10.

Price, J., & Shildrick, M. (2002). Bodies Together: Touch, Ethics, and Disability. In *Disability/ Postmodernity: Embodying Disability Theory* (pp. 62–75). Bloomsbury.

Priestley, M. (1998). Childhood Disability and Disabled Childhoods: Agendas for Research. *Childhood, 5*(2), 207–223.

Ramsey, K. A., Ranganathan, S., Park, J., Skoric, B., Adams, A. M., Simpson, S. J., Robins-Browne, R. M., Franklin, P. J., de Klerk, N. H., Sly, P. D., Stick, S. M., & Hall, G. L. (2014). Early Respiratory Infection is Associated With Reduced Spirometry in Children with Cystic Fibrosis. *American Journal of Respiratory and Critical Care Medicine, 190*(10), 1111–1116.

RCPCH. (2019). Retrieved September 09, 2021, from https://stateofchildhealth.rcpch.ac.uk/ evidence/long-term-conditions/diabetes/

Richard, A. A., & Shea, K. (2011). Delineation of Self-care and Associated Concepts. *Journal of Nursing Scholarship., 43*, 255–264.

Rodriguez, A., & King, N. (2009). The Lived Experience of Parenting a Child with a Life-limiting Condition: A Focus on the Mental Health Realm. *Palliative & Supportive Care, 7*(1), 7–12.

Rodriguez, A., & King, N. (2014). Sharing the Care: The Key-working Experiences of Professionals and the Parents of Life-limited Children. *International Journal of Palliative Nursing, 20*(4), 165–171.

Rodriguez, A., Smith, J., & McDermid, K. (2018). Dignity Therapy Interventions for Young People in Palliative Care: A Rapid Structured Evidence Review. *International Journal of Palliative Nursing, 24*(7), 339–349.

Rodriguez, E. M., Dunn, M. J., Zuckerman, T., Vannatta, K., Gerhardt, C. A., & Compass, B. E. (2012). Cancer-related Sources of Stress for Children with Cancer and Their Parents. *Journal of Pediatric Psychology, 37*(2), 185–197.

Rogosch, F. A., Dackis, M. N., & Cicchetti, D. (2011). Child Maltreatment and Allostatic Load: Consequences for Physical and Mental Health in Children from Low-income Families. *Development and Psychopathology, 23*(4), 1107–1124.

Royal College of Paediatrics and Chid Health. (2020). Retrieved August 06, 2021, from https:// www.rcpch.ac.uk/resources/impact-covid-19-child-health-services-tool

Royal College of Physicians. (2014). Retrieved October 05, 2021, from https://www.asthma.org. uk/support-us/campaigns/publications/national-review-of-asthma-deaths/

Rudolph, K. D., Dennig, M. D., & Weisz, J. R. (1995). Determinants and Consequences of Children's Coping in the Medical Setting: Conceptualization, Review, and Critique. *Psychological Bulletin, 118*(3), 328.

Ryan, P., & Sawin, K. J. (2009). The Individual and Family Self-Management Theory: Background and Perspectives on Context, Process, and Outcomes. *Nursing Outlook, 57*(4), 217–225.

Scully, J. (2008). Disability and the Thinking Body. In K. Kristiansen, S. Vehmas, & T. Shakespeare (Eds.), *Arguing about Disability: Philosophical Perspectives* (pp. 57–73). Routledge.

Shah, R., Hagell, A., & Cheung, R. (2019). *International Comparisons of Health and Wellbeing in Adolescence and Early Adulthood Research Report February 2019.* Nuffield Trust & The Association for Young People's Health.

Sieberg, C. B., Williams, S., & Simons, L. E. (2011). Do Parent Protective Responses Mediate the Relation between Parent Distress and Child Functional Disability among Children with Chronic Pain? *Journal of Pediatric Psychology, 36*(9), 1043–1051.

Sinclair, R. (2004). Participation in Practice: Making it Meaningful, Effective, and Sustainable. *Children and Society, 18*(2), 106–118.

Skinner, A. T., Godwin, J., Alampay, L. P., Lansford, J. E., Bacchini, D., Bornstein, M. H., Deater-Deckard, K., Di Giunta, L., Dodge, K. A., Gurdal, S., Pastorelli, C., Sorbring, E., Steinberg, L., Tapanya, S., & Yotanyamaneewong, S. (2021). Parent–adolescent Relationship Quality as a Moderator of Links between COVID-19 Disruption and Reported Changes in mothers' and Young Adults' Adjustment in Five Countries. *Developmental Psychology, 57*(10), 1648–1666.

Spencer, J. E., Cooper, H. C., & Milton, B. (2013). The Lived Experiences of Young People (13–16 years) with Type 1 Diabetes Mellitus and Their Parents–A Qualitative Phenomenological Study. *Diabetic Medicine, 30*(1), e17–e24.

Stevelink, S., Wu, I. C., Voorend, C. G., & van Brakel, W. H. (2012). The Psychometric Assessment of Internalised Stigma Instruments: A Systematic Review. *Stigma, Research and Action, 2*(2), 100–118.

Taft, T. H., Ballou, S., & Keefer, L. (2013). A Preliminary Evaluation of Internalized Stigma and Stigma Resistance in Inflammatory Bowel Disease. *Journal of Health Psychology, 18*(4), 451–460.

TfSL. (2021). Retrieved September 05, 2021, from https://www.togetherforshortlives.org.uk/

Thompson, R. J., Jr., & Gustafson, K. E. (1996). *Adaptation to Chronic Childhood Illness*. American Psychological Association.

Thompson, R. J., Jr., Kronenberger, W., & Curry, J. F. (1989). Behavior Classification System for Children with Developmental, Psychiatric, and Chronic Medical Problems. *Journal of Pediatric. Psychology, 14*, 559–575.

Toombs, K. (1997). Taking the Body Seriously. *In Hastings Center Report, 27*(5), 39–43.

Unicef. (2018). Children, HIV and AIDS: The World in 2030.

Vachon-Presseau, E., Roy, M., Martel, M. O., Caron, E., Marin, M. F., Chen, J., Albouy, G., Plante, I., Sullivan, M. J., Lupien, S. J., & Rainville, P. (2013). The Stress Model of Chronic Pain: Evidence from Basal Cortisol and Hippocampal Structure and Function in Humans. *Brain, 136*(3), 815–827.

Van Cleave, J., Gortmaker, S. L., & Perrin, J. M. (2010). Dynamics of Obesity and Chronic Health Conditions Among Children and Youth. *Jama, 303*(7), 623–630.

Vasquez, L., Sampor, C., Villanueva, G., Maradiegue, E., Garcia-Lombardi, M., Gomez-García, W., Moreno, F., Diaz, R., Cappellano, A. M., Portilla, C. A., Salas, B., Nava, E., Brizuela, S., Jimenez, S., Espinoza, X., Gassant, P. Y., Quintero, K., Fuentes-Alabi, S., Velasquez, T., … Gamboa, Y. (2020, June). Early Impact of the COVID-19 Pandemic on Paediatric Cancer Care in Latin America. *Lancet Oncology, 21*(6), 753–755.

Waite-Jones, J. M., & Madill, A. (2008). Amplified Ambivalence: Experiences of Having a Sibling with JIA. *Psychology and Health, 23*(4), 477–492.

Warner, E. L., Nam, G. E., Zhang, Y., McFadden, M., Wright, J., Spraker-Perlman, H., Kinney, A. Y., Oeffinger, K. C., & Kirchhoff, A. C. (2016). Health Behaviors, Quality of Life, and Psychosocial Health Among Survivors of Adolescent and Young Adult Cancers. *Journal of Cancer Survivorship, 10*(2), 280–290.

Watson, N. (2012). Theorising the Lives of Disabled Children: How can Disability Theory Help? *Children and Society, 26*(3), 192–202.

Watson, N., Shakespeare, T., Cunningham-Burley, S., Barnes, C., Corker, M., Davis, J., & Priestley, M.. (1999). *Life as a Disabled Child: A Qualitative Study of Young People's Experiences and Perspectives*. University of Edinburgh, Department of Nursing Studies. Retrieved September 12, 2021, from http://pf7d7vi404s1dxh27mla5569.wpengine.netdnacdn.com/files/2011/10/life-as-a-disabled-child-report.pdf

Watts, L., Smith, J., McSherry, W., Tatterton, M., & Rodriguez, A. (2020). Stakeholder Perceptions of Dignity Therapy for Children and Young People with Life-limiting and Life-threatening Conditions in the UK. *OBM Integrative and Complementary Medicine, 5*(1), 1–1.

Wiebe, D. J., Berg, C. A., Korbel, C., Palmer, D. L., Beveridge, R. M., Upchurch, R., Lindsay, R., Swinyard, M. T., & Donaldson, D. L. (2005). Children's Appraisals of Maternal Involvement in Coping with Diabetes: Enhancing our Understanding of Adherence, Metabolic Control, and Quality of Life Across Adolescence. *Journal of pediatric psychology, 30*(2), 167–178.

Young Minds. (2020). Coronavirus: Impact on Young People with Mental Health Needs. https://youngminds.org.uk/about-us/reports/coronavirus-impact-on-young-people-with-mental-health-needs/

Zeng, S., & Hui, X. (2018). Parents Reporting Adverse Child Experiences among Young Children with Disabilities: Informing Systems Transformation. *Topics in Early Childhood Special Education, 38*(3), 162–173.

Zhang, J., Shuai, L., Yu, H., Wang, Z., Qiu, M., Lu, L., Cao, X., Xia, W., Wang, Y., & Chen, R. (2020, June). Acute Stress, Behavioural Symptoms, and Mood States among School-age Children with Attention-deficit/Hyperactive Disorder During the COVID-19 Outbreak. *Asian Journal of Psychiatry, 51*, 102077.

Vulnerability and Resilience in Childhood and Adolescence

11

11.1 Introduction

Evidence is continually being gathered about the short- and long-term risks to health and wellbeing incurred through experiencing adverse life experiences in childhood, particularly where those adversities are prolonged, cumulative, or occurring during sensitive periods of neurobiological development. The interest in the science of resilience emerged in childhood research in the 1970s when scholars were investigating children at risk of mental health difficulties. The researchers were astounded at the variability observed between those children who had experienced multiple risks and adversities. Since then, we have maintained the aim to identify the root causes of observable variations. Why is it that some children, despite adversity, still reach developmental milestones and maintain mental wellness? These children and adolescents are possibly the key to understanding what the optimum factors are for achieving healthy childhood development. This chapter considers the development of resilience-focused research and theory in children and adolescents, highlighting promoting factors and methods to support and understand childhood and adolescent resiliency and developmental wellbeing. Contemporary topics of interest including 'poverty', 'trans youth', 'social media', and 'digital technology' and the 'COVID-19 pandemic' will be briefly discussed considering how children and adolescents may respond successfully or be vulnerable due to their context and what might help their resiliency in our contemporary Western society.

11.2 Changing Definitions of Resilience

There are different conceptualisations and definitions of resilience that depend on whether resilience is viewed as a personal trait or a dynamic process. It is a narrower definition that considers resilience as a trait. These definitions see the resilience trait as one that develops following a single event of adversity. However, over the

© The Author(s), under exclusive license to Springer Nature Switzerland AG 2022
J. M. Waite-Jones, A. M. Rodriguez, *Psychosocial Approaches to Child and Adolescent Health and Wellbeing*, https://doi.org/10.1007/978-3-030-99354-2_11

lifespan individuals can be subjected to many adversities leading to adjustment difficulties and disorders and we see some individuals cope better than others. These events may include deficient parenting, poverty, homelessness, traumatic events, natural disasters, violence, war, and physical illness. Through these experiences our environment, familial and support systems can influence outcomes and so researchers have increasingly considered the impact of systems, such as families, services, groups, and communities, in their studies and conceptualisations of resilience.

With increasing interest in resiliency and systems, the trait definition of resilience has broadened to consider the influence of culture, community, the family, and individual characteristics (Cicchetti, 2010), and some scholars have gone even broader with their definitions to suggest that resilience describes protective mechanisms which protect against significant stressors linked to psychopathology (Hjemdal et al., 2006) or resistance to environmental risks (Rutter, 2006).

These definitions highlight how many factors and systems may contribute to the interactive and dynamic process that increases a person's resilience to the adversity they experience. Resilience may also be context and time specific and implicate other qualities/characteristics. For example, 'hardiness' (a trait characterised by being able to take control, find meaning, and embrace change as a challenge), 'benefit finding' (where one can find meaning in times of adversity, identifying positive changes or development of the self), 'thriving' (where despite the adversity, the person can increase their skill set and positively improve their characteristics and relationships), and 'post-traumatic growth' (this can happen following thriving and resilience and can mean many things including increased appreciation of life, more meaningful relationships, greater sense of emotional strength, a desire for new opportunities, and increased spirituality) (Tedeschi & Calhoun, 2004).

11.3   Methods Used in Resilience Studies

Initial studies of resilience used case reports or descriptions of people identified as being at an elevated risk for difficulties but who were managing ok with their situation and compared them with others with 'at risk' profiles who were struggling (Masten, 2015). Later following the identification of factors of resilience, studies began to explore why these factors may have had influence. Then where possible, researchers started to undertake randomised controlled trials of interventions that targeted processes that may influence resilience (Fig. 11.1).

The current or fourth wave of resilience research continues to explore resilience processes, but the research undertaken is integrated with an attempt to understand how resilience can have multiple levels, be interconnected, and involve complex adaptive systems at biological, psychological, and social levels. This work has been aided by the advancement of statistical analytical methods and now also spans research looking at the epigenetics of parenting as a protective process to sociocultural influences on brain development.

Numerous child and adolescent adverse experiences have been investigated including neglect or abuse, separation and loss, family or neighbourhood violence,

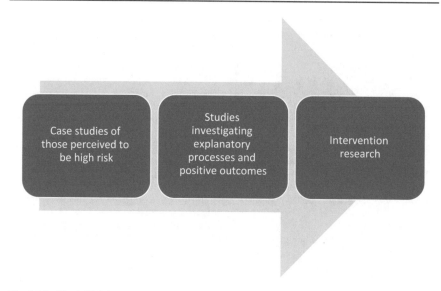

Fig. 11.1 The initial three waves of resilience research

Table 11.1 Examples of resilience study topics and constructs measured

Risk factors	Factors that highlight resilience and wellbeing	Support processes
Trauma	Achievement of developmental tasks	Neurobiological
Neglect	Mental health	Behavioural
ACEs	Physical health	Familial and relational
Poverty	Happiness	Community
Natural disaster	Work achievement	Cultural
War	Caregiving	Societal

war, natural disasters, poverty, and hospitalisation. Studies have focused on singular traumatic experiences, such as rape or being bereaved of a parent. Others have explored 'cumulative risks' or multiple negative life events otherwise termed as 'adverse childhood experiences' or ACEs (Obradović et al., 2012) (see Table 11.1 for examples of resilience study foci and constructs likely to be measured). Singular adversities unfortunately are not so common because many types of childhood adversity are often associated with persistent or repeated or combined exposure to other highly stressful experiences.

In studies exploring resilience in children and adolescents, age and developmental stage competence is measured across behavioural, emotional, and educational functioning areas. Those deemed resilient will have similar outcomes to control samples (those who have not experienced adverse events) or the wider population average. In older adolescents or young adults, unemployment, homelessness, substance abuse, and criminality are sometimes included as negative measures of resilience (Sandler et al., 2007). In addition, there are both quantitative and qualitative studies that include by-proxy or self-reports of resilience. Researchers with

Table 11.2 Resilience factors for child development (child and family)

Factor	Related family factors
Caring family	Sensitive care giving, family nurturance
Close relationships	Emotional security, family cohesion, sense of belonging
Skilled parenting	Family management
Agency, motivation to adapt	Active coping, achievement of skills
Problem solving, planning and executive functioning skills	Collaborative problem solving, flexibility within families
Self-regulation skills and emotional regulation	Co-regulation, family balance
Self-efficacy, positive sense of self and identity	Positive view of family and family identity
Hope faith and optimism	Hope faith and optimism, positive family outlook
Meaning making, belief	Coherence, family purpose, collective meaning making
Routines and rituals	Family role organisation
Engagement in a well-functioning school	School belonging
Connections with well-functioning communities	Community belonging

psychological interests are also likely to use tools that measure psychological difficulties, for example, depression, anxiety, and post-traumatic distress (PTSD) (Werner & Smith, 2001).

11.3.1 What Is Effective?

There are many resilience factors that can make a difference to the health and well-being of children, adolescents, and their families following adversity. These factors can be influenced by age and context. For example, a resilience factor for an older child will be the belief that life has meaning. This factor is irrelevant to an infant dependent on the quality of care giving they receive and the wider family resilience to support their own resilience to adversity. Table 11.2 highlights general positive and protective resilience factors related to the self and how supportive family factors can harness or boost those factors.

Psychological, biological, and environment/system or social factors can each or in combination impact on a child or adolescent's resilience to events.

11.4 Psychological Factors in Resilience

There has been much research undertaken on the psychosocial factors of stress tolerance and resilience enhancement. Personality traits (e.g. openness, extraversion, and agree-ableness), internal locus of control, mastery, self-efficacy, self-esteem, cognitive appraisal, and optimism have all been found to contribute to resilience in children and adolescents. In particular, significant correlations have been found between measures of resilience and cognitive re-appraisal (where one can monitor thoughts of events and reappraise them to form more positive evaluations of the events) (McRae et al., 2012). This ability is also known as cognitive flexibility or cognitive reframing. Viktor Frankl, the author of *Man's Search for Meaning*, famously suggested his own psychological resilience and survival of concentration camps were because of 'meaning finding'. He suggests that being able to find meaning in life can be the most important motivating factor to keep living and maintaining a positive outlook (Frankl, 2006). Internalised values and ethics can assist our resilience. Religion and spirituality can be allies to our moral compasses or belief systems. Min et al. (2012) investigated the beliefs and coping behaviours of 121 outpatients diagnosed with depression and/or an anxiety. They found participants with a lack of purpose in life had lower resilience. This finding was similar in a study of 259 primary care patients who had previous experience of trauma (Alim et al., 2008).

Attachment style may also contribute to a child or adolescent's ability to cognitively reappraise events and resilience. In a study of 632 participants, secure attachment was correlated with higher cognitive reappraisal and resilience (Karreman & Vingerhoets, 2012). Securely attached participants could reframe situations as less upsetting and did not supress their emotional response, whereas anxious attachment was correlated with lower measures of wellbeing and related to a lower use of cognitive reappraisal. A positive outlook has been found to be a protective factor against stress and correlated with more speedy recovery times and overall physical health. Similarly, optimism, which is regarded as the expectation for good outcomes, has been repeatedly correlated with the use of active coping strategies, subjective wellbeing, physical health, and larger and more supportive social networks and relationships. Indeed, social support and seeking social support is correlated with psychological hardiness and thriving despite major adverse life events. The opposite is also evidenced in that poor or a lack of social support for children and adolescents is associated with psychological difficulties including PTSD (Tsai et al., 2012). These psychological factors interact with biological factors to improve adaptation and adjustment during and following traumatic events, and influence resilience (Charney, 2004).

11.5 Biological Factors in Resilience

Stressful early environments can impact the developing brain structure, its function, and neurobiological systems. Changes have been observed in brain size, neural networks, the sensitivity of receptors, and the synthesis and reuptake of neurotransmitters (Curtis & Nelson, 2003). These changes can render individuals more vulnerable to psychological difficulties as there can be a reduced capacity to manage the emotionality of situations (Cicchetti & Curtis, 2006).

There is a substantial evidence base that highlights how supportive and responsive early care giving for infants and young children can bolster resilience and reduce the impacts of stressful or 'toxic' environments. There are also identified critical periods where interventions can be more effective (Gunnar & Fisher, 2006).

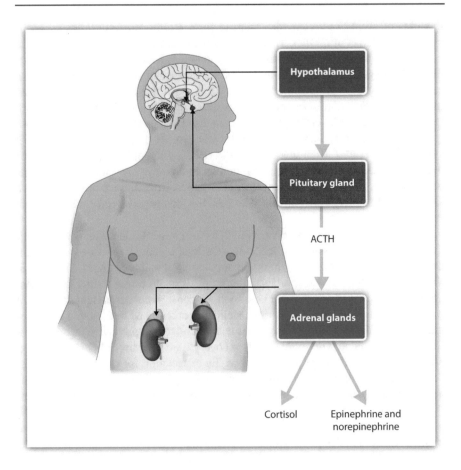

Fig. 11.2 Hypothalamic-pituitary-adrenal (HPA) axis

Animal studies have found that maternal care including licking lowers the hypotha-lamic-pituitary-adrenal (HPA) response to stress (Meaney, 2001). In humans, where the child is in receipt of good parental cares, the neurochemical oxytocin suppresses the HPA axis (a physiological response to stress involving interactions with the (H) hypothalamus, the (P) pituitary, and the (A) adrenal glands—see Fig. 11.2). This biological process can influence positive social interaction because of the lowering of the physiological experience of stress and anxiety (Carter, 2005). Where children are exposed to stressful situations, long-term alterations have been found in the HPA axis. These changes can heighten vulnerability to psychological difficulties including depression and anxiety.

Similarly, where children have survived trauma they have changes in their cen-tral nervous system (CNS) circuits (Heim et al., 2010). Prenatal stress and child-hood trauma have also been associated with a hyperactive HPA axis with attendant risk of negative effects of chronic hypercortisolaemia (referred to as Cushing syn-drome, which is resultant of the body being exposed to high levels of the hormone

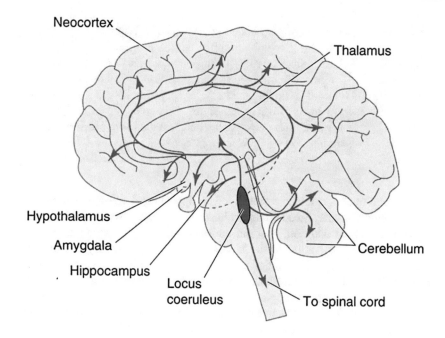

Fig. 11.3 The locus coeruleus-norepinephrine (LC-NE) system

cortisol for a long period of time) in later years (Frodl & Keane, 2013). In addition, chronic early life stress can lead to hyperfunctioning of the locus coeruleus-norepinephrine (LC-NE) system (see Fig. 11.3) in adulthood (Wu et al., 2013).

Box 11.1 Biological responses to stress

Stress activates the HPA axis which causes the anterior pituitary gland to release adrenocorticotropic hormone (ACTH). ACTH travels down to the adrenal glands above the kidneys. This then influences the release of epinephrine and norepinephrine (neurotransmitters and hormones) and cortisol (a steroid hormone, one of the glucocorticoids, made in the cortex of the adrenal glands). Epinephrine is also termed adrenaline and norepinephrine is termed as noradrenaline. Both participate in the regulation of the sympathetic nervous system which influences body's 'fight or flight' response. Increased release of cortisol exhausts stress mechanisms leading to psychological difficulties and tiredness. Persistent stress causes immune dysfunction, hypertension, chronic heart disease and has been associated with other long-term conditions (Wager & Cox, 2017).

Box 11.2 The role of the locus coeruleus in the response to stress
The locus coeruleus is the major site of the neurotransmitter norepinephrine and functions along with amygdala in the brain's pain or stress response, encouraging the 'fight-or-flight' mechanism. It activates the sympathetic nervous system. In the brain, noradrenaline (norepinephrine) is a neurotransmitter, but in the body it acts as a hormone and is released by the adrenal glands. The stress response as a result of activation here is linked to depression, panic, and anxiety disorders and PTSD (Wager & Cox, 2017).

Childhood trauma can also result in lower hippocampal volume. Lower hippocampal volume is often seen in individuals with mood disorders (Davidson & McEwen, 2012). In addition, positron emission tomography (PET) studies have identified reduced activation in the hippocampus during memory testing where patients have a history of childhood abuse (PET is a functional imaging technique which utilises radioactive substances to view and measure changes in metabolic processes, and in other physiological mechanisms, for example, blood flow, regional chemical composition, and absorption) (Heim et al., 2010). Epigenetic differences can also result from stress exposure during critical periods of development and contribute to susceptibility to psychological difficulties (Dudley et al., 2011) (epigenetics refers to how there can be functional modifications to the genome without change in the DNA sequence). Several epigenetic studies have identified correlations between epigenetic changes and risks for maladaptive stress responses and psychological difficulties (Murgatroyd & Spengler, 2012).

11.6   Social (Environment-System) Factors in Resilience

Less behavioural difficulties and greater psychological wellbeing have been observed when there is a secure attachment to a main caregiver, family stability, non-abusive parenting, good parenting skills, and no maternal depression or substance abuse even in those children who have been maltreated. At the micro environmental level, social support from positive peer relationships, supportive teachers, and other adults as well as immediate family influence resiliency. On a more macrosystemic level, community is viewed as important for good resilience outcomes. For example, good schooling, community activities, opportunities for extracurricular activities, supportive cultural traditions and rituals, spirituality and religion, and lack of exposure to violence, all influence higher levels of resilience (Luthar & Cicchetti, 2000). Despite this knowledge there remain gaps in social policies to enhance resilience in populations.

11.6.1 Intervention

Resilience frameworks are embedded in effective interventions that aim to protect or build resilience outcomes in children and adolescents. They include the following components:

- motivation for positive goals
- protective and promotive factor models
- strategies to mitigate risk, boost assets, and mobilise adaptive systems
- multidisciplinary involvement to motivate change
- identifying critical periods for change, therefore using strategic timing, and targeting methods (Masten, 2015).

Risk-focused interventions include strategies that aim to reduce risk; for example, those focused on reducing stress in pregnancy, exploring low mood symptoms in new mothers, and providing them with support and treatment, screening for family violence and child maltreatment, and acting upon issues once identified (Garman et al., 2017).

Asset-focused promotive interventions aim to enhance existent resources or assets available to children and adolescents or families. This may include adding resources or improving access to support to encourage motivation and action. For example, providing families with food and shelter necessities, parenting support, monetary help, library access, playgrounds (Reynolds et al., 2011).

Protection-focused interventions to engage or mobilise adaptive systems focus on nurturing, engaging, encouraging, or restoring individual's adaptive systems so that there can be an increase in resilience protective factors in their lives. For example, parenting classes, foster or adoptive care, play schemes, instrumental social support, youth workers, and mentorship (Sandler et al., 2011).

The interventions with the best evidence for positive outcomes are related to improving parenting or child parent–guardian relationships where there are background contexts of risk or adversity. This may include a history of abuse, divorce, bereavement, institutional or foster care. Where interventions are targeted to improve individual-level factors such as self-efficacy or emotional regulation, these are most effective for children and adolescents. Examples include promoting positive sleep habits and encouraging mindfulness skills among children and adolescents facing poverty (Sibinga et al., 2016).

11.6.2 Timing and Windows of Opportunity

The evidence base is clear in that when children are exposed to persistent stressful circumstances their development will be affected. This impacts on neurodevelopment and later health and psychosocial development. However, not all stressful situations pose negative consequences for children and adolescents. Our bodily systems that enable us to adapt to stress require us to also experience stress—so that we can learn how to cope (Masten & Cicchetti, 2015).

In addition, resilience studies argue there are windows of opportunity for supporting or promoting resilience through preventative interventions. In pre-schoolaged children we see much development in neural systems, behaviour, and social systems that support school readiness. Executive function (EF) skills develop quickly during this time, influencing early school success (Zelazo et al., 2016). Children with high-risk background contexts will show less development in terms of EF skills compared to their peers. Because this is a developmental period that can be highly malleable, interventions have been developed to promote EF skills in younger children, for example, information technology lessons, martial arts, yoga, and mindfulness sessions (Diamond & Lee, 2011).

There are also windows of opportunity in late adolescence and early adulthood where again this is a period of rapid neural development and plasticity. At this age, executive control systems that support planning and self/emotional regulation are maturing. There are also more social opportunities available at this age, including work placement, novel places of study, new mentors, and romantic relationships. Combined these factors can facilitate positive change (Masten, 2015).

11.7   Contemporary Resilience Issue Exemplars

11.7.1 Poverty

Poverty is described by Cauthen and Fass (2008, p. 1) as when *'Families and their children are unable to achieve a minimum, decent standard of living that allows them to participate fully in mainstream society.'* Poverty is not something that only impacts children in developing countries, it affects children in our own neighbourhoods, hospitals, clinics, and classrooms. In the UK between 2019 and 2020 there were approximately 4.3 million children considered to be living in poverty in the UK. This equates to around nine children in every class of thirty at school. Almost 50% of these children live in one-parent families. Single parents do not have the support of a second wage and themselves experience inequality in employment not least due to the current expense of childcare. Employment however does not always protect families from poverty, with currently 75% of children in poverty living with families where one parent works. Children from black and minority ethnic groups are more at risk of poverty with statistics highlighting that there are now 46% of black and minority ethnic children in poverty as compared to 26% of white British children (Dept for Work and Pensions, 2021).

Where children are raised in poverty, they face many potential risks to their health and wellbeing. They begin their lives most often with a lower birthweight, with mothers more likely to be experiencing poor health outcomes and who engage in risky health behaviours such as smoking (Hirsch & Spencer, 2008).

11.7.2 Impacts on Development

Children living in poverty are more likely to have developmental concerns and experience physical/mental health difficulties and have lower perceived wellbeing across their lifespans (Levin et al., 2009).

Cognitive development: Studies suggest that children in poverty have slower cognitive development. Even where young children achieve good ability scores, as they grow up in poverty, their peers advance and in comparison, achieve much better outcomes in adolescent testing (Blanden & Machin, 2010). Parents experiencing poverty are subjected to a lot of stress to make ends meet and to provide for their children; this can lead to them not having the time or mental capacity to engage much in cognitively stimulating their children through play or in-depth conversation. Fewer parent–child interactions and together time in play impact on child developmental outcomes. Where there are resultant psychological difficulties in parents such as low mood, this also negatively impacts on children's behaviour (Mensah & Kiernon, 2009).

Social, emotional, and behavioural development: Poverty is correlated with poorer social, emotional, and behavioural outcomes for children and especially adolescents. These outcomes are mediated negatively by maternal low mood or depression, low self-esteem, and low-quality parent child relationships. Negative outcomes are more prevalent in boys (Kiernan & Huerta, 2008).

11.7.3 Children's Experiences

Much of the evidence base on the impacts of living in poverty consider how living in poverty as a child or adolescent may impact on developmental trajectories and wellbeing in adulthood. Considerably less attention is focused on how living in poverty affects the child or adolescent now and how they may be experiencing their current life situations. Children and adolescents living in poverty, however, often feel marginalised as they are unable to keep up with the latest trends/fashions or participate in expensive pass times or events. This can lead to being bullied, self-stigma, and shame (Kintrea et al., 2011).

Children and adolescents living in poverty may have to undertake caring duties in the home, and their parents may find it difficult to buy learning aides such as textbooks or digital devices, thus they find it difficult to engage in homework and to achieve the grades of their peers. Children in these situations, however, display a protectiveness towards their parents and an understanding of their family financial hardship, leading them to not demand monies from their parents and instead will often themselves try to achieve employment to contribute to the family income. These actions can be positive, enabling an understanding of financial issues but again can impede schoolwork completion and educational achievements (Ridge, 2002).

Children's experiences of poverty are complex and do not always lead to an array of difficulties. Several protective factors can mediate negative influences; for example, child and adolescent relationships within their families, their inclusion in their peer group, and broader supportive communities.

11.7.4 Resilient Communities

The old African proverb reminds us that, *'It takes a village to raise a child'*. Communities that possess high levels of social capital, inferred by trust existent amongst and between households, reciprocity, and community participation, support the mental health and resiliency of children and adolescents (McKenzie & Harpham, 2006). The mental health of communities, however, can act as a risk factor (e.g. if there is social recession) and a protective factor (e.g. awareness and support for mental health) (Stewart-Brown, 2003).

Social participation and support are correlated with a lowered incidence of psychological difficulties and more frequent good self-reported health outcomes. Alternatively, social isolation is a risk factor for increasing psychological difficulties, including suicide. Unfortunately, several studies have shown that social capital (participation and support) is unable to positively mediate all the negative effects of living in poverty. When there is disruption in communities and community trust breaks down, and where there are neighbourhood difficulties, the impacts on wellbeing can result regardless of socio-economic status. However, the risk of violent discord can be heightened by economic deprivation and levels of inequality. Poor communities have higher rates of violence, but they also possess strong norms of violence. These otherwise termed 'socially disorganised areas' can lead to a significant number of offenders perhaps because crime may feel like their only option with little support in place to take alternative pathways in life (Agyemang et al., 2007).

In addition, there can be area level effects in areas of poverty which influence mortality statistics. In Scotland there are increases in death rates amongst young people in areas of high deprivation. Young people suffering from conditions such as liver disease are more frequently attempting and achieving suicide, suffering the consequences of assault, and experiencing psychological difficulties resultant of taking illegal drugs (Leyland et al., 2007). In such communities it could be that the risk factors of low self-esteem, emotional vulnerability in communities (psychological difficulties, social isolation) take precedence over the many protective factors that may still be present.

11.7.5 Resilient Individuals

Protective factors to influence resilience are more important for children and adolescents living in poverty. These include:

- nurturance and nutrition effects of breast feeding
- parental and familial beliefs and behaviours that support self-esteem
- social support and support from other adults in the broader family, for example, grandparents, aunts, and uncles
- a home environment that supports learning

Where children and adolescents live in supporting households with attentive parents, they have better outcomes than those from similar backgrounds. Where targeted interventions are put in place for pre-school children living in poverty there are positive impacts to their development and wellbeing (Schweinhart et al., 2005). This is a time of much biopsychosocial development so an important window of opportunity. In addition, we know that where there is evidence of resilience in the adolescent years this can provide them with a trajectory of escape from poverty, also lowering risks for psychological difficulties. Where there is adolescent resilience, the person will have the resources to cope well with stressors and may delay their own engagement with serious romantic relationships and parenting (Sacker & Schoon, 2007).

11.7.6 Needs

The experience of living in poverty can clearly have major impacts on the developing brain and physical maturation influencing physical and mental development and wellbeing. There is more to be done to evaluate and develop interventions, especially at sensitive points in development, for example early childhood, early and late adolescence. There is also interest around exploring multiple risk factors that exist for those living in poverty conditions. For example, a study undertaken by Shahtahmasebi et al. (2011) suggests that children with disabilities are more likely to be living in poverty. This could be resultant of poverty conditions for mothers' prenatally, genetic concerns, or it could be that the additional costs of supporting children with disabilities mean families can find themselves living in poverty. For example, parents may lose paid employment which can then lead to food insecurity, housing insecurity, health disparities, lack of transportation, increased risk of child maltreatment, and lack of enriching environments and relationships.

Government policy and community initiatives need to work harder to ensure those living in poverty are better supported to allow them the opportunities to thrive. High-quality early intervention activities for families can significantly contribute to improved child outcomes in families living in poverty. These outcomes may include educational success, responsible citizenship, and their own successful parenting. In summarised terms, *'Parents and other caregivers who are able to form close, nurturing relationships with their children can foster resilience in them that protects them from many of the worst effects of a harsh early environment'* (Tough, 2012, p. 28). If interventions are put in place that can assist parents, families, and communities to be more responsive to the needs of children and adolescents, then developmental delays, psychological difficulties, and other negative outcomes may be mitigated (Eshbaugh et al., 2011).

11.8 Trans Youth

The development of gender identity and sexuality involves physical, cognitive, social, and emotional developmental dimensions. However, each child is different and as such it is still normative for children to develop their gender identity and understanding of what that means, at different rates. Families, however, are increasingly attending primary and secondary care with children and adolescents displaying transgender preferences and related behaviours (trans or transgender are terms used to describe individuals who do not identify with their sex assigned at birth)

(Winters & Conway, 2011). There is much debate around the topic of gender identity and at what age it would be appropriate to accept that a young person understands their identity preferences enough to warrant social or medical transition. Children and adolescents living through their transgender identity trajectories may experience both risk and protective factors that can boost or undermine their resilience.

11.8.1 Gender Identity Development

Kohlberg's theory of gender identity development (see Chap. 5) considers how children begin to understand their gender identity in and amongst other developmental and daily living tasks. He highlighted three stages; firstly, in preschool years (three to four years), children begin gender labelling. They will identify boys and girls and label them as such. At this age, however, children think that gender can change and do not really grasp the notion that males and females may have different body shapes but can still have similar characteristics. As young children mature, they obtain a better understanding of gender identity. Once children reach six to seven years and are engaging in primary school socialisation processes, they understand gender consistency, that they are one gender, and that gender will remain. Still, there will be a small number of children who feel at conflict with this and will feel unsettled with their assigned gender. This struggle can continue across their lifespans.

Piaget's theory of development (see Chap. 5) can also be considered and evaluated by exploring young children's play and socialisation. Once a child reaches around five years of age, they will generally play with 'gender-specific' toys. For example, girls, even if there is an array of toys available in day care environments, will opt to play with dolls and animal toys, and boys with superhero and action figure toys. We also begin to see gender differences in play socialisation with boys playing more in groups and girls in pairs. It is at this age where children also become aware of gender typical behaviours. For example, a girl may re-enact mum caring for her siblings and a boy may re-enact his dad fixing his car. Children's early beliefs around gender and gender identity can mirror the behaviours of those close to them.

It is generally agreed, however, by both academics and health and social professionals that gender identity begins evolving around the age of two to three years, while the child is also learning to talk. Children who are transgender will often early in their years make their parents aware of their perceived transgender status. Although, when a child is very young they are unable to comprehend what their felt gender means, they will show preferences via their choice of clothes and toys (Ehrensaft, 2011). There have also been common incidences of young children expressing their gender identity via 'three early behaviours', including, 'what underwear the child selects; what swimsuits the child prefers; and how the child urinates' (Solomon, 2012, p. 616). A study was undertaken with 121 transgender adults asking them to recollect their memories of their gender identity experiences (Kennedy & Mark, 2010). Findings highlighted how most participants had experienced an indication of their transgender status by the age of five years, with over 75% of the sample suggesting that by the time they left primary school they were sure of their transgender status.

11.8.2 Multidisciplinary Insights

In drawing on the more general psycho-social theories of development it is suggested that gender development is influenced by the child's parenting, their immediate environments, and how the child is treated through their development. This notion of nurture was exemplified famously in the 1960s when Dr John Money published his John/Joan case study, suggesting a child's gender was resultant of nurturing, not nature (Goldie, 2014).

The John/Joan case study was documented as an experiment. There was an incident incurred in the circumcision surgery of a two-month-old twin boy. Following this incident Dr Money supported the twin's parents to make the decision to allow their mutilated son to undergo further surgery to appear feminine. In addition, the child would be given hormones and their nurturing be aligned with raising a girl. While Dr. Money reported this experiment as one of overwhelming success, many years later a man called David Reimer unveiled himself as the twin who had undergone the gender change surgery. He suggested the case was reported with bias and that the experiment was not a success. David had experienced many psychological difficulties in trying to come to terms with his gender and once he was told the truth about his surgery aged 14, he made the choice to then identify as male as had never felt comfortable regarding potential relationships with boys. Unfortunately, David did later commit suicide possibly because of the trauma and stress he had experienced as a child (Goldie, 2014) including the conflicts he felt due to his genetic male inheritance.

This case and following history lend us to further question if gender identity is the consequence of nature or nurture. The big question both within and outside of the transgender community is, are those who identify as transgender born transgender, or have they somehow learnt or chose to become transgender?

The Social Perspective—How we construct our identities is influenced by our socialisation, social learning, and interacting, with many parents gendering their children from birth (Kane, 2006).

Biological Perspectives—Historically, theorists suggested *'those who were born male are supposed to act masculine and be sexually attracted to women, whereas those who were born female are supposed to act feminine and be sexually attracted to men'* (Nagoshi & Brzuzy, 2010, p. 433). Following on, theorists argued where normative gender differentiation did *'not occur as expected, it is possible that some biological alterations may have occurred'* (Giordano, 2013, p. 35). This meant that if there were children identifying differently to their assigned gender, then there must be some biological 'alterations' present, that this situation would suggest a biological irregularity, therefore pathologising the difference but suggesting that gender identity does have a biological or nature basis. These biological perspectives are still maintained by some current academics (Giordano, 2013).

Neurological Perspectives—Ehrensaft (2011, p. 33) stated *'the core of our gen-der identity lies not between our legs but between our ears—in the physiology of our brains and in the working of our minds ....'* This perspective suggests gender is determined prebirth; both biological and psychological development is present prior to any social influence. To this end we are 'pre-wired' to be the gender we identify to be. It is entirely acceptable from this perspective that our gender and mental representations of such may not be congruent with our anatomical sex (Winter, 2010).

The Biopsychosocial Perspectives—Ehrensaft (2011, p. 36) states, *'gender is born, yet gender is also made. Gender is an interweaving of nature and nurture'*. To this end we can appreciate that our gender identity could be the result of interacting biological, psychological, and social factors and is a complex process, unique to everyone.

While the academic literature on gender identity and development is informed by various academic disciplines, it is important that we accept that transgender identification is a valid phenomenon. Our theoretical position or disciplinary background may influence our thoughts on whether identifying as transgender is resultant of nature or nurture or both and relatedly at what age it would be appropriate to support social or medical transition. Children and adolescents, however, who identify as transgender can incur many risk factors for resilience which suggests a need for protective factors to support children and adolescents in their gender identity experiences.

11.8.3 The Experience of Trans Youth (Children and Adolescents)

Trans youth encounter discrimination and other life barriers that impact on their wellbeing and ultimately their resilience. Although community and charitable groups have made much progress to remove discriminatory barriers for trans youth, barriers continue. Such barriers include family difficulties related to understanding and acceptance, employment discrimination, school discrimination, and health care access difficulties. These barriers are risks to wellbeing and can lead to young people playing truant from school, leaving home, substance abusing, and engaging in unsafe sex (Singh et al., 2011).

The most damaging risk appears to be that of familial non-acceptance and the lack of social support from family members and peers (Moody et al., 2015). Transgender individuals can be victimised and rejected by their own families and friends so their need for belonging is heightened. They often find solace in becoming members of lesbian, gay, bisexual, transgender, and queer (LGBTQ) communities. The transgender community connectedness is thought to buffer the negative impacts of rejection and is correlated with lower levels of anxiety and depression symptoms (Barr et al., 2016). Where there is family acceptance and understanding there is a noted increase in resilience amongst trans youth (Torres et al., 2015).

Furthermore, positive role models may be an important resilience factor for transgender children and adolescents, especially given there are fewer visible role transgender models in comparison to other marginalised groups (Bockting et al.,

2013). The influence of social media that positively represents transgender individuals is not to be underestimated for those who can benefit from positive role models and community support. Social media may give transgender children and adolescents access to more diverse representations of transgender people that are less bound by the stereotypical representations that are seen in mainstream media (Craig et al., 2015). In addition, being a role model to others is also a protective resilience factor for trans youth. Moody et al. (2015) in their study on transgender found that being a role model promoted healthy active coping and a sense of purpose and meaning to transgender individuals.

11.8.4 Individual Resilience Factors

Like other populations, where individuals maintain their self-worth, they can be more resilient to adversities. Unfortunately, a good sense of self-worth can be difficult to maintain when faced with discriminatory messages about your self-identity. Self-stigma can also play its part here. Where trans youth hold positive views of their identity (transgender is a valid aspect of your identity) and hold positive views of others who are also transgender they can have *identity pride*. Identity pride lowers psychological distress (Bockting et al., 2013). In addition, where transgender youth can describe their own identity, they can feel empowered and more able to cope with discrimination (Singh et al., 2014).

A sense of hope and possessing a positive outlook can also support transgender individuals to overcome adversities (Bry et al.', 2017). Where there is hope for the future, individuals can manage stress incurred from discrimination. A positive outlook could also be a protective factor against suicidal ideation and behaviour (Moody et al., 2015).

Lastly, experiencing transition, be this medically or socially, can also increase resilience. For those who desire medical intervention, trans-affirming medical procedures are highly correlated with positive mental health outcomes (Vance et al., 2014). Medical or social transitioning has also been found to be a major protective factor for suicide (Moody et al., 2015). A meta-analysis of 28 studies exploring hormone therapy and gender affirmative surgeries found 80% of participants had significant improvement in gender dysphoria and quality of life scores, with 78% reporting fewer negative psychological symptoms (Murad et al., 2010).

11.8.5 Individual and Group Interventions

Interventions are being targeted for trans youth at individual and group levels and to increase awareness and acceptance amongst broader communities. Educational programmes are now implemented with the aim of creating supportive environments for transgender children and adolescents in schools. Although there is a dearth of studies exploring the effectiveness of these initiatives and activities, there is anecdotal evidence that the atmosphere/culture of some schools and colleges have improved as a consequence (Poynter & Tubbs, 2008).

Recommendations for health and social care professionals supporting trans youth are highlighted in professional guidelines on practice with transgender and gender nonconforming individuals. Key recommendations include 'understanding gender as a nonbinary construct that is different but related to sexual orientation'; 'becoming aware of one's biases toward transgender individuals'; and 'working to educate oneself on transgender-related topics'. It is also relevant to acknowledge the effects of discriminatory messages and environments in supporting those experiencing difficulties (Dickey & Singh, 2017).

Most young people who engage in the transition process (social/medical) in Western contemporary society will be offered psychotherapeutic interventions. These interventions can use therapeutic techniques to target resilience. For example, drawing on the concepts of hope and purpose and positive psychology (Feldman & Dreher, 2012). In addition, self-compassion interventions can increase self-worth and self-acceptance among trans youth, acknowledging and working through feelings associated with minority stressors, societal and self-stigma. Exploring gender identity can assist self-acceptance, identity, and identity pride (Neff & McGehee, 2010). In addition, where the young person is wanting to pursue medical intervention, it is important to provide assistance in helping them gain factual knowledge on procedures and treatments (Ducheny et al., 2017).

There is a wealth of research that has explored community support for transgender individuals, showing improvements in measures of wellbeing. In relation, group therapy can lead to positive outcomes, providing individuals with peer support and role models. Peer support is also growing amongst virtual communities which may be an easier route to connecting with role model mentors (Wager & Cox, 2017). Virtual and in person (perhaps at school) mentorship programmes encourage different relationships to those of parent and child, lending young people to be able to feel more at ease to discuss issues of gender, identity, and sexuality (Mulcahy et al., Mulcahy et al., 2016). There is also scope to offer therapeutic intervention to families to encourage family acceptance. Published case studies on family therapy demonstrate benefits (Coolhart & Shipman, 2017).

11.8.6 Needs

There has been an increased interest recently in undertaking research with transgender communities. However, much more research is needed that explores the experiences of trans youth, the impacts of community, group, and individual interventions to determine the pertinent stress and resilience factors. There is still much more to be done to educate health and social care professionals and further studies to be undertaken that evaluate the effectiveness of interventions, for example the measures taken in schools. It is important that we continue where possible to train and educate communities around discriminatory and supportive behaviours towards transgendered people, to limit or prevent stressors, and to allow trans youth to feel comfortable with their identities (Moradi et al., 2016).

11.9   Social Media and Digital Technology: The Changing Landscape of Play

Over the last twenty years there has been a tidal change in how children play and how adolescents spend their leisure time. We have borne witness to the advent and increase in virtual play even for incredibly young children. As a result, there have been concerns about the involvement of children and adolescents in new forms of communication which increasingly mean that adults have less control over their activities. Concern has been expressed in the past about young people having access to books, cinema, and television. Bandura's work and that of others were undertaken to see if levels of anti-social behaviour resulted (see Chap. 3).

Children and adolescents now spend much of their free time in virtual worlds, gaming, and participating on social networking platforms targeted towards young people. What is not clear is whether children who are raised interacting regularly in virtual worlds will develop differently and if the nature of their play behaviours will also change. Technology is now a developmental norm for children, indeed young children will learn to use a keyboard and mouse as they also learn to read and write. They will also become familiar from an early age with the social norms of smart phone usage and interacting with the screens of computers and tablet devices. These multimodal experiences that children are now exposed to engage all their senses. The concern is that social media and digital technology use for the purposes of play may hinder learning and psycho-social development.

Vygotsky (1978) suggested cognitive development is associated with speech as the convergence of practical and abstract intelligence. Firstly, children's egocentric (towards the self) speech follows their actions. Then, speech accompanies those actions, describing, and speech then precedes the action, helping to plan it. The development of executive functions is associated with the ability to plan and self/emotionally regulate. Vygotsky (1978) also argued, by using language as a problem-solving tool, that children learn to master not only their environment, but also their own behaviour. The amount of speech that children use is increased as the difficulty of the task at hand increases.

Shin (2018) interested in Vygotsky's arguments explored speech, action, and planning in relation to virtual reality (VR) play, and evaluated the impact of immersive storytelling. The findings suggest that cognitive processing determines levels of empathy within VR stories. Therefore, even when the child is playing within virtual environments, using digital technology, their cognitive development follows a similar sequence and as such social-emotional development occurs with the development of cognitive skills.

Although virtual worlds are a new phenomenon, their roles in facilitating learning through play, imagination, and representative experiences are a progression of traditional play. Children can explore new virtual environments and related novel experiences. There are problem-solving strategies to develop and implement. Whether children are spending time seated playing with Lego or sitting in front of a laptop computer, the processes share many similarities (Klug & Schell, 2006). Yelland (2010, p. 18) however states that the exploratory context of young children's social media platforms, with their tools for creating characters, '*somewhat turns Piaget's ideas about egocentricity on their head*'. Digitally mediated friendships are also changing the nature of friendships, and the ways in which children and adolescents interact with each other. There is the concern though as to whether digital friendships buffer the support that in person friendships provide which can buffer influences of stress and isolation (Subrahmanyam & Šmahel, 2011).

11.9.1 Cyberbullying

In acknowledging virtual friendships, online connectivity, and networking, it is important to consider the risk of cyberbullying. *Cyberbullying* is conceptually defined as '*wilful and repeated harm inflicted through computers, cell phones, and other electronic devices*' (Hinduja & Patchin, 2015, p. 11). This definition is influenced by definitions of in person bullying at school, highlighting negative deliberate behaviours that are persistent and result in harm. In less complex terms, cyberbullying is where individuals use technology to harass, threaten, humiliate, or otherwise hassle their peers. Studies have found that cyberbullying can often result in negative emotions including sadness, anger, frustration, embarrassment, and fear. These emotions are associated with low self-esteem, depression, suicidal thoughts, academic difficulties, and allied in person school bullying (Gini & Espelage, 2014). However, a large-scale longitudinal study including 3136 adolescents aged 12–14 found that those with higher self-esteem, more social connectedness, and better family relationships had higher emotional resilience (were less depressed than would have been expected) and behavioural resilience (showed fewer behavioural manifestations than expected) (Sapouna & Wolke, 2013). In addition, supportive family relationships were significantly correlated with resilience to bullying in a UK-based longitudinal study. The study included 1116 pairs of twins aged between 10 and 12 years (Bowes et al., 2010). These findings are corroborated by the findings of a study undertaken in South Africa that included 48 families and employed mixed methods. Where families reported good communication, mutual support, cooperation, durability, and good community relations, there was evidence of resilient adaptations when their children were bullied (Greeff & Van den Berg, 2013).

11.9.2 Online Gaming and Gambling by Children and Adolescents

Most children and adolescents do engage or have engaged in online gaming. What is unclear is why some children then move on to engage with online gambling. One school of thought suggests the addictive nature of online gaming transfers to an appetite for gambling. In association, the DSM-5 recognises 'internet gaming disorder', but also acknowledges definitional issues and therefore the need for further research. Adolescents are particularly susceptible to online gambling because the games used are remarkably like none of the gambling games in their design (Petry

& O'Brien, 2013). The Gambling Commission's report on gambling in young people (2019) highlights the increase in online gambling and especially in paying for loot boxes in video gaming. At least half of 11–16-year-old have knowledge of 'in-game' items, and of those, 44% have paid money to open loot boxes and 6% have gambled with in-game items on websites outside of games or privately, but with friends. Skin gambling is a related phenomenon. Skins are virtual goods used to enhance your gaming image, for example, clothes for your character but which gives you no gaming advantage. These and other items can be obtained via the purchasing of gaming currency. As a result of these gaming features incurring expenditure, there are pressures from activists that age controls should be applied, as children become 'addicted' to these in game purchases (Griffiths, 2018).

11.9.3 Cyber Safety

Cyber safety and protection against online risks have shaped policy and research agendas. The ground-breaking EU Kids Online project (Livingstone et al., 2011) highlighted key online risks for children and adolescents as they play and build networks with others through digital technology via gaming and social media. Major risks aside from cyberbullying and gambling include exposure to adult-oriented or violent content; they can be subjected to 'grooming' or sexual exploitation or have their data misused (Livingstone et al., 2011). Belonging to a minority group is a risk factor for cyberbullying and harassment, exposure to violence, and hate speech (Leurs, 2014).

These risks inhibit the formation of socially cohesive digital environments. Study findings have increased anxieties around children and adolescents being recruited online to join high-profile global terrorist organisations such as ISIS (Talbot, 2015). Involvement in online violent extremism can be a precursor to terrorism. Lennings et al. (2010, p. 427) suggested that children and adolescents *'from backgrounds where parents may have been physically or psychologically absent'*, and/or where *'life skills and moral values were not a high priority'* are more vulnerable to extremist groups online as they strive for the sense of belonging they provide. This method of replacing the 'family' is considered *'subtle grooming.'*

There are, however, also benefits to having an online presence as a child or adolescent. These benefits are viewed to outweigh the risks. Digital media offers opportunities to play, to learn, to develop relationships and connectedness, develop resilience, and participate in a growing digital economy. As a result, there are initiatives that aim to promote digital literacy and digital resilience, as these are identified as key protective factors. Digital literacy incorporates technical and social skills used to navigate technology and related social norms and evaluate its content quality and reliability (Third et al., 2014). This leads to the increased teaching of ICT skills and knowledge in schools, helping to also boost digital resilience. Digital resilience is *'the ability to deal with negative experiences online or offline. Strategies focus on skilling users to adapt and respond effectively to potentially harmful online experiences'* (Third et al., 2014, p. 17). d'Haenens et al. (2013) suggest that peer support, teacher support, and parent mediation are key to the development of digital resilience.

11.9.4 Online Intervention

Socialisation processes help shape cultural expectations for youth, including what role technology will play in their everyday lives. In fact, people have an innate need to form networks with others. Online networks do have the capacity to encourage user compassion, empathy, and other valued constructs by providing good role models. School culture can take an active role in educating children, parents, and other adults who interact with youth as well as by providing safety training relevant to online settings. In implementing intervention and anti-bullying programmes, school representatives can incorporate training as a means of encouraging self-regulation and caring among students (Michikyan et al., 2014).

While there has been a steady increase in research examining children and adolescents use of online gaming, social media, and digital technology both in the UK and in other countries worldwide, there are large knowledge gaps, and this is exacerbated by the fact that the field is constantly evolving. Most surveys undertaken to date are cross-sectional therefore more longitudinal studies investigating relationships between variables associated with risk and protective factors among children and adolescents are needed.

11.10 The Effects of COVID-19

To consider resilience in the context of the COVID-19 pandemic we draw on life course theory (Elder, 1998). Life course theory can assist us in the understanding of how macro-level sociohistorical events can impact child and adolescent development. With current variants of the virus, children and adolescents are considered less at risk of physical illness as compared to adult populations. However, they are still susceptible to developmental risks due to the many different and stressful disruptions entering their lives. For example, children have had family disruptions due the high death rate, meaning they may have lost family members, and if not, they may have had worries because of COVID-19 illness and related hospital admissions in their families. Due to the closure of workplaces and furlough arrangements, many families have also suffered financial difficulties. There have also been many schooling disruptions, including the closure of schools and day care facilities and then the requirement to adapt to new online styles of learning with less face-to-face support from teachers. In addition, there have been public health restrictions that have meant a reduction in peer contact, and physical activities, because of distancing and isolation measures. All these issues combined provide us with concern for the psychological and physical wellbeing and safety of children and adolescents.

11.10.1   Life Course Perspective

The life course theory assists our understanding of intertwined developmental trajectories in critical transition periods (Elder, 1998). These transition periods can be typical and expected, for example, the transition to high school. However, when faced with large sociohistorical events and the impact of related social changes then the critical transition can then be unexpected, like a shock to development. As such they can lead to a turn or deflection in developmental direction (Almeida & Wong, 2009). Again, the timing of such large sociohistorical events can be impactful. Elder identified that those who experienced the Great Depression as young children, and especially if they were male, appeared to be impacted more negatively over the longer term, with lower confidence levels, and lower educational achievement as compared to those experiencing the same events in late childhood or early adolescence (Elder, 1998).

As previously stated, early childhood (prenatal to 8 years) and adolescence (from onset of puberty to early 20s) are times of rapid neurobiological and brain development, cognitive and social growth. As such, these years are sensitive periods of development and therefore children and adolescents at these ages could be more impacted by COVID-19. Young children (from birth to 4 years) may be especially vulnerable because of an array of risk factors including delayed vaccinations, health screenings, food insecurity, residential crowding, and displacement, and lost access to education and childcare (Yoshikawa et al., 2020).

Studies that have explored the effects of large-scale disasters have identified immediate and longer term effects on the mental health and wellbeing of children and adolescents. For example, studies undertaken in other pandemics (e.g. SARS, H1N1) with young people in Asia discovered adjustment and psychological difficulties in school-aged children, adolescents, and young adults (Sprang & Silman, 2013). Studies that have examined impacts of COVID-19 to date highlight similar findings. An Italian study found that children and adolescents were fearing negative educational consequences (Buzzi et al., 2020). Whereas studies undertaken in China have found higher rates of psychological difficulties and post-traumatic stress disorder (PTSD) symptoms amongst school-aged children and adolescents (Zhou et al., 2020), an adolescent study in the USA highlighted how social distancing measures have led to symptoms of anxiety and depressive symptoms (Oosterhoff et al., 2020).

These are viewed to be immediate effects, but we know through drawing on life course theory that there can also be developmental turning points that impact longer term trajectories of wellbeing. There are however no studies to our knowledge that have examined this notion in relation to pandemics and children and adolescent wellbeing. This highlights the need for longitudinal studies now we have experienced the COVID-19 pandemic so that we can examine how developmental trajectories play out over time and as a response to such a wide scale stressful event. We do however have studies of children post large-scale events. For example, following the 9/11 terrorist attacks in the USA, there were studies highlighting heightened substance abuse in adolescents, especially those who had witnessed events or were injured (Gargano et al., 2017). A qualitative study of the same event however would suggest that immediate effects were mild and transitory (Eisenberg & Silver, 2011). We are however in unknown territory with the current pandemic as it could go on for many more months yet. At the time of writing, we are witnessing a new variant 'Omicron' that may take countries back into lockdown measures. As such, effects on children and adolescents maybe different to what we have seen with events that although are large scale and are more acute and time limited in terms of stressful impact.

11.10.2   Experiencing the Pandemic with Others

Life course theory highlights how we do not live in isolation, children and adolescents are experiencing the COVID-19 pandemic with others, their families, peers, and social communities (Elder, 1998). Relationships with others through this time can serve to be supportive or strenuous. Support from others can enhance wellbeing but in these times of stress for everyone, the supportive reserves people can give to others can be limited.

Children and adolescents have had major impacts to their schooling since the start of the pandemic in January 2020. They have lived through months of lockdowns where schools were closed. This has impacted on their education with differences amongst parental capacity to provide home education. In addition, more vulnerable children lost their access to balanced meals and their school safe haven. Food insecurity is associated with poorer academic and socioemotional skills, physical and mental wellbeing. In addition, school personnel (teachers and others) are a source of support to children and adolescents, they can monitor for signs of psychological difficulty and unsafe circumstances. Since children and adolescents have returned to school, they have been subjected to staying within class or year group 'bubbles' preventing peer socialisation outside of these bubbles. Furthermore, adolescents continue two years into the pandemic to wear face coverings whilst in high school. The likely negative impact of the pandemic on children and adolescents derailed academic trajectories is clear. Based on research where children have had a delayed start to school or learning gaps, there are negative impacts on achievement and drop out, especially for those with disabilities or living in poverty (Masonbrink & Hurley, 2020).

COVID-19 has affected other areas of life for families. Working parents have needed to juggle work with caring and home-schooling demands and for some also the stress of job loss and financial insecurity. Those who are key workers (health care professionals for example) have needed to navigate health and safety considerations. All families have needed to cope with confinement-related stress. All these factors can impact family relationships with implications for children's and adolescents' wellbeing (Prime et al., 2020). The life course perspective highlights how psychological difficulties experienced by parents impact children and adolescents' physical and mental health and educational outcomes.

Where there are heightened levels of family stress close family relationships can mitigate the risks to wellbeing. In addition, a supportive relationship outside the immediate family can also act as a buffer to the effects of stress on children's functioning (Prime et al., 2020). Maternal support and positive active coping strategies are associated with better wellbeing in children and adolescents following natural disasters and terrorist attacks (Eisenberg & Silver, 2011). Research with adolescents in the USA has shown that those happy at being at home at the start of the pandemic reported less anxiety and depressive symptoms (Oosterhoff et al., 2020). To nurture children and adolescents through this pandemic it is important we try our best to offer support and positivity but also consider children and adolescents' subjective experiences, how they perceive events can be internalised differently depending on their developmental age. For example, adolescents can accommodate the implications of job loss and young children are likely to become less familiar in their behaviour towards family members they have had little contact with. They can indeed become fearful of others because they no longer 'know them'. Early evidence also suggests that the wellbeing impacts of COVID-19 will be felt more heavily in black and minority ethnic communities and among low-income families (Golberstein et al., 2020).

Summary

- Resilience is the term used to describe being able to adjust to or 'bounce back' from adversity. Stressful life events and life traumas can negatively influence brain function and structure and impede psychosocial development, leading to psychological difficulties including post-traumatic stress disorder (PTSD), anxiety, depression, and other mental health disorders. However, many children and adolescents manage to maintain wellbeing and are therefore deemed to be resilient.
- The growing understanding of resilience promoting and protecting factors (and at key developmental stages) assist health and social care professionals to create supportive interventions to heighten resilience and to mitigate negative outcomes.
- In exploring the issues of poverty, trans youth identity, social media, and digital technology we can agree that our knowledge and theorising of resiliency can extend to these topics but there is much we must not assume. A positive move forward is to consider an assets-based approach looking at children and adolescents' self-reported experiences and needs so that we as adults can scaffold their developmental wellbeing.
- The worldwide effects of COVID-19 are still unfolding. As some countries begin to release restrictions, others continue to battle containing COVID-19. Life course theory provides a framework or heuristic for considering children's and adolescents' development, understanding the importance of developmental timing and how developmental trajectories can unfold following trauma. Resilience factors can protect or exacerbate detrimental immediate and longer term effects.

Case Study Questions

Read the family case study on page 265 and consider the following:

- How can the Wilson children be helped to develop resilience to cope with some of the difficult experiences they have encountered?
- What different effects may the dependence on online communication have on Gemma, Ben, and Liam?
- How might the restrictions imposed due to COVID-19 have affected the educational opportunities for the Wilson children?

Reflective Questions:

- Why is some level of stress necessary for wellbeing?
- To what extent is the use of digital technology in childhood and adolescence a cause for concern?
- How may stress from adverse early experiences impact the future physical and mental health across an individual's life course?

References

Agyemang, C., van Hooijdonk, C., Wendel-Vos, W., Lindeman, E., Stronks, K., & Droomers, M. (2007). The Association of Neighbourhood Psychosocial Stressors and Self-rated Health in Amsterdam, The Netherlands. *Journal of Epidemiology & Community Health, 61*(12), 1042–1049.

Alim, T. N., Feder, A., Graves, R. E., Wang, Y., Weaver, J., Westphal, M., et al. (2008). Trauma, Resilience, and Recovery in a High-Risk African American Population. *American Journal of Psychiatry, 165*, 1566–1575.

Almeida, D. M., & Wong, J. D. (2009). Life Transitions and Daily Stress Processes. In G. H. Elder Jr. & J. Z. Giele (Eds.), *The Craft of Life Course Research* (pp. 141–162). The Guilford Press.

Barr, S. M., Budge, S. L., & Adelson, J. L. (2016). Transgender Community Belongingness as a Mediator Between Strength of Transgender Identity and Well-Being. *Journal of Counselling Psychology, 63*(1), 87–97.

Blanden, J., & Machin, S. (2010). Intergenerational Inequality in Early Years Assessments. In K. Hansen, H. Joshi, & S. Dex (Eds.), *Children of the 21st Century: The First Five Years*. The Policy Press.

Bockting, W. O., Miner, M. H., Swinburne Romine, R. E., Hamilton, A., & Coleman, E. (2013). Stigma, Mental Health, and Resilience in an Online Sample of the US Transgender Population. *American Journal of Public Health, 103*(5), 943–951.

Bowes, L., Maughan, B., Caspi, A., Moffitt, T. E., & Arseneault, L. (2010). Families Promote Emotional and Behavioural Resilience to Bullying: Evidence of an Environmental Effect. *Journal of Child Psychology and Psychiatry, 51*(7), 809–817.

Bry, L. J., Mustanski, B., Garofalo, R., & Burns, M. N. (2017). Management of a Concealable Stigmatized Identity: A Qualitative Study of Concealment, Disclosure, and Role Flexing Among Young, Resilient Sexual and Gender Minority Individuals. *Journal of Homosexuality, 64*(6), 745–769.

Buzzi, C., Tucci, M., Ciprandi, R., Brambilla, I., Caimmi, S., Ciprandi, G., & Marseglia, G. L. (2020). The Psycho-Social Effects of COVID-19 on Italian Adolescents' Attitudes and Behaviours. *Italian Journal of Pediatrics, 46*(1), 1–7.

Carter, C. S. (2005). The Chemistry of Child Neglect: Do Oxytocin and Vasopressin Mediate the Effects of Early Experience? *Proceedings of the National Academy of Sciences of the United States of America, 102*(51), 18247–18248.

Cauthen, N. K., & Fass, S. (2008). *Measuring Poverty in the United States*. National Centre for Children in Poverty.

Charney, D. S. (2004). Psychobiological Mechanisms of Resilience and Vulnerability: Implications for Successful Adaptation to Extreme Stress. *American Journal of Psychiatry, 161*, 195–216.

Cicchetti, D. (2010). Resilience Under Conditions of Extreme Stress: A Multilevel Perspective. *World Psychiatry, 9*, 145–154.

Cicchetti, D., & Curtis, W. J. (2006). The Developing Brain and Neural Plasticity: Implications for Normality, Psychopathology, and Resilience. In D. Cicchetti & D. Cohen (Eds.), *Developmental Psychopathology. Vol 2: Developmental Neuroscience* (2nd ed., pp. 1–64). Wiley & Sons, Ltd.

Coolhart, D., & Shipman, D. L. (2017). Working Toward Family Attunement: Family Therapy with Transgender and Gender-Nonconforming Children and Adolescents. *Psychiatric Clinics, 40*(1), 113–125.

Craig, S. L., McInroy, L. B., McCready, L. T., Di Cesare, D. M., & Pettaway, L. D. (2015). Connecting Without Fear: Clinical Implications of the Consumption of Information and Communication Technologies by Sexual Minority Youth and Young Adults. *Clinical Social Work Journal, 43*(2), 159–168.

Curtis, W. J., & Nelson, C. A. (2003). Toward building a better brain: Neurobehavioral Outcomes, Mechanisms, and Processes of Environmental Enrichment. In S. S. Luthar (Ed.), *Resilience and Vulnerability: Adaptation in the Context of Childhood Adversities* (pp. 463–488). Cambridge University Press.

d'Haenens, Vandoninck, and Donoso. (2013). How to Cope and Build Online Resilience? http://eprints.lse.ac.uk/48115/1/How%20to%20cope%20and%20build%20online%20resilience%20(lsero).pdf

Davidson, R. J., & McEwen, B. S. (2012). Social Influences on Neuroplasticity: Stress and Interventions to Promote Well-Being. *Nature Neuroscience, 15*, 689–695.

Dept for Work and Pensions. (2021). *Households Below Average Income, Statistics on the Number and Percentage of People Living in Low Income Households for Financial Years 1994/95 to 2019/20*. Department for Work and Pensions.

Diamond, A., & Lee, K. (2011). Interventions Shown to Aid Executive Function Development in Children 4 to 12 Years Old. *Science (New York, N.Y.), 333*(6045), 959–964.

Dickey, L. M., & Singh, A. A. (2017). Finding a Trans-affirmative Provider: Challenges Faced by Trans and Gender Diverse Psychologists and Psychology Trainees. *Journal of Clinical Psychology, 73*(8), 938–944.

Ducheny, K., Hendricks, M. L., & Keo-Meier, C. L. (2017). TGNC-Affirmative Interdisciplinary Collaborative Care. In A. Singh & L. M. Dickey (Eds.), *Affirmative Counselling and Psychological Practice with Transgender and Gender Nonconforming Clients* (pp. 69–93). American Psychological Association.

Dudley, K. J., Li, X., Kobor, M. S., Kippin, T. E., & Bredy, T. W. (2011). Epigenetic Mechanisms Mediating Vulnerability and Resilience to Psychiatric Disorders. *Neuroscience & Biobehavioural Reviews, 35*(7), 1544–1551.

Ehrensaft, D. (2011). *Gender Born, Gender Made: Raising Healthy Gender Non-conforming Children*. The Experiment, LLC.

Eisenberg, N., & Silver, R. C. (2011). Growing Up in the Shadow of Terrorism: Youth in America After 9/11. *American Psychologist, 66*(6), 468–481.

Elder, G. H., Jr. (1998). The Life Course as Developmental Theory. *Child Development, 69*(1), 1–12.

Eshbaugh, E. M., Peterson, C. A., Wall, S., Carta, J. J., Luze, G., Swanson, M., & Jeon, H. J. (2011). Low-Income Parents' Warmth and Parent–Child Activities for Children with Disabilities, Suspected Delays and Biological Risks. *Infant and Child Development, 20*(5), 509–524.

Feldman, D. B., & Dreher, D. E. (2012). Can Hope to Be Changed in 90 Minutes? Testing the Efficacy of a Single-Session Goal-Pursuit Intervention for College Students. *Journal of Happiness Studies, 13*(4), 745–759.

Frankl, V. E. (2006). *Man's Search for Meaning*. Simon and Schuster.

Frodl, T., & O'Keane, V. (2013). How Does the Brain Deal with Cumulative Stress? A Review with Focus on Developmental Stress, HPA Axis Function and Hippocampal Structure in Humans. *Neurobiology of Disease, 52*, 24–37.

Gargano, L. M., Welch, A. E., & Stellman, S. D. (2017). Substance Use in Adolescents 10 Years After the World Trade Centre Attacks in New York City. *Journal of Child & Adolescent Substance Abuse, 26*(1), 66–74.

Garman, M., Rinke, M. L., Gurney, B. A., Gross, R. S., Bloomfield, D. E., Haliczer, L. A., Colman, S., Racine, A. D., & Briggs, R. D. (2017). Comparing Two Models of Integrated Behavioural Health Programs in Paediatric Primary Care. *Child and Adolescent Psychiatric Clinics of North America, 26*, 815–828.

Gini, G., & Espelage, D. L. (2014). Peer Victimization, Cyberbullying, and Suicide Risk in Children and Adolescents. *Jama, 312*(5), 545–546.

Giordano, S. (2013). *Children with Gender Identity Disorder: A Clinical, Ethical and Legal Analysis*. Routledge.

Golberstein, E., Wen, H., & Miller, B. F. (2020). Coronavirus Disease 2019 (COVID-19) and Mental Health for Children and Adolescents. *JAMA Paediatrics, 174*(9), 819–820.

Goldie, T. (2014). *The Man Who Invented Gender: Engaging the Ideas of John Money*. UBC Press.

Greeff, A. P., & Van den Berg, E. (2013). Resilience in Families in Which a Child Is Bullied. *British Journal of Guidance & Counselling, 41*(5), 504–517.

Griffiths, M. D. (2018). Is the Buying of Loot Boxes in Video Games a Form of Gambling Or Gaming? *Gaming Law Review, 22*(1), 52–54.

Gunnar, M. R., & Fisher, P. A. (2006). Bringing Basic Research on Early Experience and Stress Neurobiology to Bear on Preventive Interventions for Neglected and Maltreated Children. *Development and Psychopathology, 18*, 651–677.

Heim, C., Shugart, M., Craighead, W. E., & Nemeroff, C. B. (2010). Neurobiological and Psychiatric Consequences of Child Abuse and Neglect. *Developmental Psychobiology, 52*(7), 671–690.

Hinduja, S., & Patchin, J. W. (2015). *Bullying Beyond the Schoolyard: Preventing and Responding to Cyberbullying* (2nd ed.). Sage.

Hirsch, D., & Spencer, N. (2008). Unhealthy Lives: Intergenerational Links Between Child Poverty and Poor Health in the UK. In Poverty. (ed.). End Child Poverty.

Hjemdal, O., Friborg, O., Stiles, T. C., Martinussen, M., & Rosenvinge, J. H. (2006). A New Scale for Adolescent Resilience: Grasping the Central Protective Resources Behind Healthy Development. *Measurement and Evaluation in Counselling and Development, 39*(2), 84–96.

Kane, E. W. (2006). "No way my boys are going to be like that!" Parents' Responses to Children's Gender Nonconformity. *Gender and Society, 20*(2), 149–176.

Karreman, A., & Vingerhoets, A. J. (2012). Attachment and Well-being: The Mediating Role of Emotion Regulation and Resilience. *Personality and Individual Differences, 53*(7), 821–826.

Kennedy, N., & Mark, H. (2010). Transgender Children: More Than a Theoretical Challenge. *Graduate Journal of Social Science, 7*(2), 25–43.

Kiernan, K. E., & Huerta, M. C. (2008). Economic Deprivation, Maternal Depression, Parenting and Children's Cognitive and Emotional Development in Early Childhood. *British Journal of Sociology, 59*, 783–806.

Kintrea, K., St Clair, R., & Houston, M. (2011). *The Influence of Parents, Places and Poverty on Educational Attitudes and Aspirations*. York.

Klug, G. C., & Schell, J. (2006). Why People Play Games: An Industry Perspective. *Playing Video Games, Motives, Responses, and Consequences*, 91–100.

Lennings, C. J., Amon, K. L., Brummert, H., & Lennings, N. J. (2010). Grooming for Terror: The Internet and Young People. *Psychiatry, Psychology & Law, 17*(3), 424–437.

Leurs, K. (2014). Digital Thrown Togetherness: Young Londoners Negotiating Urban Politics of Difference and Encounter on Facebook. *Popular Communication, 12*(4), 251–265.

Levin, K. A., Currie, C., & Muldoon, J. (2009). Mental Well-Being and Subjective Health of 11 to 15-Year-Old Boys and Girls in Scotland, 1994–2006. *European Journal of Public Health, 19*, 605–610.

Leyland, A. H., Dundas, R., McLoone, P., & Boddy, F. A. (2007). Cause-Specific Inequalities in Mortality in Scotland: Two Decades of Change. A Population-Based Study. *BMC Public Health, 7*(1), 1–12.

Livingstone, S., Haddon, L., Görzig, A., & Ólafsson, K. (2011). Risks and Safety on the Internet: The Perspective of European Children: Full Findings and Policy Implications from the EU Kids Online Survey of 9–16-Year-Olds and Their Parents in 25 Countries. EU Kids Online, Deliverable D4. EU Kids Online Network, London, UK.

Luthar, S. S., & Cicchetti, D. (2000). The Construct of Resilience: Implications for Intervention and Social Policy. *Development and Psychopathology, 12*, 857–885.

Masonbrink, A. R., & Hurley, E. (2020). Advocating for Children During the COVID-19 School Closures. *Pediatrics, 146*(3), e20201440.

Masten, A. S. (2015). *Ordinary Magic: Resilience in Development*. Guilford Publications.

Masten, A. S., & Cicchetti, D. (2015). Resilience in Development: Progress and Transformation. In D. Cicchetti (Ed.), *Developmental Psychopathology* (Vol. 1, 3rd ed., pp. 215–263). John Wiley & Sons, Inc.

McKenzie, K., & Harpham, T. (2006). *Social Capital and Mental Health*. Jessica Kingsley Publishers.

McRae, K., Gross, J. J., Weber, J., Robertson, E. R., Sokol-Hessner, P., Ray, R. D., … Ochsner, K. N. (2012). The Development of Emotion Regulation: An fMRI Study of Cognitive Reappraisal in Children, Adolescents, and Young Adults. *Social Cognitive and Affective Neuroscience, 7*(1), 11–22.

Meaney, M. J. (2001). Maternal Care, Gene Expression, and the Transmission of Individual Differences in Stress Reactivity Across Generations. *Annual Review of Neuroscience, 24*, 1161–1192.

Mensah, F. K., & Kiernan, K. E. (2009). Parents' Mental Health and Children's Cognitive and Social Development: Families in England in the Millennium Cohort Study. *Social Psychiatry and Psychiatric Epidemiology, 45*, 1023–1035.

Michikyan, M., Subrahmanyam, K., & Dennis, J. (2014). Can You Tell Who I Am? Neuroticism, Extraversion, and Online Self-presentation Among Young Adults. *Computers in Human Behavior, 33*, 179–183.

Min, J., Silverstein, M., & Lendon, J. P. (2012). Intergenerational Transmission of Values Over the Family Life Course. *Advances in Life Course Research, 17*(3), 112–120.

Moody, C., Fuks, N., Peláez, S., & Smith, N. G. (2015). "Without this, I would for sure already be dead": A Qualitative Inquiry Regarding Suicide Protective Factors Among Trans Adults. *Psychology of Sexual Orientation and Gender Diversity, 2*(3), 266–280.

Moradi, B., Tebbe, E. A., Brewster, M. E., Budge, S. L., Lenzen, A., Ege, E., … Flores, M. J. (2016). A Content Analysis of Literature on Trans People and Issues: 2002–2012. *The Counseling Psychologist, 44*(7), 960–995.

Mulcahy, M., Dalton, S., Kolbert, J., & Crothers, L. (2016). Informal Mentoring for Lesbian, Gay, Bisexual, and Transgender Students. *The Journal of Educational Research, 109*(4), 405–412.

Murad, M. H., Elamin, M. B., Garcia, M. Z., Mullan, R. J., Murad, A., Erwin, P. J., & Montori, V. M. (2010). Hormonal Therapy and Sex Reassignment: A Systematic Review and Meta-analysis of Quality of Life and Psychosocial Outcomes. *Clinical Endocrinology, 72*(2), 214–231.

Murgatroyd, C., & Spengler, D. (2012). Genetic Variation in the Epigenetic Machinery and Mental Health. *Current Psychiatry Reports, 14*(2), 138–149.

Nagoshi, J. L., & Brzuzy, S. (2010). Transgender Theory: Embodying Research and Practice. *Affilia, 25*(4), 431–443.

Neff, K. D., & McGehee, P. (2010). Self-compassion and Psychological Resilience Among Adolescents and Young Adults. *Self and Identity, 9*(3), 225–240.

Obradović, J., Shaffer, A., & Masten, A. S. (2012). Risk in Developmental Psychopathology: Progress and Future Directions. In Cambridge Handbooks in Psychology. The Cambridge Handbook of Environment in Human Development. In C. Mayes & M. Lewis (Eds.), (Vol. 2012, pp. 35–57). Cambridge University Press.

Oosterhoff, B., Palmer, C. A., Wilson, J., & Shook, N. (2020). Adolescents' Motivations to Engage in Social Distancing During the COVID-19 Pandemic: Associations with Mental and Social Health. *Journal of Adolescent Health, 67*(2), 179–185.

Petry, N. M., & O'Brien, C. P. (2013). Internet Gaming Disorder and the DSM-5 [Editorial]. *Addiction, 108*(7), 1186–1187.

Poynter, K. J., & Tubbs, N. J. (2008). Safe Zones: Creating LGBT Safe Space Ally Programs. *Journal of LGBT Youth, 5*(1), 121–132.

Prime, H., Wade, M., & Browne, D. T. (2020). Risk and Resilience in Family Well-Being During the COVID-19 Pandemic. *American Psychologist, 75*(5), 631.

Reynolds, A. J., Temple, J. A., White, B. A., Ou, S. R., & Robertson, D. L. (2011). Age 26 Cost-Benefit Analysis of the Child-Parent Centre Early Education Program. *Child Dev, 82*, 379–404.

Ridge, T. (2002). *Childhood Poverty and Social Exclusion: From a Child's Perspective.* Policy Press.

Rutter, M. (2006). Implications of Resilience Concepts for Scientific Understanding. *Annals of the New York Academy of Sciences, 1094*, 1–12.

Sacker, A., & Schoon, I. (2007). Educational Resilience in Later Life: Resources and Assets in Adolescence and Return to Education After Leaving School at Age 16. *Social Science Research, 36*(3), 873–896.

Sandler, I. N., Schoenfelder, E. N., Wolshick, S. A., & MacKinnon, D. P. (2011). Long-Term Impact of Prevention Programs to Promote Effective Parenting: Lasting Effects But Uncertain Processes. *Annual Review of Psychology, 62*, 299–329.

Sandler, I. N., Wolchik, S. A., & Ayers, T. S. (2007). Resilience Rather Than Recovery: A Contextual Framework on Adaptation Following Bereavement. *Death studies, 32*(1), 59–73.

Sapouna, M., & Wolke, D. (2013). Resilience to Bullying Victimization: The Role of Individual, Family, and Peer Characteristics. *Child Abuse & Neglect, 37*(11), 997–1006.

Schweinhart, L. J., Barnes, H. V., & Weikhart, D. P. (2005). Significant Benefits: The High/Scope Perry Preschool Study Through Age 27. In *Child Welfare: Major Themes in Health and Social Welfare* (pp. 9–29).

Shahtahmasebi, S., Emerson, E., Berridge, D., & Lancaster, G. (2011). Child Disability and the Dynamics of Family Poverty, Hardship and Financial Strain: Evidence from the UK. *Journal of Social Policy, 40*(4), 653–673.

Shin, D. (2018). Empathy and Embodied Experience in Virtual Environment: To What Extent Can Virtual Reality Stimulate Empathy and Embodied Experience? *Computers in Human Behaviour, 78*, 64–73.

Sibinga, E. M. S., Webb, L., Ghazarian, S. R., & Ellen, J. M. (2016). School-Based Mindfulness Instruction: An RCT. *Pediatrics, 137*, e20152531.

Singh, A. A., Hays, D. G., & Watson, L. S. (2011). Strength in the Face of Adversity: Resilience Strategies of Transgender Individuals. *Journal of Counselling & Development, 89*(1), 20–27.

Singh, A. A., Meng, S. E., & Hansen, A. W. (2014). "I am my own gender": Resilience Strategies of Trans Youth. *Journal of Counselling & Development, 92*(2), 208–218.

Solomon, A. (2012). *Far from the Tree: Parents, Children, and the Search for Identity*. Scribner.

Sprang, G., & Silman, M. (2013). Posttraumatic Stress Disorder in Parents and Youth After Health-Related Disasters. *Disaster Medicine and Public Health Preparedness, 7*(1), 105–110.

Stewart-Brown, S. (2003). Research in Relation to Equity: Extending the Agenda. *Pediatrics, 112*(Supplement 3), 763–765.

Subrahmanyam, K., & Šmahel, D. (2011). Constructing Identity Online: Identity Exploration and Self-presentation. In *Digital Youth* (pp. 59–80). Springer.

Talbot, D. (2015). The Lonely Efforts to Counteract ISIS's Mastery of Social Media. MIT Technology Review, September.

Tedeschi, R., & Calhoun, L. (2004). Posttraumatic Growth: Conceptual Foundations and Empirical Evidence. *Psychological Inquiry, 15*(1), 1–18.

The Gambling Commission. (2019). Young People and Gambling. Birmingham: Gambling Commission 2019. https://www.gamblingcommission.gov.uk/pdf/survey-data/youngpeople-and-gambling-2018-report.pd

Third, A., Bellerose, D., Dawkins, U., Keltie, E., & Pihl, K. (2014). Children's Rights in the Digital Age: A Download from Children Around the World. Retrieved November 20, 2021, from http://www.uws.edu.au/__data/assets/pdf_file/0003/753447/Childrens-rights-in-the-digital-age.pdf

Torres, C. G., Renfrew, M., Kenst, K., Tan-McGrory, A., Betancourt, J. R., & López, L. (2015). Improving Transgender Health by Building Safe Clinical Environments That Promote Existing Resilience: Results from a Qualitative Analysis of Providers. *BMC Paediatrics, 15*(1), 1–10.

Tough, P. (2012). *How Children Succeed: Grit, Curiosity, and the Hidden Power of Character.* Houghton Mifflin Harcourt.

Tsai, J., Harpaz-Rotem, I., Pietrzak, R. H., & Southwick, S. M. (2012). The Role of Coping, Resilience, and Social Support in Mediating the Relation Between PTSD and Social Functioning in Veterans Returning from Iraq and Afghanistan. *Psychiatry: Interpersonal & Biological Processes, 75*(2), 135–149.

Vance, S. R., Ehrensaft, D., & Rosenthal, S. M. (2014). Psychological and Medical Care of Gender Nonconforming Youth. *Pediatrics, 134*(6), 1184–1192.

Vygotsky, L. (1978). Interaction Between Learning and Development. *Readings on the Development of Children, 23*(3), 34–41.

Wager, K., & Cox, S. (2017). *The Limbic (Emotional) System (Chap 6) (pp57–67) Auricular Acupuncture and Addiction; Mechanisms, Methodology and Practice.* The Choir Press.

Werner, E. E., & Smith, R. S. (2001). *Journeys from Childhood to Midlife: Risk, Resilience and Recovery.* Cornell University Press.

Winter, C. R. (2010). *Understanding Transgender Diversity: A Sensible Explanation of Sexual and Gender Identities.* CreateSpace Independent Publishing Platform.

Winters, S., & Conway, L. (2011). How Many Trans* People Are There? A 2011 Update Incorporating New Data. http://web.hku.hk/~sjwinter/TransgenderASIA/paper-how-many-trans-people-are-there.htm

Wu, G., Feder, A., Cohen, H., Kim, J. J., Calderon, S., Charney, D. S., & Mathé, A. A. (2013). Understanding Resilience. *Frontiers in Behavioural Neuroscience, 7*, 10.

Yelland, N. (2010). New Technologies, Playful Experiences, and Multimodal Learning. In I. R. Berson & M. J. Berson (Eds.), *High-Tech Tots: Childhood in a Digital World* (pp. 5–22). Information Age Publishing.

Yoshikawa, H., Wuermli, A. J., Britto, P. R., Dreyer, B., Leckman, J. F., Lye, S. J., … Stein, A. (2020). Effects of the Global Coronavirus Disease-2019 Pandemic on Early Childhood Development: Short-and Long-Term Risks and Mitigating Program and Policy Actions. *The Journal of Pediatrics, 223*, 188–193.

Zelazo, P. D., Blair, C. B., & Willoughby, M. T. (2016). Executive Function: Implications for Education; NCER 2017-2000; National Centre for Education Research, Institute of Education Sciences, U.S. Department of Education: Washington, DC, USA, 2016. Retrieved November 20, 2021, from https://eric.ed.gov/?id=ED570880

Conclusion

12

Given the complexity of human social and emotional development, it has only been possible within this book to explore a selection of significant influences on the health and wellbeing of children and adolescents. Explaining how perceptions of 'childhood' and 'adolescence' change over time and between cultures offered a base from which to examine individual experiences within their social context in the chapters that followed. As the intention was to concentrate on Western society, and particularly the UK, this included evidence of post-industrialisation legal changes including child employment, education, rights, and the juvenile justice system. As a result of this exploration, it became obvious that, despite impressive improvements to the lives of children and adolescents, there still exists a need to reduce social inequalities, child abuse/maltreatment, and further emerging threats to their mental and physical health and wellbeing created by technology and social media.

The brief description of theories from psychology and sociology provided an initial understanding of theoretical references within later chapters. For example, evidence cited from neuroscience helped in appreciating future reference to complex, 'pre-wired' biological processes during child and adolescent development. The introduction to psychodynamic, social/cognitive, and behavioural theories suggested how unconscious mental processes can be made intelligible and information processed from learned association and observation. Descriptions of interactionist theories, feminist theory, and functionalism helped explain how the constraints of existing social structures on individual interactions impact upon children and adolescents' health and wellbeing.

The exploration of attachment theory provided an essential starting point in understanding the influence of social experiences, given that early, secure relationships aid the future development of children and adolescents and help them develop an 'internal working model' of their world. An explanation of the potential for 'separation anxiety' and insecure attachments to create difficulties with future relationships offered a base for understanding problematic behaviour covered in later chapters. Despite criticism of the universal application of this UK-based theory, which initially marginalised mothers from the 'outer world' and fathers from family life, it became clear that it now forms an essential base for institutional care and therapeutic methods using a family-centred approach.

An inherited, biological preparedness to form attachments and engage in social interactions was explained as important in the development of sociability and a positive self-identity. That individual differences exist in the ability to adapt to the needs of others, feel empathy, and develop a 'theory of mind' was discussed to enhance appreciation of problematic behaviour discussed in later chapters. Influences on self-esteem (the level of self-worth in children and adolescents develop from interactions with others) were found to include ethnicity, class, and gender. Conclusions drawn suggested that, whilst the welcome increased acceptance of more varied gender identities within current Western society was appreciated, concerns may exist about recent medical approaches to 'gender realignment' for children and adolescents.

The exploration of the role of play on children and adolescent's learning as well as their social and physical development highlighted the benefits of rough and tumble play, outdoor play, pretend play, playing alone, and with others. Symbolic play and activities such as music, drawing, and writing were shown to enhance language and cognitive development. The importance of play in helping children and adolescents cope with adversity, deprivation, restrictions, and atypical development was noted along with the important role of adult participation in play. The importance of understanding cultural, institutional, and societal challenges to play was emphasised along with the need to address recent barriers created by new forms of media.

Having covered essential features of child and adolescent development the impact of different socialising agencies was explored, starting with ambiguities within family life due to changes in the function and structures of families within Western culture. The dichotomy between the ideal harmonious, nuclear family and the economically driven mundane features of family life was pointed out, along with how families that are considered 'safe-havens' yet can contain domestic violence and abuse. Important changes in family roles were considered, including mothers working outside the home, greater father participation in childcare, and siblings' and grandparent's contributions. Benefits and potential stress within families became apparent due to changing family roles and increased diversity within family structures. Recognition of such changes was seen within the family systems approach currently adopted within legislation, policies, and initiatives guiding health and social care provision.

Having considered the impact of family life on children and adolescents it was important to recognise the way that their behaviour is judged within wider society. Although aided by inherited human cognitive abilities in categorisation and affiliation, any behaviour termed deviant was seen to be socially constructed as it resulted from social rules which could change depending upon what was required to ensure group survival. The impact on young lives once their appearance and/or behaviour is labelled as deviant was seen to lead to stereotyping, prejudice, discrimination, and sanctions. It was concluded that as specific social contexts in which deviant acts take place can create moral panics and become self-fulfilling prophecies, there is a need to question assumptions made at societal and individual levels to avoid unfair discrimination.

As within Western society deviancy is increasingly seen as a health issue creating greater medicalisation of children and adolescents' lives, it was questioned whether it is kinder to see such behaviour as 'mad' or 'bad'. Applying Parsons' (1951) sick role theory to parents and their children suggested that both take on a medical career once a diagnosis is given. Reference to the three forms of iatrogenesis identified by Illich (1977) helped to illustrate the potentially detrimental effects of over-reliance on medicine at both individual and societal levels. Concern was raised about the impact of the increasing culture of 'healthism', including diet, exercise, and appearance based on some ideal perfectionism along with the numerous newly discovered health and behavioural 'conditions'. Ethical dilemmas due to potential conflict between the views of parents, children, adolescents, and professionals were considered. Having discussed the impact of wider social forces on individual behaviour it became apparent that despite improved therapeutic approaches, injustices and inequalities within existing power relationships need addressing.

The socially constructed nature of deviance and medicalisation became particularly well illustrated when considering the experiences of children and adolescents diagnosed with long-term and complex conditions. Such experiences were also seen to impact on family and peer relationships. Exploration of early theories of disabling pain helped in understanding the limitations of taking a purely biomedical approach. The need to appreciate psychological factors and adopt a transactional model of disability, including attachment security, became clear, especially when considering the social model of disability and concept of ableism. Revisiting issues of legal rights and power relationships between professionals, patients, and carers in practice reinforced the importance of promoting patient and carer empowerment. This was seen especially important within therapeutic interventions and when supporting those with life-limiting conditions in a death denying culture.

Drawing together and exploring further some of the examples of vulnerability to child's and adolescent's health and wellbeing referred to in previous chapters offered the opportunity to underline further the detrimental effects of social inequalities, poverty, conflict, trauma, and neglect. The need to consider the wellbeing of carers became clear. Consideration of social media and digital technology enabled appreciation of how potential excessive consumerism, gaming, gambling, and cyber bullying threatened mental wellbeing. However, this had to be balanced against the 'gateways' to opportunities afforded by technology, such as through distance-learning. Considering vulnerability in more depth offered an even deeper appreciation of the need to examine essential features of resilience. Examination of concepts and theories of resilience enabled appreciation of ways in which resilience emerges within individual characteristics as well as through protective mechanisms within family life.

To ensure that the most recent influences on child and adolescent health and wellbeing were covered, the impact of the 2020+ COVID-19 virus pandemic has been consistently considered throughout this book. The powerful force of social structures on individual lives, referred to within previous chapters, became clear from the start of the pandemic. Tensions emerged between responses from those responsible for health, politics, and the social sciences. Confusion resulted from new, often contradictory advice and laws enforced which proved impossible to police. Economic considerations have often been found to override health decisions, for example, the reticence to restrict air traffic and overseas visitors. The rationale provided for the high-level decisions have been over-zealously publicised as based on the 'certainty' of medical science whilst ignoring existing differences in thinking between those most experienced in their field.

All this has increased levels of anxiety and created a culture of uncertainty to the detriment of the lives of children and adolescents. Reports of domestic abuse involving children and adolescents have increased dramatically over the periods of 'lockdown'. There are also fears and uncertainty about potential negative long-term effects on children and adolescents' physical and mental health and wellbeing due to both the virus and the enforced restrictive preventative measures they have experienced. Children and adolescents' education has been seriously disrupted and their social development severely restricted. It is impossible to measure the detrimental effects of the constraints on family life and children's ability to form secure attachments and have access to family support from grandparents and nurseries. Even when childcare facilities were open again preventative measures against COVID-19 transmission meant that there was no form of parental involvement or adequate preparation when handing children over to 'mask wearing' staff. All this harks back to pre-Bowlby days in institutional care and potential emotional damage recognised and recorded by Robertson referred to earlier within this book.

Whilst it is too early to know the full extent of the impact of the pandemic, The Children's Society and York University (2001) estimates that a quarter of a million children and adolescents struggled due to being isolated from friends and their wider family. Their report also refers to the current plans within the National Health Service to vaccinate all children aged twelve years and above. It is particularly concerning, given the examination of child and parents' rights within this book, that, if they agree, these children could be vaccinated without parental consent.

The new 'post-COVID' era, which appears to be emerging, seems to be creating a deep sense of uncertainty in children and adolescents' view of their future. The Children's Society and York University found that although many adolescents were optimistic, they expressed concerns about money, school grades, the environment, and further pandemics. Such uncertainty can impact on future mental health which is concerning as the report notes that those found to be unhappy with their lives at fourteen years were likely to present later with mental health issues including self-harm and suicide attempts. Conclusions drawn in the report demonstrate the importance of offering emotional and educational support, physical care, supervision, and supporting parents.

There is still much to learn about the full extent to which the pandemic has changed the lives of all those likely to be reading this book. However, it is hoped that what has been covered proves useful in appreciating the need to reduce vulnerability and promote resilience in children and adolescents. This will also involve finding ways to support them by fostering a family-based approach along with addressing the material disadvantage so highly influential on their health and well-being within the UK.

References

Illich, I. (1977). *Limits to Medicine – Medical Nemesis. The Expropriation of Health.* Hamondsworth. Penguin.

Parsons, T. (1951). *The Social System.* London: Routledge and Kegan Paul.

The Children's Society and York University. (2001). The Good Childhood Report. Retrieved November 7, 2021, from https://www.childrenssociety.org.uk/good-childhood

Appendix—Case Study

The Wilson Family

Lily (Mother) is black British, thirty-one years old and works as a care assistant in a local council-run residential home for the elderly. Lily came to Britain with her mother from the Caribbean when she was a small child. After her mother's death she was taken into care. She conceived her first child whilst still at school due to a relationship with a boy in her class.

Damian (Lily's husband) is thirty years old and white British. He married Lily once aware that she was pregnant with their first child. He was made unemployed due to the closure of the supermarket where he had worked since leaving school. Damian left the family home after their second child was born to live in London with a new male partner he met online.

Stuart (Lily's recent ex-partner) is forty years old, white British, and unemployed. He suffers from long-term problems due to alcohol addiction.

Gemma (Lily's first child) is sixteen years old, and never knew her biological father. She is studying for the GCSE exams to be taken later in the year. Gemma hopes to go on to study A levels as she is keen to become a doctor. Before the Covid-19 outbreak she had just started dating Ryan, a sixth-former from her school. Gemma suffers from asthma and is also concerned about the amount of weight she has gained recently through lack of exercise.

Ben (Lily's first son with Damian) is twelve years old. After a long time and many medical examinations, he was finally diagnosed with juvenile arthritis when he was five years old. Ben constantly truants from school and has started to mix with a group of boys who are considered troublemakers. He was recently brought home by the police as he had been caught shoplifting with two of these boys.

Liam (Lily's second son with Damian) is six years old. He is considered a handful as full of energy, can be defiant, and has poor concentration. Teachers at Liam's school want to have him statemented as requiring additional support, but the family social worker has suggested that a course of play therapy may help improve his behaviour.

Chrissy (Lily's daughter to Stuart) is two years old and has normally attended nursery since being a few months old.

© The Author(s), under exclusive license to Springer Nature Switzerland AG 2022
J. M. Waite-Jones, A. M. Rodriguez, *Psychosocial Approaches to Child and Adolescent Health and Wellbeing*, https://doi.org/10.1007/978-3-030-99354-2

Family History

Lily became involved in a relationship with Damian when they both worked at the same supermarket. They married once she realised that she was pregnant with Ben. Although Damian left soon after Liam was born, he has kept in touch with the family, and he and his partner now plan to move back to the North East so that Damian can be in closer contact with his children.

After Damian left the family, Lily began a relationship with Stuart, and he moved into the family home. When Lily became pregnant with Chrissy, she asked the family social worker to help her to find a place for herself and her children to live as Stuart's alcohol problems had increased and she feared for their safety. The social worker helped Lily and the children secure the council flat in which they now live.

Lily and her children live in a town within the North East of England. Due to the decline of the mining industry, there is high unemployment in the area, and many shops and businesses have closed and are now boarded up.

Due to the recent 'lockdown' because of the Covid-19 pandemic, the schools are closed, and children are having to be taught at home. Gemma and Ben have been lent iPads by their school so that they can join the daily online classes provided. Lily has borrowed a laptop for Liam to use so that he can access the online meetings and work set by his school. Lily cannot afford to stop working as she receives little money from Damian and none from Stuart, who persists in coming to the flat to demand money. She is forced to leave Gemma in charge of the younger children whilst she is at work and is constantly worried about catching Covid-19 and passing this on to her family.

Index

Printed in the United States
by Baker & Taylor Publisher Services